# Telemedicine Technologies: Information Technologies in Medicine and Telehealth

# Telemedicine Technologies: Information Technologies in Medicine and Telehealth

Editor: Brittany McGrath

FOSTER ACADEMICS

www.fosteracademics.com

www.fosteracademics.com

FOSTER ACADEMICS

**Cataloging-in-publication Data**

Telemedicine technologies : information technologies in medicine
and telehealth / edited by Brittany McGrath.
p. cm.
Includes bibliographical references and index.
ISBN 978-1-64646-600-9
1. Telecommunication in medicine. 2. Medical telematics. 3. Medical informatics.
4. Medical technology. 5. Information storage and retrieval systems--Medicine.
6. Information storage and retrieval systems--Health. I. McGrath, Brittany.
R119.9 .T45 2023
610.285--dc23



Foster Academics,
118-35 Queens Blvd., Suite 400,
Forest Hills, NY 11375, USA

ISBN 978-1-64646-600-9 (Hardback)

# Contents

# Preface

It is often said that books are a boon to mankind. They document every progress and pass on the knowledge from one generation to the other. They play a crucial role in our lives. Thus I was both excited and nervous while editing this book. I was pleased by the thought of being able to make a mark but I was also nervous to do it right because the future of students depends upon it. Hence, I took a few months to research further into the discipline, revise my knowledge and also explore some more aspects. Post this process, I begun with the editing of this book.

Telemedicine (TM) refers to the usage of telecommunication technology to treat patients in a remote place. It uses advanced technological innovations to transfer medical information and data from one location to another. It gathers medical data and information that can be used to improve the patient's care. Telemedicine uses virtualized treatment methods for patients. It enables doctors to treat patients in less time and increase access to more patients. It also decreases the cost related with each patient visit. Telemedicine comprises the clinical care of specific patients and it also ensures the exchange of information in a protected environment. Various technologies that are contributing in shaping the future of telemedicine include Internet of things (IoT) and nanotechnology, augmented and virtual reality, 3D printing, artificial intelligence and tele-robots. This book unravels the recent studies on telemedicine technologies. Those in search of information to further their knowledge will be greatly assisted by it.

I thank my publisher with all my heart for considering me worthy of this unparalleled opportunity and for showing unwavering faith in my skills. I would also like to thank the editorial team who worked closely with me at every step and contributed immensely towards the successful completion of this book. Last but not the least, I wish to thank my friends and colleagues for their support.

**Editor**

Section 1

# Telemedicine: Use in Different Scenarios

# 1

# Better Ways to Cope with Increasingly Common Diseases: The Impact of Telemedicine on the Management of Pregnancy Complicated by Diabetes

Nino Cristiano Chilelli, Maria Grazia Dalfrà and
Annunziata Lapolla

## 1. Introduction

Diabetes is the most common complication of gestation, and this condition is associated with a higher frequency of maternal and fetal complications. Gestational diabetes mellitus (GDM), defined as glucose intolerance with onset or first recognition in pregnancy that is not clearly overt diabetes (ADA, Standards of Medical Care, 2013), is responsible for the majority of these complications and affects 1–14% of all pregnancies, becoming a growing health concern (Albrecht et al, 2010). Although diabetes types 1 and 2 are proportionally smaller contributors to this problem, the prevalence of pregnancies complicated by pregestational diabetes is rising as a result of certain environmental risk factors and the exponential increase in obesity (Wendland et al, 2011).

There is a well-documented relationship between a good glycemic control in healthy or diabetic pregnant women and lower rates of congenital malformations and perinatal complications (Ballas et al, 2012). On the other hand, despite the increasing number of pregnant women with diabetes, there has been a gradual decline in the amount of attention paid by specialists to the follow-up of these patients, and the dwindling economic resources allocated to public health services mean that access to specialized healthcare facilities is becoming more difficult. Attending a metabolic care unit can prove difficult for other reasons too (e.g. for women living too far away, or with no independent means of transportation, or needing to rest to avoid preterm delivery). In this complex and worrying scenario, exploiting new technologies may be a ploy to ensure the effective management of these patients.

Telemedicine, or the use of information and communication technology (ICT) to provide medical care at a distance, is one such opportunity, in its various applications that differ mainly in terms of the mode of interaction, the monitoring method, and the types of device involved (Klonoff DC, 2012).

The basic principle behind telemedicine is to use ICT to facilitate the interaction between health professionals and patients. The current inability to assure certain patients a regular, direct contact with their healthcare providers can be offset by using telemedicine applications, teleconsultations and videoconferencing. Using telemedicine to support pregnant women with diabetes could have an impact not only on the classical maternal-fetal outcomes, but also on other aspects not always taken into due account in the management of these patients, i.e. their quality of life, their perception of the effectiveness of care ("diabetes self-efficacy"), and their glycemic variability (Mastrogiannis et al, 2013).

Little research has been conducted on the impact of telemedicine systems on clinical outcomes in women with pregnancies complicated by diabetes. In this chapter we analyze the currently available evidence regarding the use of telemedicine in this scenario (Table 1 and Table 2), trying to highlight the main limitations of the trials performed to date and possible strategies to overcome them with a view to improving the efficacy of future clinical interventions involving these medical applications.

| | N° of partecipants (intervention/control) | Clinical outcome (metabolic/QoL) | Behavioural outcome | Care coordination outcome |
|---|---|---|---|---|
| **Wójcicki JM, 2001** | 15/15 | ↑/nv | nv | nv |
| **Ładyżyński P, 2001** | 15/nv | ↑/nv | ↑ | nv |
| **Ładyżyński P, 2007** | 15/15 | =/↑ | nv | nv |
| **Di Biase N, 1997** | 10/10 | ↑/nv | nv | nv |
| **Frost D, 2000** | 11/10 | ↑/nv | nv | nv |
| **Dalfrà MG, 2009** | 17/15 | =/↑ | ↑ | nv |

For more details about the "clinical, behavioral and care coordination" outcomes, refer to Verhoeven et al, 2010

**Table 1.** Brief summary of the main outcomes of the studies conducted in pregnants with type 1 diabetes. QoL: quality of life; nv: not valued

| | N° of partecipants (intervention/control) | Clinical outcome (metabolic/QoL) | Behavioural outcome | Care coordination outcome |
|---|---|---|---|---|
| **Pérez-Ferre N, 2009** | 49/48 | =/nv | nv | ↑ |
| **Pérez-Ferre N, 2010** | 49/48 | =/↑ | ↑ | ↑ |
| **Homko CJ, 2007** | 32/25 | =/↑ | ↑ | nv |
| **Homko CJ, 2012** | 40/40 | =/↑ | ↑ | nv |
| **Dalfrà MG, 2009** | 88/115 | ↑/↑ | ↑ | nv |

For more details about the "clinical, behavioral and care coordination" outcomes, refer to Verhoeven et al, 2010

**Table 2.** Brief summary of the main outcomes of the studies conducted in pregnants with GDM. QoL: quality of life; nv: not valued

## 2. Goals of telemedicine: pregnancy and fetal outcome

Maternal hyperglycemia prompts the passage of more glucose to the fetus, causing fetal hyperinsulinemia and an overgrowth of insulin-sensitive (especially adipose) tissue, which lead to an unbalanced growth of the fetus and the consequent risk of greater trauma at birth, shoulder dystocia and perinatal death. Hyperinsulinemia can also cause numerous neonatal metabolic complications, such as hypoglycemia, hyperbilirubinemia, hypocalcemia, hypomagnesemia, polycythemia, respiratory distress syndrome, and a higher long-term risk of diabetes mellitus and obesity in the child. Diabetes in pregnancy is related to maternal complications too, such as hypertension, pre-eclampsia, a greater need for caesarean delivery, and a higher risk of developing diabetes mellitus later on. Pregnancy complicated by obesity is characterized by higher adverse maternal and fetal outcome rates too, especially in GDM patients (Lapolla et al, 2009). Education for women at risk and regular visits to an antenatal clinic are important potential modifiers of most of these factors.

In this setting, the HAPO Study enrolled more than 23,000 women attending 15 antenatal centers all over the world, considerably improving our understanding and demonstrating that even mild degrees of hyperglycemia in pregnancy are associated with increased fetal fatness, cesarean delivery and neonatal hypoglycemia, all against a background of a biological increase in fetal insulin production. The HAPO study was supported by two recent randomized trials (Crowther CA, 2005; Landon MB, 2009) confirming that treatment for mild hyperglycemia (largely by means of changes in lifestyle) is effective in improving a number of maternal and fetal outcomes. In both the latter trials, birth weights and the frequency of large for gestational age (LGA) babies and pre-eclampsia were all reduced by treatment (McCance DR, 2011).

The best approach to women with pregnancies complicated by diabetes is therefore intensive, involving frequent glucose self-monitoring and dietary restrictions and/or adequate insulin therapy (Landon MB, 2011). Using telemedicine can facilitate the management of pregnancy complicated by diabetes, being applicable to all the above-mentioned areas of intervention. The great challenge now is to demonstrate the efficacy of this innovative tool in terms of maternal-fetal outcome and an advantageous cost/benefit ratio.

## 3. Telemedicine and its applications to diabetes care in pregnancy

The main applications of telemedicine relate to educating patients to manage their chronic diseases, making it easier for them to contact their healthcare providers, and enable the collection of information and its transfer to clinical databases. ICT can help in the management of diabetic patients by providing additional clinical support, which is now increasingly difficult to achieve in the classical face-to-face interaction due to the limited health resources available (Lapolla A, 2011). The most encouraging technology nowadays is teleconsultation, involving telemonitoring schemes that include asynchronous exchanges between patients and their healthcare providers (e.g. e-mails, text messages on mobile phones, automated messaging, or other methods requiring no face-to-face contact), or synchronous communications in the form of face-to-face contact using videoconferencing equipment (television, digital camera, webcam, videophone) to connect healthcare providers to one or more patients at the same time, also for the purpose of providing education and training (Kern J, 2006).

These systems are designed basically as a means to improve the quality of care through closer communications between patients and professionals, in an effort to create a more dynamic and motivating exchange, involving patients to a greater extent in their own care, and making the monitoring of their disease more compatible with their lifestyle (Verhoeven F, 2007; McMahon GT, 2005). This applies in particular to the management of diabetes (Franc S, 2011) and especially in pregnancy complicated by diabetes, given the drastically reduced time available for examining and educating these patients who need short-term adjustments to their therapy and reassurance concerning an appropriate diet, as well as routine care (Lapolla et al, 2011). Combining the applications of telemedicine with programs for managing diabetes in pregnancy seems to be a fundamental step to combine the need for an intensive approach to these patients with the containment of the associated costs.

Studies evaluating these applications must take into account both clinical aspects, including those related to the effects on quality of life, both behavioral outcomes and finally economic/social issues, especially related to health care costs (Verhoeven F et al, 2010).

### 3.1. Evidence of the use of telemedicine in pregnant women with type 1 diabetes

Wojcicki et al analyzed the effectiveness of an automated telematic intensive care system for transferring all of patients' glucose measurements taken during the course of a day to a central clinical unit. The patients' mean blood glucose (MBG) and an indicator of glucose variability (the J-index) were used to monitor their glycemic control. The authors demonstrated a better glycemic control in the experimental group by comparison with a control group, based on the average differences in the patients' MBG and J indices, calculated weekly

($\Delta$MBG = -3.2 +/- 4.3 mg/dL, p = 0.0016, $\Delta$J = -1.4 +/- 2.3, p = 0.0065). They also found a tendency for a better glycemic control in patients with a lower intelligence quotient (IQ < 100) supported by the telematic system by comparison with all the other groups of patients, though this difference lacked statistical significance. The telematic intensive care system improved the efficacy of diabetes treatment during pregnancy (Wójcicki JM, 2001).

Ladyzynsky et al developed a system for supporting intensive insulin treatment in pregnant women with type 1 diabetes. The system consists of a patient teletransmission module (PTM) and a central clinical control unit (CCU). The PTM comprises a box containing a blood glucose meter and an electronic logbook, a modem for dial-up internet or a cellular phone set. The CCU consists of a PC with a modem and DIAPRET software – a dedicated program designed to monitor the intensive insulin treatment. The system was tested on 15 pregnant type 1 diabetic women for 166±24 days. Its total effectiveness was 69.3±13.0% and its technical effectiveness was 91.5±6.1%, and was not significantly influenced by the patients' IQ, formal education or place of residence, while it turned into a better metabolic control (Ładyżyński et al, 2001).

The same authors also assessed the influence of the greater frequency of data reporting on diabetic patients' metabolic control. Data were reported via a home telecare system that stored blood glucose levels and was integrated with a simple electronic logbook. The data collected by patients were automatically transmitted via the telephone network every night. The study population consisted of 30 patients with type 1 diabetes, who were randomly allocated to the home telecare group or a control group. The control group's treatment was based on clinical examinations performed every three weeks. For the home telecare group, the data recorded by patients were transmitted to the hospital daily, enabling doctors to intervene more frequently. The average duration of the study was 180 days (standard deviation, SD 22) in the home telecare group and 176 days (SD 16) in the control group. The mean level of metabolic control and the insulin dose adjustment patterns were very similar in the two groups despite the much greater (15-fold) reporting frequency in the home telecare group. The data collected by patients were not fully usable, mainly because of an excessively high within-day variability in glycemic control and the high workload for the hospital staff performing the daily data analysis. On average, for the home telecare group, the patients' data were collected about 0.7 times per day (i.e. 15 times more often than in the case of routine treatment), although average metabolic control was found only slightly better for the home telecare group than for controls, and the number of adjustments to patients' insulin doses was very similar in the two groups. Both general compliance issues (relating to the considerable effort needed to analyze the daily data) and clinical problems (e.g. a high intraday glycemic variability) probably contributed to the lack of any significant differences between the two groups. These findings prompted the authors to conclude that remote systems used at home by patients with type 1 diabetes on intensive insulin therapy improves their glycemic control, but needs to support real-time data transmission and be combined with appropriate data analysis and subsequent decision-making for it to achieve any real improvement in the quality of care (Ładyżyński et al, 2007).

Di Biase et al also investigated whether telemedicine could be useful in the management of pregnant type 1 diabetic women. A fully automated system (the DIANET system) was used and 20 type 1 pregnant women took part in the study: 10 were treated using the telemedicine system, the other 10 using the conventional approach. The DIANET system was adopted at 4 different times, termed as: "entry" (at 9.5 weeks of gestation); "basal" (9.5-16.8 weeks); "1st month" of investigation; and "end" (near delivery). All the women adopted intensified insulin administration protocols. Judging from the profiles of the women's absolute blood glucose values, the DIANET ensured a better metabolic control than the conventional approach. These results were associated with higher insulin doses being used by the women in the DIANET group. There was a significant reduction in both groups' hypoglycemic episodes at the "end", "1st month" and "basal" study points by comparison with the situation at "entry". Based on their results, the authors suggest that telemedicine (DIANET) is a practical way to provide specialist care in pregnancy (Di Biase et al, 1997)

Frost et al used a remote data management system (CareLink; Abbott-MediSense, New Bedford, MA) to monitor 11 pregnant women with type 1 diabetes (all on intensive insulin therapy) from the 15th gestational week onwards, comparing them with controls receiving routine diabetes care, which consisted of visits every 2-3 weeks. The controls were 10 pregnant women with type 1 diabetes matched for age, history of diabetes, and expertise with self-monitoring and insulin regimens. The average time between two visits was 3.3 weeks for the CareLink group and 2.9 weeks for the control group. There was an improvement in HbA1c in both the CareLink group (from 6.1±1.0 to 5.4±0.3) and the control group (from 6.2±0.8 to 5.7±0.6), though the differences were not statistically significant. MBG levels dropped in the CareLink group from 141±90 to 110±18 mg/dl, and fasting glucose from 111±17 to 101±23 mg/dl ($p < 0.05$). Glycemic variability was also significantly reduced in both groups: the standard deviation of the MBG levels in individual patients fell from 51.6 to 44.4 mg/dl ($p < 0.01$), while for mean fasting blood glucose the SD decreased from 41.4 to 31.0 mg/dl. There was no significant reduction in the number of hypoglycemic episodes in either of the groups. The authors concluded that the system was easy to use and helpful in the treatment of diabetic women during pregnancy, enabling fewer outpatient visits. This aid would therefore be particularly suitable for women who have difficulty attending the prescribed regular check-ups at the clinic (Frost et al, 2000).

### 3.2. Evidence of the use of telemedicine in pregnant women with GDM

Dalfrà et al enrolled a total of 235 pregnant women (203 with GDM and 32 with type 1 diabetes mellitus) and assigned them sequentially to a telemedicine or a control group. Women with type 1 diabetes were enrolled in the study immediately after conception, while women with GDM were included one week after their GDM was diagnosed (at a mean 28±1 weeks of gestation). The pregnant women in the telemedicine group were trained to monitor their blood glucose levels with a glucometer (One Touch Ultra-Lifescan) and send their blood glucose profiles to Glucobeep by means of a standard phone call. These women also attended 1 outpatient visit per month. The women in the control group only had a medical examination every two weeks. All patients could contact the physician whenever they wished.

Clinical and non-clinical outcomes were evaluated: the former included mode and timing of delivery, macrosomia, maternal and fetal morbidity; the latter were deduced using questionnaires, i.e. the CES-D for depression, the SF-36 for health-related quality of life (QoL), the Stress and Distress or the impact of diabetes. The telemedicine GDM group achieved a better metabolic control in the third trimester (p=0.008) and a lower rate of cesarean sections (p=0.02) and macrosomia (p=n.s.). The women in the telemedicine group also had lower levels of frustration and concern about their diabetes, and a better acceptance of their diabetic condition. A strength of this study lies in that the authors adopted a straightforward telemedicine system (using the telephone) that was easy for all patients to handle, demanding no IT expertise or computer literacy (Dalfrà et al, 2009).

Pèrez-Ferre et al studied 97 women with GDM to ascertain the feasibility of a telemedicine system based on the Internet and text messaging, and its influence on delivery and neonatal outcomes (HbA1c values < 5.8%, normal vaginal deliveries, and LGA babies). Forty-eight women attended traditional face-to-face visits and 49 formed the experimental group using the telemedicine system to send capillary glucose data and short text messages, receiving professional feedback weekly. There was no significant difference between the two groups in terms of the outcomes considered, despite the experimental group's significantly reduced number of visits to the clinic, particularly among the insulin-treated women. The authors concluded that the telemedicine-based system achieved similar pregnancy, delivery and newborn outcomes to the traditional treatment approach, while significantly reducing the need for outpatient clinic visits (Pérez-Ferre N, 2009)

More recently, the same authors demonstrated that, compared with a control group, a telemedicine group reduced the number of unscheduled face-to-face visits by 62% (and by 82.7% for the subgroup of insulin-treated patients), improving patient satisfaction and achieving comparable pregnancy and newborn outcomes (Pérez-Ferre N, 2010).

In a study by Homko et al, women with GDM were randomized to either an Internet group (n = 32) or a control group (n = 25). Patients in the Internet group were given computers and/or Internet access as necessary. A website was established for recording glucose levels and for communications between patients and the health care team. Women in the control group kept paper logbooks, which were reviewed at each prenatal visit. Maternal feelings about diabetes self-efficacy were assessed at study entry and again before delivery. Women in the Internet group accessed the system and sent a mean 21.8 (±16.9) sets of data. There was no difference between the two groups' fasting or post-prandial blood glucose levels, although more women in the Internet group were on insulin therapy (31% vs. 4%; P <0.05). There were also no significant differences in pregnancy and neonatal outcomes between the two groups. The women in the Internet group demonstrated a significantly stronger sense of self-efficacy at the end of the study. The potential benefits of monitoring blood glucose via the Internet in indigent women with GDM was limited by their infrequent use of the telemedicine system. While using the system was not associated with better pregnancy outcomes, the diabetic women in the telemedicine group did experience a better sense of psychosocial self-efficacy (Homko CJ, 2007).

In a subsequent study, these authors tested a more advanced telemedicine system, which included automated reminders to patients to send their data. Eighty GDM women were randomized to join an intervention group using telemedicine to send blood glucose recordings obtained 4 times a day via the Internet or telephone, or a control group using paper logbooks. Although there were no significant differences in the outcomes considered (glucose control and birth weight of offspring), this type of telemedicine approach improved the contact between patients and healthcare professionals, making the use of technology for monitoring of diabetes in pregnancy more familiar (Homko CJ, 2012).

Finally, in GDM patients one study showed that integrating telemedicine applications and involvement of the nursing staff turns into better fetal outcome and adhesion to glucose monitoring. With this respect Ferrara et al demonstrated that higher referral frequency to telephonic nurse management for gestational diabetes mellitus decreased risk of macrosomic infant and increased postpartum glucose testing (Ferrara et al, 2012).

## 4. Conclusion

Recent reports in the literature have addressed several aspects of telemedicine applied to the treatment of diabetes in pregnancy. The use of telemedicine appears to be not only feasible, but also capable of achieving the same glycemic control and perinatal outcomes as conventional care, with fewer visits to the clinic. This would naturally be appreciated by patients, but there is also the economic impact on the physician's side to consider. Fewer visits to the doctor would cut costs while assuring the same level of care, even after the costs of creating a telemedicine system have been taken into account. If telemedicine applied to the treatment of diabetes during pregnancy can benefit both parties (patients and doctors), it could drastically change current treatment methods (ATTD 2010 Yearbook, 2011). The implementation of telemedicine in the clinical management of GDM also supports the greater involvement of figures, such as nurses and dietitians (Figure 1), whose support can help in saving time and resources in the follow-up of these patients (García-Patterson, 2003).

The present review raises a number of questions about the intrinsic value of telemedicine in the management of chronic disease. It would be useful if future studies were designed very carefully in order to identify the true value of remote patient support systems. It would also be valuable to future reviewers if a minimum dataset were adopted to measure outcomes. Quantitative indices, from which pooled estimates of effect can be calculated, include:

- quality of life (measured on scales appropriate to the diseases in question);
- cost to society;
- emergency department visits;
- days in hospital.

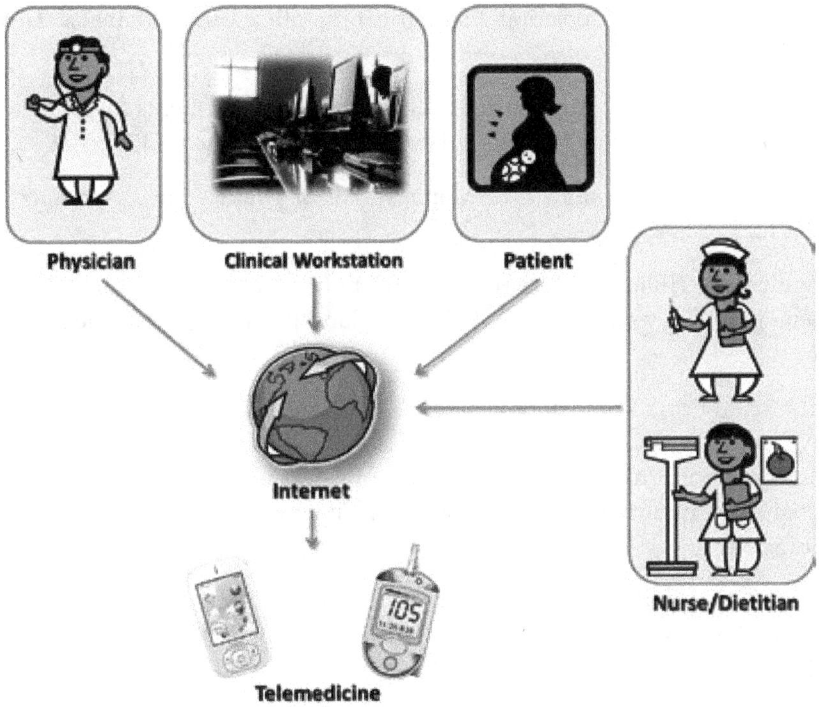


**Figure 1.** Schematic representation of the interconnection between patients, specialists and technologies supported by telemedicine.

Finally, it seems unlikely that any intervention on chronic diseases can have much effect unless it is applied over a lengthy period of time (Wootton R, 2012). Future studies might consider testing telemedicine schemes for years rather than months.

## Author details

Nino Cristiano Chilelli, Maria Grazia Dalfrà and Annunziata Lapolla

Department of Medicine (DIMED), University of Padova, Italy

## References

[1] Albrecht SS, Kurlina EV, Bansil P, Jamieson DJ, Whiteman MK, Kourtis AP, Posner SF, Callaghan WM. Diabetes Trends Among Delivery Hospitalizations in the U.S., 1994–2004. Diabetes Care 2010; 33:768–773

[2] American Diabetes Association. Standards of medical care in diabetes. Diabetes Care 2013; 36, S11-S66

[3] ATTD 2010 Yearbook: Advanced Technologies and Treatments for Diabetes. International Journal of Clinical Practice 2011; 65, Issue Supplement s170:55–60

[4] Ballas J, Moore TR, Ramos GA. Management of Diabetes in Pregnancy. Curr Diab Rep 2012; 12:33–42

[5] Crowther CA, Hiller JE, Moss JR et al. Effect of treatment of gestational diabetes mellitus on pregnancy outcomes. The New England Journal of Medicine 2005; 352: 2477–2486

[6] Dalfrà MG, Nicolucci A, Di Benedetto A, Di Cianni G, Dolci MA, Franzetti I, Galluzzo A, Napoli A, Salietti G, Santini C, Torlone E, Tortul C, Vitacolonna E, Lapolla A. Telemedicine in Pregnancy Complicated by Diabetes. The effect of telemedicine on outcome and quality of life in pregnant women with diabetes. J Telemed Telecare 2009;15:238-42.

[7] Di Biase N, Napoli A, Sabbatini A, Borrello E, Buongiorno AM & Fallucca F. Telemedicine in the treatment of diabetic pregnancy. Annali dell'Istituto Superiore di Sanità 1997; 33: 347-351

[8] Ferrara A, Hedderson MM, Ching J, Kim C, Peng T, Crites YM. Referral to telephonic nurse management improves outcomes in women with gestational diabetes. Am J Obstet Gynecol. 2012 Jun;206: e1-5

[9] Franc S, Daoudi A, Mounier S, Boucherie B, Dardari D, Laroye H, Neraud B, Requeda E, Canipel L, Charpentier G. Telemedicine and diabetes: achievements and prospects. Diabetes Metab. 2011;37:463-76

[10] Frost D & Beischer W. Telemedicine in the management of pregnancy in type 1 diabetic women. Diabetes Care 2000; 23: 863-864

[11] García-Patterson A, Martín E, Ubeda J, María MA, Adelantado JM, Ginovart G, de Leiva A, Corcoy R. Nurse-based management in patients with gestational diabetes. Diabetes Care. 2003:998-1001

[12] Homko CJ, Santamore WP, Whiteman V, Bower M, Berger P, Geifman-Holtzman O, Bove AA. Use of an Internet-based telemedicine system to manage underserved women with gestational diabetes mellitus. Diabetes Technology & Therapeutics 2007;9: 297-306

[13] Homko CJ, Deeb LC, Rohrbacher K, Mulla W, Mastrogiannis D, Gaughan J, Santamore WP, Bove AA. Impact of a telemedicine system with automated reminders on outcomes in women with gestational diabetes mellitus. Diabetes Technol Ther. 2012 Jul;14(7):624-9

[14] Kern J. Evaluation of teleconsultation systems. Int J Med Inform. 2006;75(3-4):330-4.

[15] Klonoff DC. Improved Outcomes from Diabetes Monitoring: The benefits of better adherence, therapy adjustments, patient education, and telemedicine support. J Diabetes Sci Technol 2012;6(3):486–490

[16] Ładyżyński P, Wójcicki JM, Krzymien J, Blachowicz J, Jozwicka E, Czajkowski K, Janczewska E & Karnafel W. Teletransmission system supporting intensive insulin treatment of out-clinic type 1 diabetic pregnant women. Technical assessment during 3 years' application. Int J Artif Organs 2001; 24: 157-163

[17] Ładyżyński P & Wójcicki M. Home telecare during intensive insulin treatment – metabolic control does not improve as much as expected. Journal of Telemedicine and Telecare 2007; 13: 44-47

[18] Landon MB, Spong CY, Thom E et al. A multicenter randomized trial of treatment for mild gestational diabetes. The New England Journal of Medicine 2009; 361: 1339–1348.

[19] Landon MB, Gabbe SG. Gestational diabetes mellitus. Obstet Gynecol. 2011;118:1379–93

[20] Lapolla A, Dalfrà MG, Fedele D. Management of gestational diabetes mellitus. Diabetes, Metabolic Syndrome and Obesity: Targets and Therapy 2009; 2: 73–82

[21] Lapolla A, Chilelli NC, Dalfrà MG. Telemedicine in Pregnancy Complicated by Diabetes, Advances in Telemedicine: Applications in Various Medical Disciplines and Geographical Regions (2011), Prof. Georgi Graschew (Ed.), ISBN: 978-953-307-161-9, InTech, DOI: 10.5772/13865

[22] Mastrogiannis DS, Igwe E, Homko CJ. The role of telemedicine in the management of the pregnancy complicated by diabetes. Curr Diab Rep. 2013 Feb;13(1):1-5

[23] McCance DR. Pregnancy and diabetes. Best Practice & Research Clinical Endocrinology & Metabolism 2011; 25: 945–958

[24] McMahon GT, Gomes HE, Hohne SH, Hu TMJ, Levine BA, Conlin PR. Web-based care management in patients with poorly controlled diabetes. Diabetes Care 2005; 28:1624–1629

[25] Pérez-Ferre N, Galindo M, Fernàndez Mª D, Velasco V, de la Cruz Mª J, Martìn P, del Valle L, Calle-Pascual AL. A telemedicine system based on Internet and short message service as a new approach in the follow-up of patients with gestational diabetes. Diabetes Research and Clinical Practice 2009, 87, e15-e17

[26] Pérez-Ferre N, Galindo M, Fernàndez Mª D, Velasco V, de la Cruz Mª J, Martìn P, del Valle L, Calle-Pascual AL. The outcomes of gestational diabetes mellitus after a telecare approach are not inferior to traditional outpatient clinic visits. International Journal of Endocrinology 2010, 2010:386941. doi: 10.1155/2010/386941

[27] Verhoeven F, Van Gemert-Pijnen L, Dijkstra K, Nijland N, Seydel E, Steehouder M.

The contribution of teleconsultation and videoconferencing to diabetes care: a systematic literature review. Journal of Medical Internet Research; 9: e37, 2007.

[28] Verhoeven F, Tanja-Dijkstra K, Nijland N, Eysenbach G, van Gemert-Pijnen L. Asynchronous and synchronous teleconsultation for diabetes care: a systematic literature review.J Diabetes Sci Technol. 2010 May 1;4(3):666-84.

[29] Wendland EL, Torloni MR, Falavigna M, Trujillo J, Dode MA, Campos MA, Duncan BB, Schmidt MI. Gestational diabetes and pregnancy outcomes – a systematic review of the World Health Organization (WHO) and the International Association of Diabetes in Pregnancy Study Groups (IADPSG) diagnostic criteria. BMC Pregnancy and Childbirth 2012, 12:23

[30] Wójcicki JM, Ładyżyński P, Krzymien J, Jozwicka E, Blachowicz J, Janczewska E, Czajkowski K & Karnafel W. What we can really expect from Telemedicine in intensive diabetes treatment: results from 3-year study in type 1 pregnant diabetic women. Diabetes Technology & Therapeutics 2001; 3: 581-589

[31] Wootton R. Twenty years of telemedicine in chronic disease management--an evidence synthesis. J Telemed Telecare. 2012;18: 211-20.

# 2

# Telemedicine: Reducing Trauma in Evaluating Abuse

Sunshine Arnold and Debra Esernio-Jenssen

## 1. Introduction

The increases in child abuse reporting and shortage of medical experts in the child abuse field have fueled the need to implement telemedicine programs that provide timely expert examinations to children. Also driving this need is that some of the highest rates of child abuse and neglect occur in rural areas [1]. Without the access to trained practitioners children may not receive complete or accurate examinations. This inexperience may possibly lead to misdiagnosis, unnecessary treatment, incomplete care and follow up, and ultimately may leave the child at risk for further maltreatment. When a qualified medical practitioner is located a great distance from where the child resides or a child travels hours for an examination this is a burden to an already traumatized child. As well, the investigative professionals from law enforcement and child protective services are also inconvenienced, as they are likely to be responsible for transporting the child to the site for evaluation. In addition, the exam may be delayed for a period of time due to the travel involved leaving child protective services, law enforcement, and ultimately a child waiting in limbo for a safety decision.

## 2. Florida's child protection team telemedicine network

In 1998, Children's Medical Services (CMS) in Florida implemented a real-time telemedicine project, linking "hub" sites with "remote" or satellite service locations such as public health departments and child advocacy centers (Figure 1). The purpose of this telemedicine network was to improve access for children suspected to be victimized who resided in rural areas to the Child Protection Team medical evaluations. The telemedicine network facilitates child abuse assessments via telecommunications technology. Hub sites are comprehensive medical facilities with a wide range of medical and multidisciplinary staff while remote sites are limited in diversity and medical expertise in evaluating suspected cases of child abuse. Medical providers located at hub sites have the expertise needed to evaluate this population. The physician, physician assistant, or Advanced Registered Nurse Practitioner, the medical provider of record, is located at the hub site while a registered nurse and social worker engage with the child at the remote site during the medical evaluation. Computer integration allows for the storage of images taken by either the hub or remote site. A telemedicine exam follows the same general protocol as a traditional face-to-face medical examination provided by the Child Protection Team. Thus, the medical evaluation includes the child's birth, past and current medical, developmental, and family history, an assessment of the child's behavior and social risk factors and obtaining photographs; all the components of a comprehensive abuse assessment. Examinations are utilized to assess physical abuse, sexual abuse, and medical neglect cases.

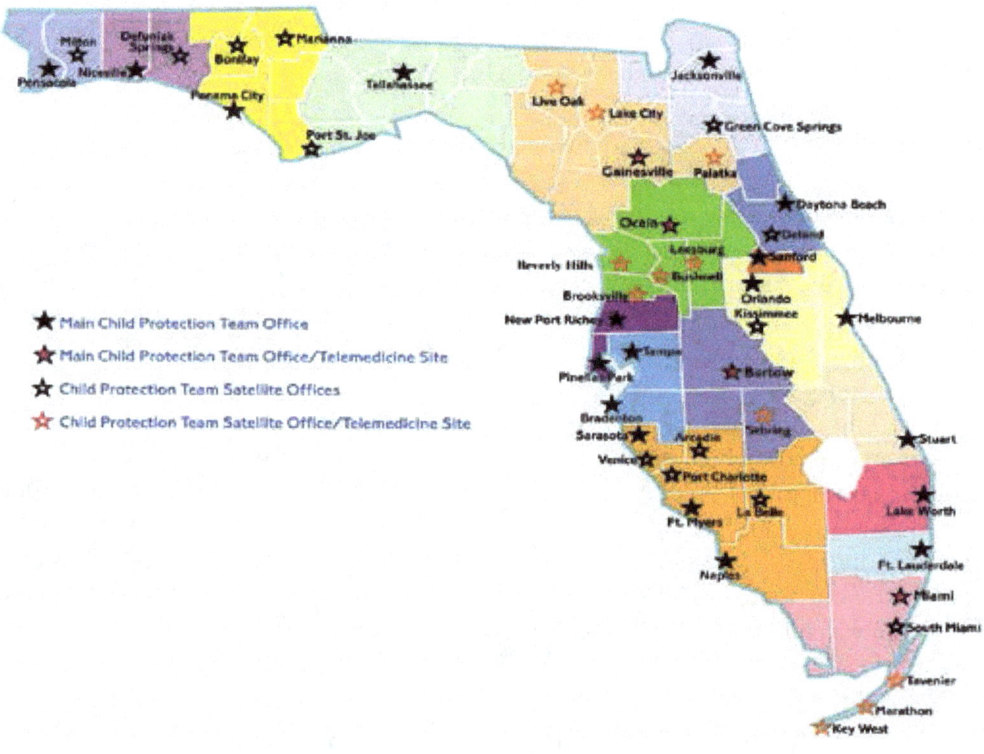


**Figure 1.** Florida Child Protection Team Map noting Main "Hub" Sites and telemedicine sites

The Child Protection Team (CPT) program at the University of Florida is a medically directed, multidisciplinary program based on the idea that child abuse and neglect involve complex issues and require the expertise of many professionals to protect children. It is one of twenty-four legislatively mandated teams of its kind throughout the state of Florida. The University of Florida Child Protection Team (UFCPT) is unique in that it serves a twelve county area in North Central Florida working in coordination with multiple community partners and localized Child Advocacy Centers (CAC) to provide CPT services in child-friendly settings. Established within the University of Florida College of Medicine, Department of Pediatrics and headquartered in Gainesville, the team has the privilege of serving children and families in Alachua, Bradford, Citrus, Columbia, Dixie, Gilchrist, Hernando, and Hamilton, Lafayette, Levy, Suwannee, and Union counties. Expert medical consultation and evaluations can occur in four different clinic settings throughout the twelve counties on a given day. This is made possible through the utilization of telemedicine examinations at two of the sites; Citrus and Hernando counties. During 2011, the UF Child Protection Team provided over 300 medical exams by telemedicine; January through July 31, 2012, the Team has already provided over 250 exams via telemedicine. This medical component is supported and enhanced by psychosocial assessments, psychological evaluations, forensic interviews, expert court testimony, multidisciplinary case staffing, and coordination of services which assist community agencies in diagnosis and treatment planning.

## 3. Applications of telemedicine in child abuse

In addition to using telemedicine for real-time child medical evaluations, the technology can also be useful for peer review and consultation. Several Child Protection Teams in Florida also use the technology to conduct quarterly peer review of complex cases among the child abuse experts at various sites. The providers are able to present cases, share images of physical findings and participate in discussion simultaneously without delay. While these peer reviews are conducted in real-time, another application known as store and forward consultations, involves the transmission of still images from a practitioner to a data storage device which can then be retrieved by the expert medical professional and reviewed at a later time. The expert can then view the images remotely to give his/her opinion.

Live telemedicine consultations are another option for remote providers to access child abuse experts at a distance. Providers at remote sites where a patient presents with an allegation of abuse can connect with experts at a tertiary care center agreeing to provide the consultation. Live consultations have shown to reduce cost in other types of medical conditions by reducing the number of patients taken by aeromedical transport to larger medical centers [2]. The use of live consultation in sexual abuse examinations has been shown to improve a rural provider's accuracy in terms of findings and the completeness of the examination [3]. Berkowitz has suggested telemedicine could even be utilized to address underreporting of child abuse by children's primary care providers [4]. Primary care providers would be able to consult on a case with a child abuse expert prior to making a report to their state central register. Physicians may feel more comfortable consulting with an expert before reporting as some fear their suspicion may be wrong.

Live, simultaneously transmitted telemedicine exams are preferable compared to the store and forward application. While both methods accomplish the goal of having a child's injuries evaluated by an expert in the field of child abuse live examinations allow the medical provider access to information that can not be captured by a still image. During the live telemedicine evaluation the medical provider is able to observe the child's body language, interact with the child, observe the child's reactions to the physical examination, and is able to ask additional questions of the child and/or non offending caregiver if needed.

Although Florida was the first state to use telemedicine, child abuse professionals throughout the United States have utilized this technology. The Southwest Alabama Abuse Network, Support for Health Involved Professionals in Children's Safety Centers (SHIPS) network, The University of Utah Child Advocacy Centers, and University of California-Davis also rely on the application of telemedicine to provide assessments and conduct reviews in child abuse cases [5]. These and other programs utilize the various telemedicine applications described previously and have had positive results [5].

## 4. Establishing a telemedicine program

### 4.1. Equipment

Telemedicine requires very specific equipment, software, and network capability. The UFCPT's current network is Secure Integrated Services Digital Network operating at 384kbps transmission speed. A Tandberg Intern was previously used and the Polycom Practitioner Cart is now located at the remote sites (Figure 2 and 3). The hub site also requires a Polycom Practitioner Cart with integrated computer and software. Second Opinion Professional is the current software being used. An AMD General Exam Camera with 50X magnification and a Welsh-Allyn or Leisgang colposcope is used to capture physical findings. The Florida Department of Health Information Technology personnel provide technical support to the CPT Telemedicine program statewide. Consultation with IT support familiar with telemedicine should be initiated in the very early stages of planning.

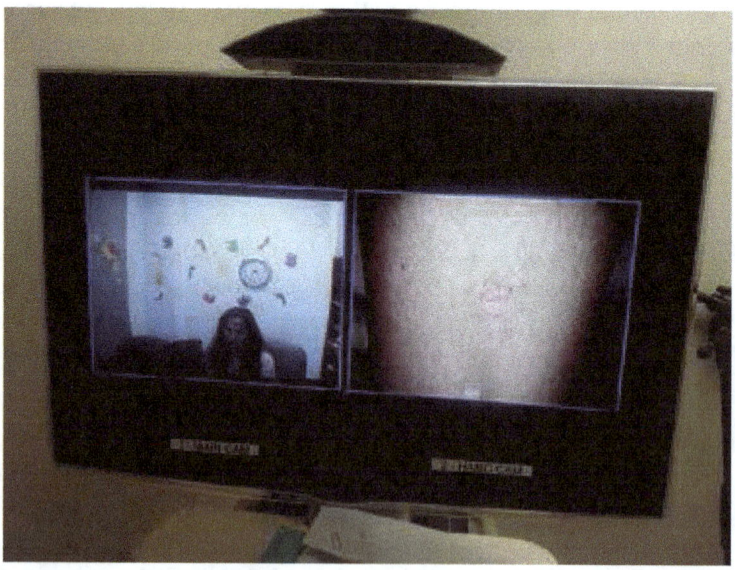

**Figure 2.** Polycom Practitioner Cart with side-by-side simultaneous view of hub site provider (left) and injury being captured (right) by AMD General Exam Camera with 50x magnification.

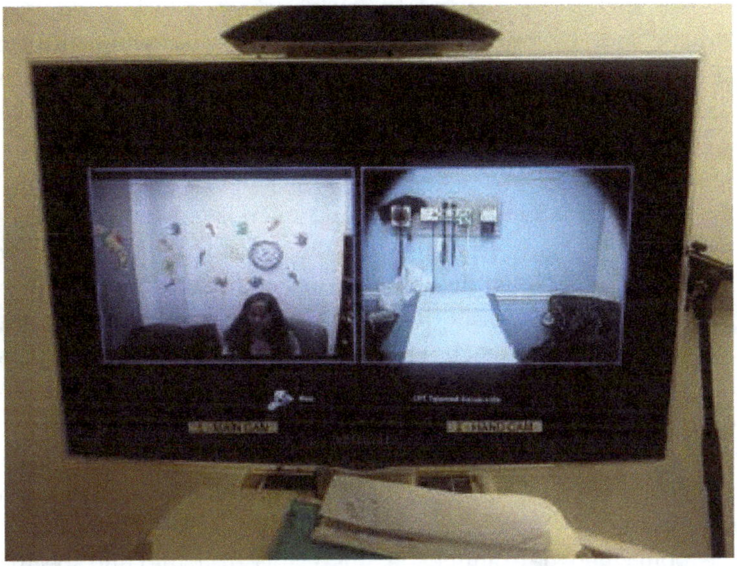

**Figure 3.** Side-by-side view of both hub site (left) and remote site (right).

### 4.2. Community support

In establishing a telemedicine program several key partners should be involved in this process outside of the obvious medical staffing needs. The pilot telemedicine project in Florida found that a key to successful establishment of a telemedicine program is a complete understanding and "buy-in" from the local agencies. An essential part of the planning process is involving these professionals early through a community meeting. This group should include, but is not limited to, hub site medical personnel, local child protective services personnel, local law enforcement investigating crimes involving children, state or district attorney involved in prosecution, local health department and hospital personnel, and the local Child Advocacy Center. The community meeting should explore the benefits of telemedicine to the children being served and the professionals involved in the investigative process. The local community members can assist in identifying viable remote site locations in the area and those best located to serve the greatest number of children. Early on, it is expected that this introduction of technology may meet with some reluctance. Providing documentation of successful programs and caregiver and victim testimonials are often helpful in allaying concerns.

### 4.3. Staffing needs

The performance of a telemedicine exam requires a minimum of two medical professionals who have specific child abuse training and training in conducting telemedicine examinations; the medical provider of record (physician, physician assistant, or ARNP) and a registered nurse. The University of Florida Child Protection Team also has a social worker present during the medical evaluation. This individual has usually already conducted a thorough forensic interview with the child prior to the medical examination unless due to the child's young age/

development this was not feasible. The social worker's presence during the exam helps to make the child comfortable and also provides continuity for the child while at the clinic or Child Advocacy Center. In addition, the social worker operates the hand held camera that captures the images in order to allow the registered nurse to act as the medical provider's "hands" during the examination. All images and video are available to the medical provider simultaneously. All personnel located at the remote site act under the direction of the medical provider. The history provided to the social worker is relayed to the medical provider via telephone before the exam begins. Prior to the child's examination the registered nurse will explain to the child and family how the exam will be conducted and provide an opportunity for questions to be asked. Families and the child most often want to be reassured that the examination is confidential and cannot be observed by an outside party. The personnel explain that the examination is conducted over secure telecommunications lines and that only the examiner at the hub site is being transmitted the encounter. The child and caregiver are shown the telemedicine equipment and explained that the utilization of the equipment avoids lengthy travel and provide them access to an expert more easily. The child's medical history is gathered from the caregiver accompanying the child to the appointment, if available. The caregiver is asked to leave the room when the examiner obtains history from the child specific to the alleged abuse. Following the medical history, the child is asked whom if any of the individuals that accompanied them to the appointment would they prefer to remain with them during the medical examination. The UFCPT program has found that often with adolescents they prefer to be examined alone.

### 4.4. The medical evaluation

The child abuse medical evaluation includes a complete physical examination. Height and weight are measured and if the child is 2 years old or younger, a head circumference is obtained. The child's face is photographed for identification. Afterwards, in older children and adolescents, the nurse proceeds to examine the child from the head to the feet. The nurse will comment on body and oral hygiene and any unusual odors in addition to cutaneous manifestations of abuse. In younger children, examination of the heart and lungs may precede eye and ear examination due to the child's inherent fear and stranger anxiety. Any noted marks, scars, or bruises are identified, measured and photographed. If there are allegations of sexual abuse, then a thorough anogenital exam is also performed. Depending on the age of the child, various positions are used to view the anogenital area. For younger females, frog leg supine position is often used to view the genitalia. Labial separation and/or traction are used to examine the urethra, hymen, fossa navicularis, and posterior fourchette. The knee-chest supine or lateral decubitus positions may be used to view the anus. Boys may be examined in similar positions. Adolescent females are often examined in the lithotomy position. When hymenal injury is detected, to confirm the findings, the nurse can run the hymenal edge with a cotton swab or position the child into knee chest prone, which enables the best view of the posterior hymen. Photographs of the anogenital exam are also obtained, especially any pertinent findings. For acute sexual assaults a forensic evidence kit is completed and given to the accompanying law enforcement officer. Site-specific cultures and/or nucleic acid amplification tests, or any other laboratory tests are obtained as per CPT protocol. The medical provider may determine that additional testing or dispensing of medication is necessary. Any child suspected to have sustained serious injuries is referred to the nearest Pediatric Emergency Department.

### 4.5. Legal consideration

For the other medical specialties utilizing telemedicine, when the examination is completed and the hub and remote sites disconnect the encounter has also ended. However, for child abuse cases when the medical provider's assessment reveals abuse, there may be criminal and civil court action. Some skepticism about the quality of the photographs that would ultimately need to be presented as evidence in court has been voiced from time to time. To date, since the Florida program's inception in 1998, there have been no legal challenges in court to the thousands of telemedicine images captured by Florida Child Protection Teams. The CPT telemedicine examinations and photos have been utilized hundreds of times in successful criminal prosecutions and dependency trials.

## 5. Case study

A 4 11/12 year old male was evaluated on 2/18/2011 via telemedicine for concerns of physical abuse due to multiple bruises. This was the fourth time in 17 months that Child Protective Services (CPS) referred him for concerns of physical abuse. There were multiple prior reports for this family including verified reports for family violence and physical injury. The child resided with his mother, four half-siblings and his stepfather. His mother reported that his older sibling (age 10) caused the injuries. The child did not disclose the true etiology of his injuries until this visit when he reported that he was punched, kicked, beaten, and dragged by his mother's paramour and hit by his mother. Physical examination revealed over 40 bruises on multiple body planes. According to a systematic review of bruising in childhood, bruises concerning for physical abuse include those located away from bony prominences, are located on the face, back, buttocks and abdomen, and are multiple occurring in clusters [6]. Please note the following images were taken using the previous Tandberg Intern. UFCPT began using the Polycom Practitioner Cart August 2012 and images for a case study were not yet available. There is much improved quality of the still images captured using the new equipment

After a thorough law enforcement investigation, his sibling disclosed that he and this child were instructed by their mother to lie and state that the injuries resulted from fights between them. Additionally, it was revealed that this child was specifically targeted by his mother. She beat him, burned him with cigarette lighters, cut his hands, locked him outside their home in the cold and rain, and forced him to remain in a dark closet for hours. In June 2012, his mother pled guilty to 9 felonies, including six counts of child abuse. She was sentenced to 20 years. His stepfather pled guilty to 4 felonies, including one count of child abuse. He was sentenced to 5 years.

Prior to the criminal case, a Dependency Trial successfully terminated the mother and stepfather's parental rights to each of their children. The telemedicine images were accepted into evidence and were an invaluable component of the child abuse medical professional's expert testimony.

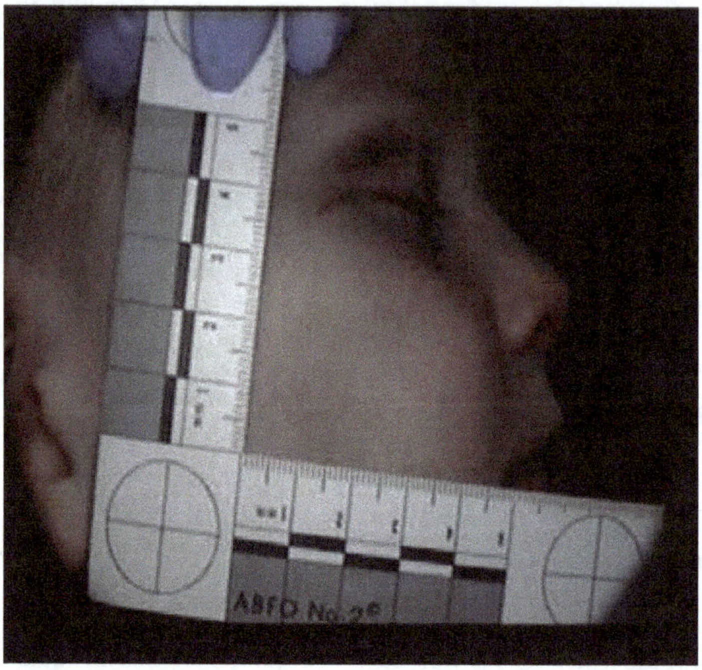


**Figure 4.** Multiple bruises and abrasions are noted on the forehead, eye, cheek, chin and neck

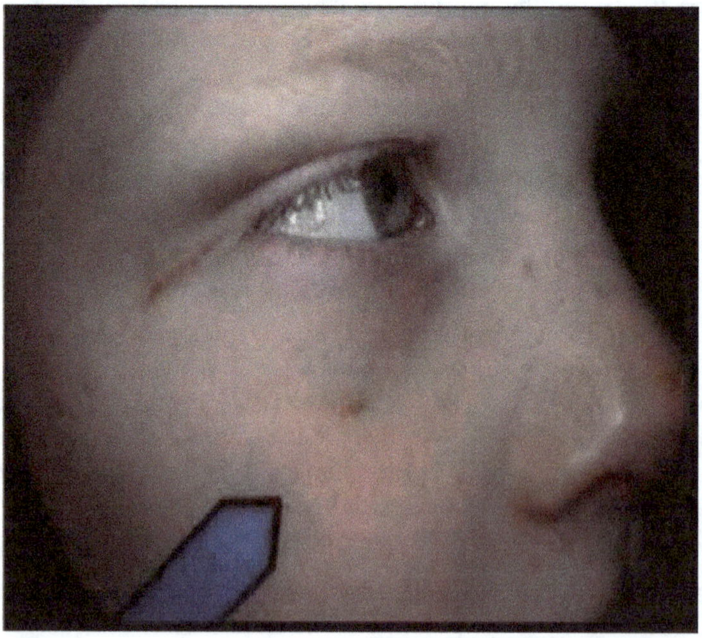

**Figure 5.** Multiple bruises and abrasions are noted on the forehead, eye, cheek, chin and neck

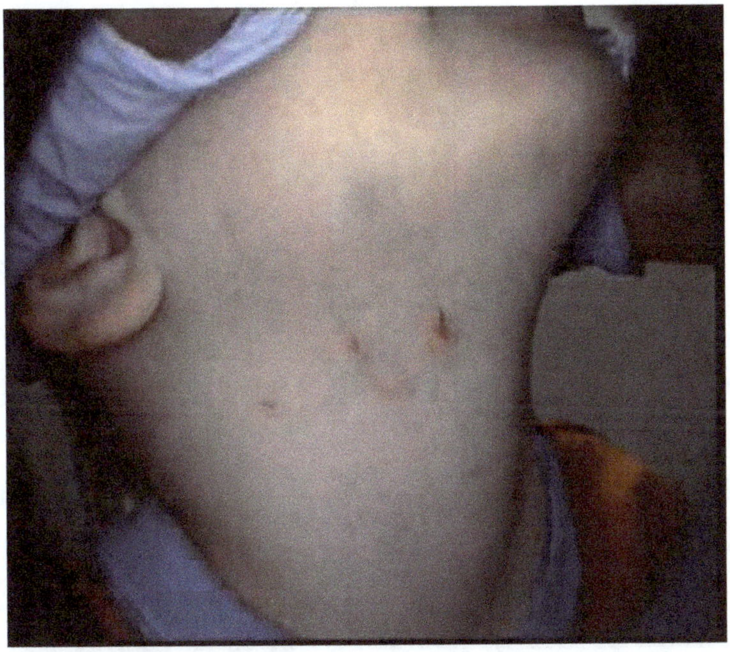

**Figure 6.** Multiple bruises and abrasions are noted on the forehead, eye, cheek, chin and neck

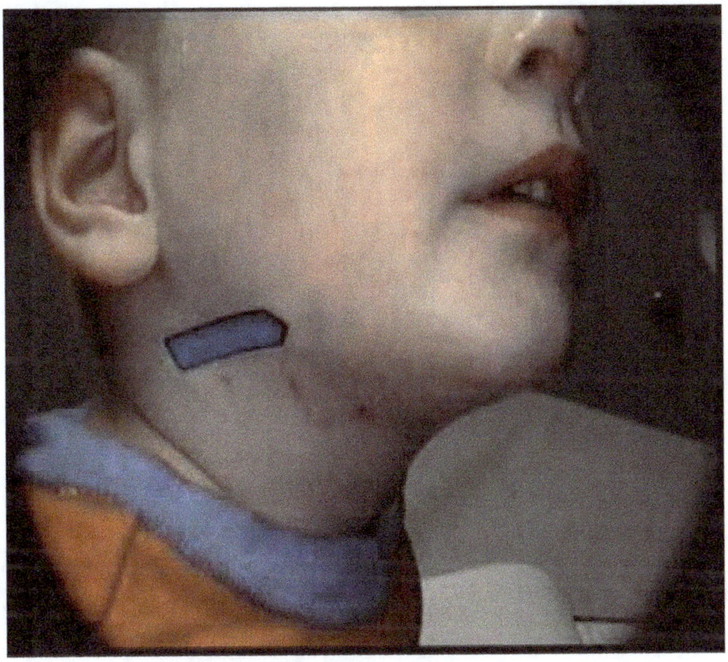

**Figure 7.** Multiple bruises and abrasions are noted on the forehead, eye, cheek, chin and neck

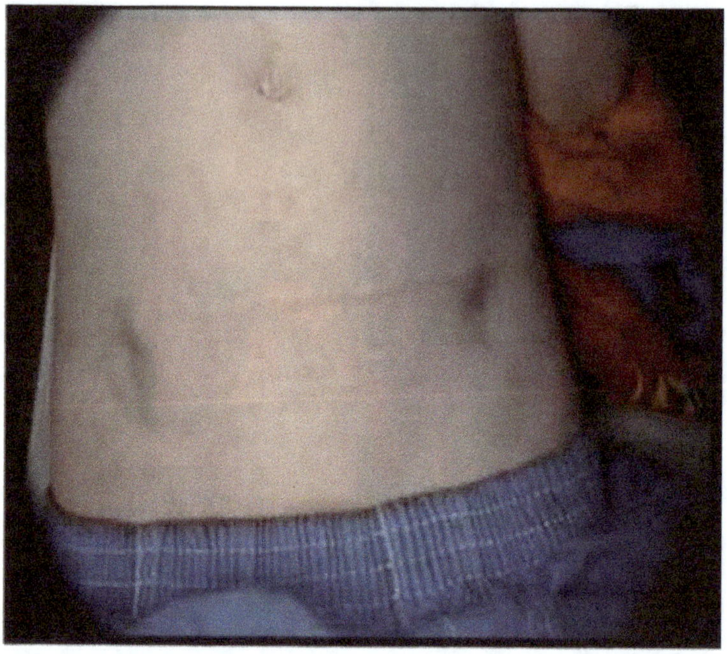

**Figure 8.** Large lower abdominal bruises are evident. An abdominal CT obtained 4 days later was reported as normal.

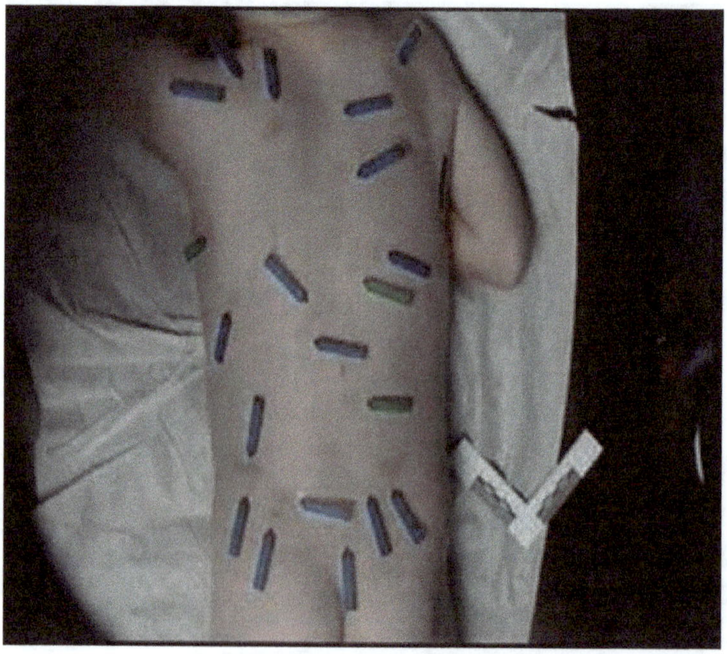

**Figure 9.** Extensive bruising is noted on his back.

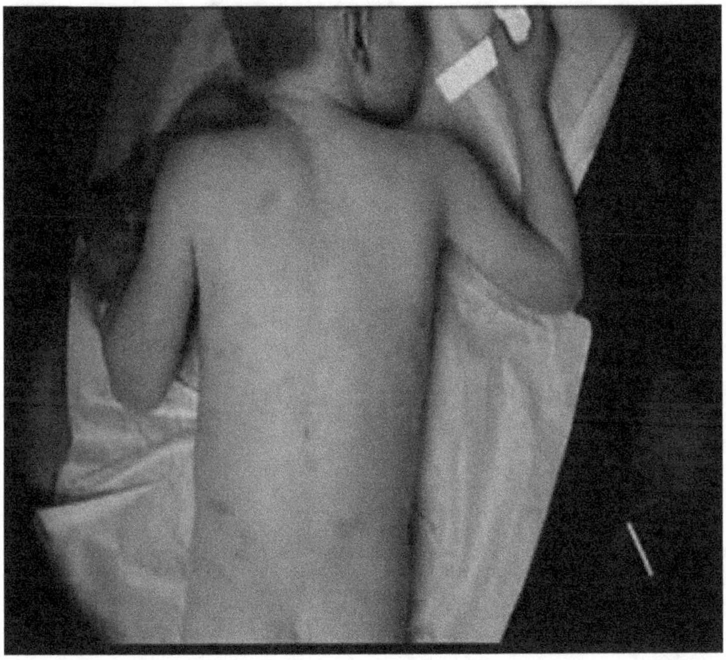

**Figure 10.** Extensive bruising is noted on his back.

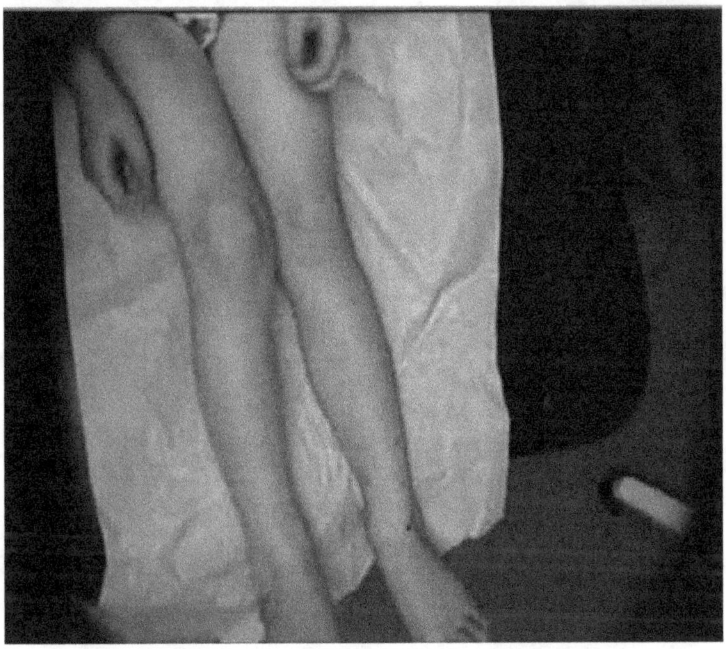

**Figure 11.** The child did not have any bruises on his anterior legs, the typical location for bruising in an active child his age.

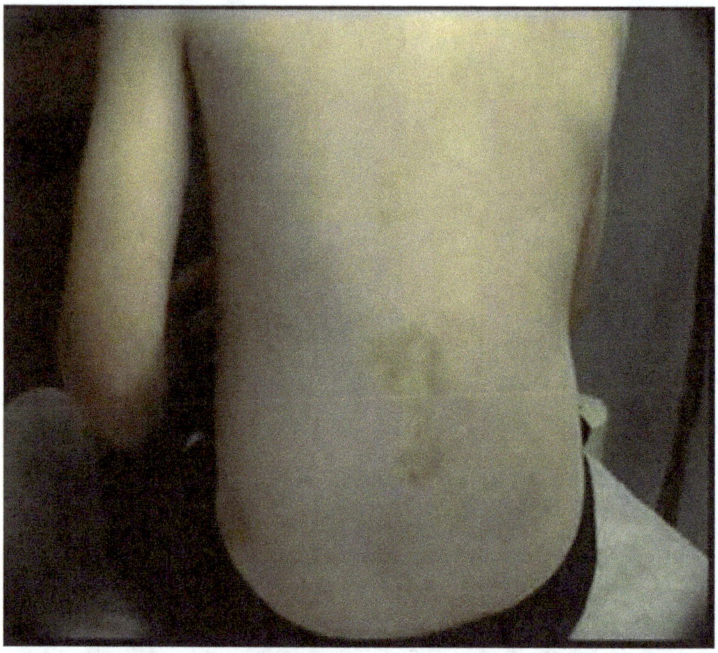

**Figure 12.**

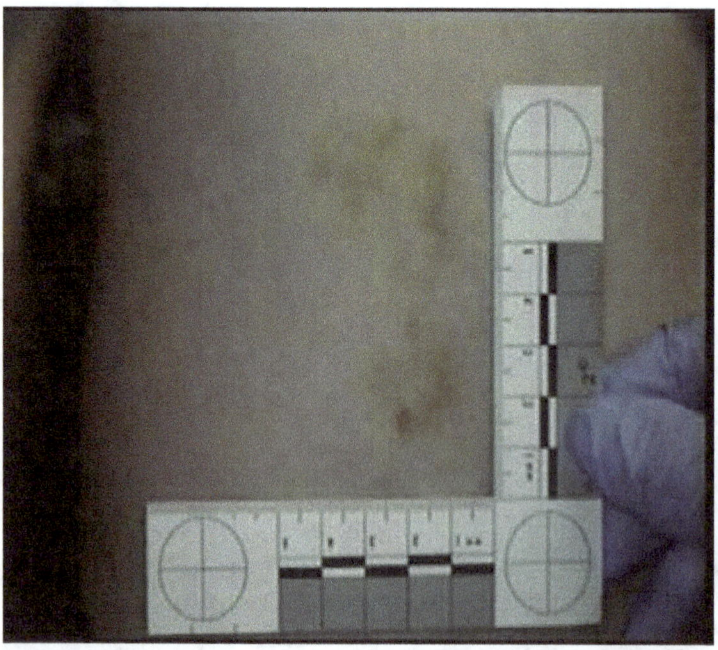

**Figure 13.**

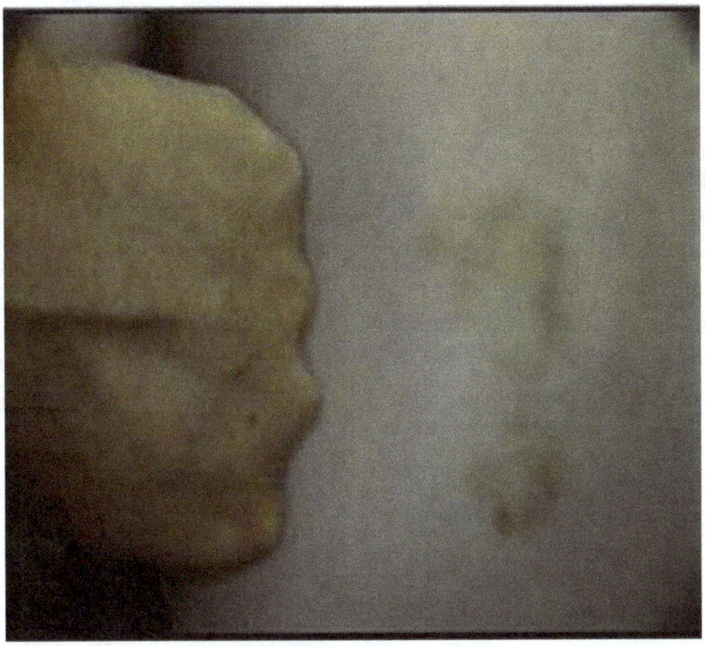

**Figure 14.** Three months prior, he was evaluated for large back and flank bruising. There is a large patterned bruise along his spine which appears to have been inflicted from a punch. Once again, the child disclosed that his 10 year old brother hurt him. Figure 14 represents an adult female fist.

## 6. Future

To our knowledge, no study has evaluated the child and non-offending caregivers' satisfaction with telemedicine for child abuse evaluations. However, child and parent satisfaction with telemedicine utilized by other medical subspecialties has been promising. A self-report questionnaire administered to patients receiving psychological intervention for childhood depression via telemedicine over an 8 week period revealed that the participants and their caregivers had very high satisfaction with the services received and had similar rates of attendance when compared to the control group receiving the same services face-to-face [7]. The authors also noted that due to the children's previous experiences with other forms of technology, they appeared to adapt easily to the use of the equipment used in the study [7]. Satisfaction surveys distributed to burn center physicians, referring MD or RN providers, and patients/family members where teleconsultation was utilized, also revealed that all involved in the process, including the patient and family, felt the encounter was helpful and that they were comfortable with the technology [8]. During an initial review of Florida's program between1999 and 2000, medical personnel reported that the children had a very high comfort level with the equipment involved [9]. With the ever growing technology present in children and parent's everyday lives, it is likely that there will be both a relatively high comfort level with the equipment and high satisfaction with the overall assessment conducted via telemedicine.

## 7. Conclusions

Telemedicine has proved to be a very useful method in conducting child abuse assessments to rural areas in the absence of local child abuse experts. The increases in child abuse reporting and lack of experts qualified to medically assess abuse cases further support the use of telemedicine. A variety of applications and uses provides a wide range of possibilities at varying costs that can be adapted by other child welfare programs throughout the world and have been demonstrated nationwide in the U.S. Telemedicine assessments and evidence obtained during the examinations have been successfully used in criminal and civil court without legal challenge. The use of telemedicine in child abuse will ensure accurate diagnosis by an expert, appropriate treatment and follow up, and reduce risk of future maltreatment.

## Author details

Sunshine Arnold[1] and Debra Esernio-Jenssen[2]

1 Team Coordinator of the Child Protection Team, University of Florida, USA

2 Medical Director of the Child Protection Team, Department of Pediatrics, University of Florida, USA

## References

[1] Menard, K. S, & Ruback, R. B. Prevalence and processing of child sexual abuse: a multi-data-set analysis of urban and rural counties. Law Hum Behav. (2003). , 27(4), 385-402.

[2] Tsai, S. H, Kraus, J, Wu, H. R, Chen, W. L, Chiang, M. F, Lu, L. H, Chang, C. E, & Chiu, W. T. The effectiveness of video-telemedicine for screening patients requesting emergency air medical transport (EAMT). Journal of Trauma (2007). , 62, 504-511.

[3] MacLeod KJMarcin JP, Boyle C, Miyamoto S, Dimand RJ, Rogers KK. Using telemedicine to improve care delivered to sexually abused children in rural, underserved hospitals. Pediatrics (2009). , 123, 223-228.

[4] Berkowitz, C. D. Child abuse recognition and reporting: supports and resources for changing a paradigm. Pediatrics (2008). SS12., 10.

[5] Alexander, R, & First, K. Telemedicine and child abuse examinations. Pediatric Annals October (2009). , 38(10), 574-578.

[6] Maguire, S, Mann, M. K, Sibert, J, & Kemp, A. Are there patterns of bruising in childhood which are diagnostic or suggestive of abuse? A systematic review. Arch Dis Child (2005). , 90, 182-186.

[7] Nelson, E. L, Barnard, M, & Cain, S. Treating childhood depression over videoconferencing. Telemedicine Journal and e-health (2003). , 9(1), 49-55.

[8] Saffle, J. R, Edelman, L, Theurer, B. S, Morris, S. E, & Cochran, A. C. Telemedicine evaluation of acute burns is accurate and cost-effective. The Journal of Trauma (2009). , 67(2), 358-365.

[9] Pammer, w, Haney, M, Wood, B. M, Brooks, R. G, Morse, K, Hicks, P, Handler, E. G, Rogers, H, & Jennett, P. Use of telehealth technology to extend child protection team services. Pediatrics (2001). , 108(3), 584-590.

# 3

# Mental Health Services for California Native Americans — Usual Service Options and a Description of Telepsychiatric Consultation to Select Sites

Donald M. Hilty, Peter M. Yellowlees, Nicole Tarui,
Steven R. Viramontes, Margo D. Kerrigan,
David L. Sprenger and Jay Shore

## 1. Introduction

### 1.1. Culture and health disparities for Native Americans

The culture of the patient refers to a set of beliefs, norms, and values (Surgeon General Report (SGR) 2001). This affects symptoms, presentation, meaning, understanding, family issues, coping styles, treatment seeking, trust, stigma, and overall health status. A clinic and its clinicians also have a culture that affects communication and care. Native Americans continue to suffer disproportionately from a variety of illnesses and diseases, despite the funds for health care services, resulting in higher death rates (age 71, nearly 5 years below average) than the rest of the U.S. population (Office General Council 2004). Some of these disparities are directly related to, or significantly affected by individual behavior and lifestyle choices (Office General Council 2004).

The Office of the General Counsel and IHS outlined the causes of the disparities for Native Americans. Racial discrimination, which introduces unique emotional variables, has been noted (NIH 2001), and the Institute of Medicine established that whites are more likely to receive more thorough, diagnostic work and better treatment and care than people of color, even when controlling for income, education, and insurance (Vernellia Randall Institute of Racism 2002). Current research indicates that there are five, non-mutually exclusive, primary five primary contributors to disparities in health status and outcomes for Native Americans. For example, a person may arrive at a health facility only to find a lack of necessary services or that there is an extended waiting period before services will be available (e.g., the Oglala Sioux has one of the best rehabilitation centers, but it does not have sufficient funding to staff the facility properly).

The five primary contributors to disparities in health status and outcomes for Native Americans are:

1. Limited access to appropriate health facilities.
2. Poor access to health insurance, including Medicaid, Medicare, and private insurance.
3. Insufficient federal funding.
4. Quality of care issues.
5. Disproportionate poverty and poor education.

The Indian Health Service (IHS) has been given primary responsibility to decrease disparities, as the primary source of biomedical services in many reservation communities, but is dramatically underfunded (Manson 2000), particularly with respect to mental health services (Nelson et al 1992). The IHS but Native Americans continue to experience significant rates of diabetes, mental health disorders, cardiovascular disease, and injuries. Native Americans are 770% more likely to die from alcoholism, 650% more likely to die from tuberculosis, 420% more likely to die from diabetes, and 280% more likely to die from accidents (Indian Health Care Improvement Act Amendments of 2003).

## 2. Mental health disparities for Native Americans: U.S., California and rural trends

**General issues.** The SGR of 2001 offered general definitions of mental health, mental illness, and mental health problems. It described mental health as important for personal well-being, family and interpersonal relationships, and successful contributions to community or society. These elements are jeopardized by mental health problems and mental illnesses. While these elements of mental health may be identifiable, mental health itself is not easy to define more precisely because any definition is rooted in value judgments that may vary across individuals and cultures. The Report outlines risks and protective factors (e.g., community or social factors are schools, availability of health and social services, and social cohesion).

The SGR of 2001, found that racial and ethnic minorities bear a greater burden from unmet mental health needs, ranking second only to cardiovascular disease in their impact on disability (Murray and Lopez 1996; Manson, 1996a). The foremost barriers include the cost of care, societal stigma, and the fragmented organization of services. Additional barriers include clinicians' lack of awareness of cultural issues, bias, or inability to speak the client's language, and the client's fear and mistrust of treatment. More broadly, disparities also stem from minorities' struggles with racism and discrimination, which affect their mental health and contribute to their lower economic, social, and political status.

**U.S. Native Americans**. Most Native Americans live in Western States, including California, Arizona, New Mexico, South Dakota, Alaska, and Montana, with 42% residing in rural areas, compared to 23% of whites (Rural Policy Research Institute, 1999). The number of Native Americans who live on reservations and trust lands has decreased substantially in the past few decades. Some events affecting Native American families parallel trends of other populations. Native American families maintained by a single female increased by 27% between 1980 and 1990, compared to the national figure of 17%. In addition, the removal of Native Americans from their lands, as well as other policies summarized above, has resulted in the high rates of poverty that characterize this ethnic minority group.

The Native American Service Utilization, Psychiatric Epidemiology, Risk and Protective Factors Project (AI-SUPERPFP) was designed to compare findings with the results of the baseline National Comorbidity Survey (NCS). It determined the lifetime prevalence of common mental disorders to be 35.7% for Southwest women to near 50% for men (Beals et al 2005a; Beals et al 2005b). Alcohol abuse and dependence were the most common disorders for men, with posttraumatic stress disorder most prevalent for women, with cultural and perhaps regional variations (Spicer et al 2003). A current study of lifetime and current physical and sexual abuse among Native American women found: 1) a significant relationship between childhood abuse, substance abuse/dependence, and adult re-victimization; and 2) a significant relationship between cumulative lifetime abuse events, substance abuse/dependence, and depression (Bohn 2003). Older Native Americans report that over 30% of older Native American adults visiting one urban IHS outpatient medical facility reported significant depressive symptoms; this rate is higher than most published estimates of the prevalence of depression among older whites with chronic illnesses (9%- 31%) (Manson 1992).

Two studies have assessed children and adolescents. The Great Smoky Mountain Study assessed psychiatric disorders among 431 youth ages 9 to 13 (Costello et al 1997). Overall, Native American children were found to have fairly similar rates of disorder (17%) in comparison to white children from surrounding counties (19%) (SGR 2001). The second study reported a follow-up of a school-based psychiatric epidemiological study involving Northern Plains youth, 13 to 17 years of age (Beals et al 1997). Altogether, more than 15% of the students qualified for a single diagnosis; 13% met criteria for multiple diagnoses. In terms of the broad diagnostic categories, 6% of the sample met criteria for an anxiety disorder, 5% for a mood disorder (either major depressive disorder or dysthymia), 14% for one or more of the disruptive behavior disorders, and 18% for substance abuse disorders.

**California Native Americans.** There are over 100 federally recognized tribes in California with 69,238 active health service users, defined as a visit in the last year (U.S. Census Bureau 2000). Native Americans constitute approximately 1% of the California population, 1.9% when the definition includes Native American/Alaskan Native in combination with other race, and are considered among the nation's most vulnerable populations due to high rates of psychiatric, medical, and substance use disorders (U.S. Census Bureau 2000). One study with a 20-year follow-up found the lifetime prevalence of mental disorders to be 70% (U.S. Department HHS, SAMSHA 2004).

Population dispersion of tribal groups in California makes it unlikely that a hospital-based service program will develop or support the members, meaning many rural and even some urban clinics depend on specialists outside the IHS. High costs associated with distance, time, and a shortage of primary care physicians in rural areas put Native Americans at high risk for suicide, trauma, and diabetes. Native Americans often do not obtain treatment due to barriers to care, differences in help-seeking behaviors, and higher dropout rate for mental health outpatient services than Caucasians (Weinick et al 2000).

### 2.1. Substance, rural health and Native Americans

A few studies have been completed regarding substance issues in Native Americans. A previously mentioned study that examined the relationship of substance abuse and psychiatric disorders among family members (Robin et al 1997) also considered their use of mental health services. Of those with a mental disorder, only 32% had received mental health or substance abuse services. The AI-SUPERPFP showed that Native American men were more likely than those in NCS to seek help for substance use problems from specialty providers; Native American women were less likely to talk to nonspecialty providers about emotional problems (Beals et al 2005b). Help-seeking from traditional healers was common in both Native American populations and was especially common in the Southwest.

There are many serious manifestations of untreated mental illness in Native Americans, particularly in rural areas. The prevalence rate of suicide for Native Americans is 1.5 times the national rate, particularly higher rates for males aged 15-24 and women aged 25-44 (U.S. HHS 2004; National Women's Health Information Center 2006). More Native Americans live in rural areas compared to Caucasians (42% to 23%) (U.S. HHS 2004). These areas have a shortage of mental health services and inadequate treatment (e.g., 70% of patients have an inadequate antidepressant dose for depression) (Unutzer et al 2002), and rural depressed patients have three times more hospitalizations and higher suicide rates than suburban patients (Rost et al 1999; Rost et al 1998). On the whole, rural communities are experiencing an acute shortage of adult, adolescent, and child psychiatric providers and those skilled in culturally appropriate care (Am Acad Child Adol Psychiatry 2004; Martinez 1993).

## 3. Primary care, mental health and telemedicine

### 3.1. Mental health services in primary care

Primary care medicine is crucial to mental health care delivery in the United States, for over half of those suffering from mental disorders (Regier et al 1978), particularly in rural areas where access to specialists is a greater problem. This lack of mental health services leads to poor outcomes, such as higher rates of homicide and suicide, as well as increased use of emergency services, hospitalizations, and placement in mental health institutions (Lishner et al 1995; Health Data Summaries 2000). Primary Care Providers (PCPs) in rural areas also report having inadequate skills to manage mental health issues, and they would benefit from assistance (Geller and Muus 2002; Geller 1999). However, rural areas inherently have provider shortages, particularly with regard to consultation-liaison psychiatrists.

Health providers use a number of psychiatric, health service and disease management models to reach primary care patients, predominantly in suburban and urban locales (Katon et al 1995; Pincus 1987; Strathdee 1987). The traditional referral or replacement model uses the psychiatrist as the principal provider of mental health services. The consultation care model includes the PCP as the principal provider of mental health services, after a psychiatric consultation. The collaborative care model involves mental health services jointly provided by the PCP and psychiatrist, including frequent communication between providers. Variations on these models also include use of mental health extenders and a stepped care to judiciously use scarce psychiatric resources (Katon et al 1997). Quality improvement programs also improve treatment rates and outcomes for depressed patients with comorbid medical illness in primary care (Koike et al 2002) and are cost-effective, too (Wells et al 2001).

These models have been evaluated both in the United States and Great Britain. In Great Britain, the majority of psychiatrists function in the traditional referral model (Strathdee 1987). The majority of PCPs, though, favored the collaborative care model, as having the psychiatrist located in the primary care clinic setting versus an offsite mental health clinic greatly improved the consultation process (Katon et al 1995; Bailey et al 1994). Such research shows that those PCPs patients are more likely to receive adequate doses of antidepressants and recover from depression (Simon et al 2000). But in rural areas, there is a dearth of specialists (Off Tech Assessment 1990), resulting in travel for patients or providers. In addition, some rural sites have unique needs and issues (e.g., high rates of substance disorders and few treatment options at an Native American reservation; enmeshed small communities, wherein patients want an objective person from the outside).

### 3.2. Telemedicine history

Telemedicine, defined as the use of technology to deliver health care (usually through videoconferencing), is one strategy to improve the accessibility of mental health care, particularly to areas underserved by physicians (Preston et al 1992; Hilty et al 2004a; Hilty et al 2013a). Telecommunications technology has been used to link specialists at academic health centers with health care professionals in rural areas for the management of patients (Hilty et al 1999). Videoconferencing, telephone and computer-based (e.g., e-mail) connect specialists with PCPs for patient care (Nesbitt et al 2000; Levine and Gorman 1999; Dick et al 1999; Hilty et al 2004b).

Medical home, home health and other mobile technology methods are in development and need to be better studied, although costs are dramatically decreasing. The patient-centered medical home (PCMH) is a concept founded on the presence of inadequate treatment in primary care and/or an inability to access needed services (Rosenthal 2008). PCMH allows telepsychiatric input at home, still under the general purview of the primary care provider, and it has been shown to improve patient care and health (Hollingsworth et al 2011). Desk-mounted video systems offer great convenience for therapy to cancer patients to avoid travel, but the cost used to be prohibitive for most consumers (Cluvey et al 2005). Internet-based video technology via personal computers and mobile devices must be HIPAA-adherent. Use of these technologies is increasingly becoming available, and will support the move of telepsychiatry to the home, such as programs that are now being implemented by the Veteran's Health Administration (Shore 2011).

Telemedicine was first used for medical purposes for psychiatric consultation (i.e. telepsychiatry) in the 1950's and 1960's to help the Nebraska Psychiatric Institute provide education, patient care, and consultation to a variety of sites (Wittson et al 1961). In the 1960s, telemedicine was also used to connect academic centers with urban populations (Straker et al 1976). Over the past several decades, academic health systems consisting solely of the medical center, are reaching out with telemedicine to rural clinics by using a consultation model of care. The University of California Davis Health System (UCDHS) connects the Medical Center with approximately 50 suburban and rural primary care clinics, up to 300 miles away, with telepsychiatric care (Nesbitt et al 2013; Hilty et al 2004a).

Telepsychiatry, in the form of consultation to primary care, and psychiatric management, has been well-received, enables valid and reliable evaluations, has good (preliminary) outcomes, and empowers parties using it (Hilty et al 2004a). PCPs in rural areas also have reported inadequate skills to manage mental health issues, and benefit from assistance (Geller 1999; Geller and Muus 2002). Telemedicine has been shown to improve medication adherence, depression severity, mental health status, health-related quality of life, and satisfaction for patients being treated for mental illnesses in primary care practices lacking on-site psychiatrists (Hilty et al 2006a; Hilty et al 2007a). The American Telemedicine Association has published telemental health practice guidelines (Yellowlees et al 2010) as has the American Association of Child and Adolescent Psychiatry (AACAP 2007).

### 3.3. Models of care for rural populations (Hilty et al 2006b)

**Model 1:** Randomized controlled trial (RCT) for depression in adults. A RCT recruited depression patients through self-report and structured psychiatric interviews (Hilty et al 2007b). Subjects were randomized to: 1) usual care with a disease management module (DMM) using telephone and self-report questionnaires; or 2) a DMM using telephone, questionnaires, and repeated televideo psychiatric consultation coupled with training of the PCP. Subjects' depressive symptoms, health status, and satisfaction with care were tabulated at 3, 6, and 12 months after study entry. There was significant clinical improvement for depression in both groups, with a trend toward significance in the more intensive module. Satisfaction and retention were statistically superior in the intensive group; there was no change in overall health functioning.

**Model 2:** Formal, multi-specialty phone and email physician-to-physician consultation. The UCDHS and California Department of Developmental Services (CDDS) developed the Physician Assistance, Consultation and Training Network (PACT Net) to assist PCPs in the treatment of patients with developmental disabilities in rural California (Hilty et al 2004b). PACT Net was a 24-hour warm-line in design and was funded from CDDS at approximately $450,000 over three years. Thirty consultations were completed: 28 by telephone and 2 by e-mail; 24 of those consultations were able to be responded to within one business day of the referral. The average duration of consultation was 47 minutes, and the consultation was accompanied with a 4-page summary/case for the referring physician. The top three services requested for consultation were psychiatry (e.g., management of behavioral disturbance), medical genetics (e.g., diagnosis), and gastroenterology. PCPs rated items baseline satisfaction on a 7-point Likert scale: 1) pre-existing local services at 3.37; 2) timeliness of the PACT Net consultation at 5.45; 3) quality of the communication at 6.3; and 4) overall quality and utility of the consultation at 6.2. Specialists rated the quality of the communication at 6.45, and the ease of the service at 6.46. While phone and e-mail consultation was effective, it was not used as much as expected.

**Model 3:** An integrated program of mental health screening, therapy on site, and telepsychiatric (video, phone, e-mail) consultation to rural primary care. The UCDHS and Northern Sierra Rural Health Network collaborated to develop a program for rural Northeastern California, funded by the California Endowment. Over a three-year period, 10 rural sites learned how to utilize screening instruments for multiple disorders (e.g., depression, alcoholism, and anxiety disorders), and collect basic outcome measures for depression at regular intervals, in concert with telepsychiatric consultations and on site therapy visits. The number of consultations per year increased by 120%. Continuing medical education (CME) was provided annually for PCPs and other providers. Services included a telepsychiatric consultant / therapist on site 25% for specific brief therapy and integrated planning meetings between rural primary and mental health care staff. Outcomes were that most children were seen only once, but a statistically significant improvement between initial evaluation and three-month follow-up in the convenience sample was seen in the Affect and Oppositional domains of the Child Behavioral Checklist (CBCL) for girls and boys, respectively; incorporating standardized checklists, may assist in diagnosis and treatment of rural children (Neufeld et al 2007).

**Model 4:** Cultural consultation to rural primary care using telemedicine. Early in the telepsychiatry service of UC Davis Department of Psychiatry and Behavioral Sciences in 1996, culturally informed consultation became incorporated into the telemedicine rural primary care collaboration. Some rural patients faced language and cultural barriers to seeking and receiving care from their local primary care physician. For example, a 56 year-old Mexican American female who became depressed following the sudden death of her husband of thirty years, was diagnosed with major depression, and started on an antidepressant but did not improve despite 4 months of treatment (Cerda et al 1999). She did not take medication as recommended and did not communicate concerns to the PCP because of the stigma and cultural reasons. A 60-minute telepsychiatric evaluation was conducted by a Mexican American psychiatrist, who met with the PCP and patient. At follow-up the patient reported daily compliance with medication thereafter, the depression had remitted and the frequency of medical visits decreased from one-to-two times per month over a one-year period to only a single visit in the six months since the consultation.

**Model 5:** Collaborative care via telepsychiatry. This model is co-provision of medication for primary care patients by the telepsychiatrist and primary care provider in rural communities, based on the earlier models of in-person care to achieve national standards of antidepressant prescriptions (Fortney et al 2013; Katon et al 1997).This model is often integrated with stepped models of care, which similar to above use 'less intensive or expensive interventions' first then if patients fail to improve, 'step it up' to more intensive services, and

**Model 6:** Asynchronous telepsychiatry. Traditionally, there have been two main types of telemedicine: *synchronous*, which typically relies on live, two-way interactive video to a remote area, and *asynchronous* (store-and-forward), which transmits clinical information via email or web applications for later review by a specialist. Broadly speaking, synchronous communication by phone or with video allows synthesis of information and easy exchange of information, with in -the-moment questions by PCPs. *Asynchronous* telemedicine has been commonly used and well-received for pathology, cardiology, radiology, dermatology and other fields. A study of synchronous telepsychiatry, including Native American patients, revealed that PCPs are highly satisfied with the service, with 100% of the respondents noting the consultation as fast as from a regular face-to-face visit, was able to meet their patient's needs and lead to an improvement in the management of their patient; 64% thought the ATP consultant was able to completely meet their patient's needs and the feedback they received over ATP was as good as from a regular face-to-face visit (Yellowlees et al 2010; Butler and Yellowlees 2012).

### 3.4. Telepsychiatry and cultural populations

Ethnicity, culture and language issues affect health (Office of Surgeon General, 2001) and there is often inadequate access to specialists (Moreno et al 2012) —inroads to patient needs and preferences that can be met by telemental health are progressing. A recent study of nearly 40 rural health clinics compared impressions of 25 primary care providers and 32 staff impressions of factors important to care: using providers who value differences (5.4/7.0), quality of the provider's care (4.9/7.0), access to care in general (4.5/7.0) and availability of trained interpreters for use with patients (4.4/7.0) (Hilty et al 2013). Others are studying the specific needs of Hispanics/Latinos (Moreno et al 2012; Nieves et al 2007, Chong et al 2012), Asians (Ye et al 2011), Native Americans (Weiner et al 2005, Shore et al 2007, Shore et al 2008), Eastern Europeans (Mucic, 2004), and those using sign language (Lopez et al 2004) —all using telepsychiatry for service provision. With patients of different cultural backgrounds, using the patients' primary language allows for a more comfortable atmosphere where they may express their genuine feelings and emotions.

### 3.5. Telepsychiatry to Native Americans

Northern Plains Native Americans were very satisfied and comfortable with telepsychiatric treatment for post traumatic stress disorder (Shore and Manson 2004a; Shore and Manson 2004b; Shore et al 2006). In fact, location, communication, trust, and confidentiality were equally satisfactory for treatment in-person versus videoconferencing. Even Native American children and families are receptive to telepsychiatric consultation (Savin et al 2006).

#### U. Colorado.

Over the past decade the University of Colorado's Center for American Indian and Alaska Native Health (CAIANH) has collaborated on multiple telepsychiatry services targeted at American Indian and Alaska Native populations (Shore et al 2006; Savin et al 2006; Shore et al

2012a). These services have occurred in a number of Western States (Alaska, Colorado, Montana, New Mexico, South Dakota, Wyoming), involved both consultative and direct service models in a range of settings (community clinics, hospitals) and spanned age ranges from children and adolescents to geriatric population. These services have helped to demonstrate the feasibility of telepsychiatry with native populations, various models of clinical structure and integration and the importance of cultural adaptation.

A recent review (Shore et al 2012a) summarizes 10 years of CAIANH work with rural Native Veterans, of rural American Indian Veterans who serve at the highest rate per capita in the military, and who have the highest rates of posttraumatic stress disorder and substance abuse related to their military service. These clinics represent a unique multi-organizational collaboration between the Department of Veterans Affairs, the Indian Health Service, the University of Colorado and Tribal partners. Outcomes provide strong evidence of the positive impact of improved access and quality of care to rural Native veterans. For example a recent published report described the increase in service utilization and appropriate medications for patient in these clinics (Shore et al 2012b). The clinics utilize a model that includes culturally knowledgeable providers, onsite clinic tribal outreach workers and collaboration with local services including as appropriate traditional medicine. This work strongly suggests the importance of the development and use of an appropriate telepsychiatry clinic model for Native patients that accommodates cultural issues, maintains overall fidelity of approach but can be adapted to best fit local services and culture.

## 4. UC Davis telepsychiatric Native American study

### 4.1. Overview

This article is a description of the patients seen from three California Native American IHS sites using a telepsychiatric consultation program from the academic medical center. Its objectives were to: a) describe the population's demographics and illnesses, b) identify needs of patients and physicians, c) report the services delivered to this patient population, and d) examine the quality of psychopharmacologic services. Patient, clinic, and system factors related to telepsychiatric consultation, which have important implications for federal health policy toward Native Americans, will be noted (Dixon 2001).

### 4.2. Methods

The University of California Davis Health System (UCDHS) is based in Sacramento, California, and serves a 33-county area to the Oregon state border. Since 1995, UCDHS has provided telemedical consultations since 1995 in 28 specialties to 42 clinics (26 rural, 16 prisons) between 100 and 350 miles away (Nesbitt et al 2013). The telepsychiatry service has provided over 4,000 consultations, using a variety of models (Hilty et al 2006b).

### 4.3. Technology

UCDMC and remote sites use dial-up integrated service digital network (ISDN) lines, transmission speeds of 384 Kbps and a CODEC (COder-DECoder). The hourly rate for lines ranges from $30-$60 depending on the distance and long-distance carrier, for each hourly consultation. Round Valley and K'ima:w use Internet Protocol (IP) with transmissions speeds of 384 Kbps, carried over a dedicated link (either Frame Relay or a T-1 connection) into the UC Davis network. The monthly cost is approximately $500/clinic, but there is no per-use charge as with ISDN. The total capital cost of these units is approximately $8,000 at all sites.

### 4.4. IHS clinics and patients

K'ima:w Medical Center (Hoopa, Karuk, and Yurok tribes), Round Valley Indian Health Center, Inc. (Round Valley Indian Tribes) and Pit River Health Service, Inc. (Big Bend, Montgomery Creek, Pit River Tribe, Roaring Creek, Smith Camp) receive specialty services from UC Davis Medical Center (UCDMC) and are officially rural areas as defined by non-metropolitan statistical criteria (Off Tech Assessment 1990). All have a population under 500 and patients travel 3-6 hours for specialty service on roads that are hard to access or treacherous to travel. Each city has an IHS primary care clinic. Most of these clinics have part-time substance abuse/dependence counseling and groups; none have a full-time psychotherapist and there are no mental health clinics or day treatment programs; psychiatric hospitalization is 3-6 hours away. California IHS has used telepsychiatric, tele-endocrinology and tele-ophthalmology since 1999. They use a specialist consulting by video to a primary care provider at the IHS site, who provides the actual care. Consecutive initial and follow-up telepsychiatric consultation from UCDMC to the IHS sites from January 2004 to December 2004 were reviewed. Data from IHS patients around the state, rural Northern California telepsychiatry sites and the California census were used as comparisons (Tables 1 and 2).

| Characteristic | Study CA IHS Patients | IHS Community | | | Rural Northern CA (eMH)[5] | CA (via US Census) |
|---|---|---|---|---|---|---|
| | | Total CA IHS patients | Native American IHS Pts. | Non-AI CA IHS Pts. | | |
| N | 45 | 7472 | 4071 | 3401 | 122 | 24,621,819[1] |
| Age | | | | | | |
| 18-30 | 35.5% | 30.1% | 36.3% | 22.7% | 27.9% | 26.4% |
| 31-45 | 37.0% | 26.6% | 28.7% | 24.1% | 29.5% | 32.5% |
| 46-65 | 20.0% | 29.8% | 24.7% | 35.8% | 36.9% | 27.2% |
| > 65 | 6.6% | 13.5% | 10.3% | 17.4% | 4.1% | 13.8% |
| Ethnicity | | | | | | 33,871,648[2] |
| Caucasian | 17.8% | 19.5% | 0% | 42.8% | 96.7% | 63.4% |

| Characteristic | Study CA IHS Patients | IHS Community | | | Rural Northern CA (eMH)[5] | CA (via US Census) |
|---|---|---|---|---|---|---|
| | | Total CA IHS patients | Native American IHS Pts. | Non-AI CA IHS Pts. | | |
| Amer. Indian | 80.0% | 52.5% | 100% | 0% | 0.8% | 0.7% |
| Latino | 2.2% | 1.4% | 0% | 3.0% | 0.8% | 32.4% |
| Afr. Amer. | 0% | .2% | 0% | 0.5% | 1.6% | 7.4% |
| Asian | 0% | 0% | 0% | 0% | 0% | 12.3% |
| Other | 0% | 26.4% | 0% | 53.6% | 0% | 20.1% |
| Gender: % Female | 66.7 | 51.9% | 52.9% | 50.6% | 58.2% | 49.3%[1] |
| Marital Status | | | | | | 26,076,163[3] |
| Married | 40.0 | | | | 39.3% | 54.9% |
| Single | 28.9 | | | | 41.8% | 30.1% |
| Divorced | 17.8 | | | | 9.0% | 9.5% |
| Widowed | 4.4 | | | | 3.3% | 5.6% |
| Not Noted | 8.9 | | | | 6.6% | |
| Unemployed | 53.3% | | | | | 15,829,202[4] |
| Not Noted | 24.4% | | | | | 7.0% |
| Prev. attempted | 28.8% | | | | | |
| suicide (1+) | 28.8% | | | | | |
| Prev. hospitalized | | | | | | |
| Current nicotine users | 35.5% | | | | | |

[1]Source: U.S. Census Bureau (USCB), Census 2000 Summary File 1, 100-% Data, DP-1. Profile of General Demographic Characteristics: 2000.

[2]These numbers reflect total population, inclusive of those under the age of 18.

[3]Source: USCB, Census 2000 Summary File 3, Matrices PCT1, PCT7, and PCT8.

[4]Source: USCB, Census 2000 Summary File 3, Matrices P43 and PCT35.

[5]Rural comparison sample of adult patients over same period of time from10 northern rural clinics.

Source: USCB, Current Population Survey, 2004 Annual Social and Economic Supplement. Table HI05. Health Insurance Coverage Status and Type of Coverage by State and Age for All People: 2003.

@ (Numbers in thousands)

**Table 1.** A Comparison of Patient Characteristics: Study CA IHS vs. All IHS vs. Rural CA vs. General CA.

| | N | Current CA IHS | N | Rural CA[1] | Chi Square Analysis | Significance |
|---|---|---|---|---|---|---|
| Total Axis I Diagnoses | 92 | 45 patients 2.04 dx/pt. | 203 | 122 patients 1.66 dx/pt. | | |
| Mood | 31 | 69% | 100 | 82% | (1, N = 167) = 3.92 | $p < 0.05$ |
| Depression | 22 | 49% | 56 | 45.9% | | |
| Bipolar Disorder | 9 | 20.0% | 44 | 36.1% | | |
| Anxiety[2] | 25 | 55.5% | 45 | 36.9% | (1, N = 167) = 4.71 | $p < 0.05$ |
| Impulse | 5 | 11.1% | 0 | 0% | (1, N = 167) = 13.97 | $p < 0.001$ |
| Substance (abuse/ dependence) | 25 | 55.5% | 22 | 18.0% | (1, N = 167) = 14.79 | $p < 0.001$ |
| Alcohol | 10 | 22.2% | 11 | 9.0% | (1, N = 167) = 5.21 | $p < 0.05$ |
| Drug | 15 | 33.3% | 11 | 9.0% | (1, N = 167) = 14.79 | $p < 0.001$ |
| Cognitive/ Dementia | 1 | 2.2% | 5 | 4.1% | | |
| Psychosis | 5 | 11.1% | 11 | 9.0% | | |
| Childhood | 0 | 0% | 8 | 6.6% | | |
| Somatoform d/o | 0 | 0% | 5 | 4.1% | | |
| Eating | 0 | | 7 | 5.7% | | |
| Unknowns | 0 | 0% | 0 | 0% | | |
| Total Axis II[3] Diagnoses | 5 | 11.1% | 11 | 9.0% | | |
| Total Axis V - GAF | Mean = 60.71; SD = 5.040; Range 50-70 | | Mean = 60.10; SD = 8.756; Range 35-85 | | | |

[1]Rural comparison sample of adult patients over same period of time from 10 northern rural clinics.

[2] PTSD nearly 2/3 of all disorders.

[3] Provisional

**Table 2.** Primary Diagnosis for Native American Telepsychiatry Consultations.

## 4.5. Teleconsultation procedures

Consultations started with a PCP referral, with an assistant faxing a one-page consultation request and, when available, information on the patient's history, medication log, and medical disorders one week prior to the consultation. All consultations were performed by psychiatric faculty in English. A consultation care model was used, in which the PCP was the provider of mental health services. Patients signed a consent form that described the nature of the consultation, personnel involved, and their option to see someone in person. Patients who presented with a medical emergency (e.g., suicidal or homicidal ideation or acute psychoses) were referred to local mental health services in lieu of telemedicine consultation, unless the presence of a staff member was sufficient to stabilize them for the appointment. If an emergency developed, the UCDMC clinic called the IHS clinic to have staff and law enforcement assist. An appointment consisted of 45 minutes for the psychiatrist to conduct the patient evaluation and 5-10 minutes for the PCP to join at the end of the evaluation to discuss options for treatment.

Diagnosis was made by a semi-structured interview, using the mood, anxiety and substance sections of the Structured Clinical Interview for DSM-IV-TR, and supplemented with the following: screening questions for other psychiatric diagnosis(es); history of abuse or domestic violence; hospitalizations; past suicide attempts and present suicidal or homicidal ideation; current and past medication; 1st and 2nd-degree family member history of psychiatric disorders; and the PCP reasons for referring for consultations (diagnostic assessment, medication management, psychological assessment or triage); this is the PCPs' understanding for the referral rather than what turned out to be true by psychiatric evaluation. On the day of the consultation, a one-page fax was sent from the psychiatrist to the rural site to summarize findings and present three treatment options per problem. The PCP would choose what he/she thought was the best option; the others automatically served as back-up plans. A dictation was sent one week thereafter.

### 4.6. Data collection

Data were collected on each consultation from telemedicine staff at the rural site (RPMS above), the patient, the PCP, and the psychiatrist. The IHS community data were retrieved from the IHS Resource and Patient Management System (RPMS). RPMS is a decentralized automated information system of over 50 integrated software applications that supports the provision of healthcare at Indian Health facilities. RPMS is a repository of patient data that can be manipulated by applications to support healthcare planning, delivery, management, and research. At UCDMC, paper protocols steered research assistants to collect information from patient registration forms, the electronic medical record and additional paper forms to log any data not usually included in a standard interview; the information was de-identified. Patient sociodemographic information included age, ethnicity, gender, marriage status, education, and employment. Comments by patients and staff were logged for informal analysis of themes that arose, in a qualitative sense, in case future evaluation might be indicated.

### 4.7. Diagnostic clustering

Due to numbers, mood disorders were spelled out, but otherwise, broad grouping of diagnostic categories was done due to small numbers and general clustering of the diagnoses, following DSM-IV-TR categorization (e.g., anxiety, psychotic and impulse control disorders). Substance use disorders were differentiated into either alcohol or drug, regardless of abuse or dependence. Provisional Axis II diagnoses were grouped together due to the fact that few were confirmed on one-time evaluation. Family members' diagnoses were not confirmed; report was considered positive if they had medication treatment, hospitalization or a long history known to family (e.g., social disturbance by alcohol).

### 4.8. Quality of medication trial

Dosing was assessed by chart review and in line with national guidelines, with adjustments made for projected age, culture and drug interactions (Depression in Primary Care. Volume 2 1993; APA Practice Guideline 2002; APA Practice Guideline 2006). The criteria vary on dosage vary according to disorder (e.g., depression, paroxetine, initial 10-20mg bedtime, initial 4-week trial, dose increase and so on). The chart was checked for a disorder in which the medication would be used, to determine if it was "Not needed" or "Needed"; since therapy is available in some sites and not others, and if available, usually used no more than one time per month, medication is more needed than not. Ancillary use of medications at low dose (e.g., for sleep) was excluded. Dosage and duration were reviewed per chart and per patient interview of how it was prescribed, in the event that the dosage was changed or new medications were not reflected in the chart. Medication was categorized as adequate, partially adequate (e.g., adequate dosage or too short of a period) or inadequate (e.g., none given, too little given to affect change). Non-adherence with medication, by self-report and by questioning by the telepsychiatrist, was excluded as a confounder.

### 4.9. Data analysis

Descriptive statistics and chi-square tests were run for the following: a) IHS vs. other socio-demographics; b) IHS vs. others' diagnoses; c) past and present diagnoses; d) present diagnoses (if more than one); e) present diagnoses and family member diagnoses; and f) dosing adequacy and ethnicity, gender, and presence of a diagnosis of substance abuse/dependence.

### 4.10. IRB approval

This project was approved by the Committee on the Protection of Human Subjects at UCDMC.

### 4.11. Results

Over the one-year period, 45 different IHS patients were seen; 80% were Native American, and 67% were female. Initial evaluations were done for 32 and 13 had follow-up visits from prior initial telepsychiatry consultations. The mean age was 39.71 (SD = 14.83). For comparison, other samples were of similar ages, though the California rural comparison sample was 97% Caucasian and 58% female; overall, Californians were 63.4% Caucasian, 49.3% female (see Table 1).

PCP reasons for consultations were consistent with primary care practice, and included depression and anxiety (40%), general medication evaluation (38%), mood disorders (11%), disability evaluation (4%), and gastric bypass psych evaluation (7%). The most common services provided were medication management (96%), diagnostic clarification (89%), psychological assessment (36%), and patient triage (18%).

The total number of Axis I diagnoses was 92 (range, 0-4), with an average of 2.04 per patient (SD = 1.06) (see Table 2). A total of 31 patients were diagnosed with mood disorders (9 bipolar/22 depression); 13 (42%) of those individuals had 1st and 2nd-degree family members with a mood disorder. Fifteen (48.3%) of the patients with mood disorders had comorbid anxiety disorders. Notably, 55% of the patients seen had a current substance abuse/dependence diagnosis, mainly methamphetamine (42% of the 55%) and marijuana (40% of the 55%). Chi-square tests revealed the IHS sample to have higher rates of anxiety, impulse, alcohol abuse/dependence, and drug abuse/dependence disorders than the rural California samples (Table 2). The average Global Assessment of Function (GAF) was 60.71 (SD 5.040).

There appeared to be a significant relationship of diagnoses to past personal and family history. High rates of disorders were found between mood, abuse/trauma, and substances. The overall sexual abuse rate at 22% (10/45) and these patients had high rates of other disorders (see Table 3). Data suggested a relationship between 1st and 2nd-degree family members using substances and patients using alcohol, as well as between mental and emotional abuse and a diagnosis of depression, but statistical differences were not found. Patients with bipolar or substance disorders commonly had a family member with bipolar disorder. As shown in Table 4, the IHS subgroup with mental and emotional abuse also showed higher of depression rates than the overall sample.

In terms of dosing and dosing adequacy, of the 45 patients, 73% had a medication indicated for their primary disorder; 60% of those were at an adequate dose. When it was looked at per group and medication, antidepressants were given adequately 50.0% of the time and sub-adequately for 63.3% of patients (Table 5). This was in stark contrast to mood stabilizers and antipsychotics adequately used 23.1% and 25.0%, respectively, mainly being under-dosed more than antidepressants; they were not erroneously prescribed, though. A chi-square analysis found a significant relationship between inadequate dosing of antipsychotics and gender (women) ($p < 0.01$). No other biases were found with inadequate dosing.

Qualitative analysis revealed that patients reported comments in several theme areas: a) gratitude for the availability of care in general, and care without the stigma of mental health services, in particular, as many do not have transportation to urban centers; b) preference for telepsychiatric consultation, since they fear stigma locally and are unsure if confidentiality can be maintained in small rural centers; c) appreciation of their clinics' initiative in helping them; and 4) initial anxiety about using the technology and surprise that it seemed to work. Staff at IHS sites felt positive about care being available, high patient satisfaction, and some frustration about making the clinic schedule "fit" the rural and cultural environment. Staff at the UCDMC Center for Health and Technology reported that IHS sites seemed to value the service as much or more than other rural sites.

### 4.12. Discussion of findings

These clinics of the IHS found more patients to be female and Native American than in other populations, and to have 2+ psychiatric disorders (mainly depression and anxiety). The main services conducted for IHS patients by telepsychiatry are medication management and diagnostic clarification. The adequacy of medication treatment was better for disorders requiring antidepressants than for those requiring mood stabilizers or antipsychotics. Patients with a personal or family history of trauma, mood or substance disorders, had higher rates of psychiatric and specifically substance disorders. As found in a previous study, relationships appear to exist between trauma history, substance abuse/dependence, mental illness, and higher rates of suicide attempts and hospitalizations (Bohn 2003). The sexual abuse rate that we found in our IHS sample–22%–is consistent with national rates estimating that 15-33% of females have experienced sexual abuse (Bohn 2003). Based on national studies, higher rates of substance abuse/dependence in the Native American sample vs. rural California were not unexpected, though this did not generalize into more overall pathology based on GAF scores.

There are many clinical implications of these data, particularly the high rates of comorbidity between mood, anxiety, substance, and other disorders. In particular, bipolar disorder and substance disorders quite commonly co-exist, and a positive family history may be helpful in diagnosis (APA Practice Guideline 2002). Clinicians may need to evaluate Native American patients differently than other rural populations. Treatment plans with a strong biopsychosocial approach are indicated in light of stress and trauma, but therapy resources are limited. Best practices and Treatment Intervention Protocols to identify and treat comorbidities are available through the Substance Abuse and Mental Health Services Administration (SAMSHA) Center for Substance Abuse Treatment (SAMSHA Subst Treatment 2002), but these protocols are complex and require more resources than many rural sites have available, or the specialist services are again not available.

Rates of medication dosing adequacy upon referral indicate that PCPs are more likely to *not* prescribe than to inaccurately prescribe psychiatric medications, which is consistent with national trends (Hilty and Servis 1999). From a programmatic point of view, if medication dosing is falling short for bipolar and psychotic disorders, disease management interventions may be indicated (Hilty et al 2007b). No major ethnic biases or gender biases were found regarding dosing, except inadequate dosing of antipsychotics in females; numbers were small and should only be interpreted as a trend.

## 5. Discussion and conclusions

Native Americans have significant needs for health care and are at significant risk for many health and mental health problems. Without attention to both health and mental health needs, patients and their families face compounded problems of health, money, access and other social problems.

| Subgroups Current / Past Drug Usage | Family N = 11 % | Sexual Abuse N = 10 % | Non-Physical, Emotional Abuse N = 4 % | Physical Abuse N = 11 % | Overall Sample N = 45 % |
|---|---|---|---|---|---|
| Alcohol | 100 | 90.0 | 25.0 | 81.1 | **64.4** |
| Amphetamines | 36.4 | 50.0 | 0 | 27.2 | **42.2** |
| Cocaine | 18.2 | 10.0 | 0 | 18.3 | **8.9** |
| Opioids | 36.7 | 20.0 | 25.0 | 27.2 | **22.2** |
| Marijuana | 45.5 | 50.0 | 75.0 | 50.0 | **40.0** |
| Suicide attempts | 27.3 | 30.0 | 75.0 | 36.3 | **28.8** |
| ? Hospitalizations | 27.3 | 30.0 | 75.0 | 28.8 | **28.8** |
| **Diagnoses** | | | | | |
| Bipolar | 27.3 | 20.0 | 0 | 9.1 | **20.0** |
| Depression | 63.6 | 60.0 | 100 | 54.5 | **49.0** |
| Anxiety | 63.6 | 60.0 | 25.0 | 63.6 | **55.5** |
| Substance | 54.5 | 30.0 | 25.0 | 54.5 | **55.5** |
| Alcohol | 18.1 | 30.0 | 0 | 18.1 | **22.2** |
| Cognitive | 0 | 0 | 0 | 0 | **2.2** |
| Psychosis | 0 | 20.0 | 0 | 2 | **11.1** |
| **Primary Family Members** | | | | | |
| Bipolar | 36.7 | 20.0 | 25.0 | 18.1 | **13.3** |
| Depression | 18.2 | 10.0 | 75.0 | 9.1 | **20.0** |
| Anxiety | 9.1 | 30.0 | 25.0 | 27.2 | **11.1** |
| Substance Abuse/ Dependence | 100.0 | 30.0 | 25.0 | 45.4 | **24.4** |
| Cognitive | 9.1 | 0 | 0 | 0 | **6.6** |
| Psychosis | 9.1 | 10.0 | 0 | 0 | **8.8** |
| Childhood | 9.1 | 10.0 | 0 | 18.1 | **6.6** |
| Unknown | 0 | 10.0 | 0 | 0 | **8.8** |

[1] Family defined as 1st and 2nd-degree members.

**Table 3.** Relationship of Patient Psychiatric Diagnoses with Personal and Family[1] Histories.

| Subgroups | Bipolar | Depression | Anxiety | Psychosis | Etoh | Drug | Overall |
|---|---|---|---|---|---|---|---|
| **Current / Past Drug Use** | **(n = 9) %** | **(n = 22) %** | **(n = 21) %** | **(n = 4) %** | **(n = 10) %** | **(n = 14) %** | **(N =45) %** |
| Alcohol | 77.8 | 59.1 | 28.6 | 0 | 100.0 | 78.6 | **64.4** |
| Amphetamines | 88.9 | 22.7 | 23.8 | 75.0 | 60.0 | 71.4 | **42.2** |
| Cocaine | 11.1 | 9.1 | 4.7 | 25.0 | 20.0 | 21.4 | **8.9** |
| Opioids | 33.3 | 18.2 | 19.0 | 50.0 | 40.0 | 42.8 | **22.2** |
| Marijuana | 44.4 | 45.4 | 23.8 | 50.0 | 60.0 | 64.3 | **40.0** |
| Suicide attempts | 33.3 | 27.3 | 23.8 | 75.0 | 40.0 | 21.4 | **28.8** |
| ?Hospitalizations | 11.1 | 31.8 | 23.8 | 75.0 | 40.0 | 35.7 | **28.8** |
| **Cormorbidity** | | | | | | | |
| Bipolar | - | 0 | 14.3 | 0 | 20.0 | 35.7 | **20.0** |
| Depression | 0 | - | 57.1 | 0 | 50.0 | 35.7 | **49.0** |
| Anxiety | 30.0 | 54.5 | - | 25.0 | 50.0 | 35.7 | **55.5** |
| Psychosis | 0 | 0 | 4.8 | - | 20.0 | 14.3 | **11.1** |
| Alcohol | 22.2 | 22.7 | 23.8 | 50.0 | - | 28.6 | **22.2** |
| Drug | 55.5 | 41.7 | 23.8 | 50.0 | 40.0 | - | **33.3** |
| Cognitive | 0 | 0 | 0 | 0 | 0 | 0 | **2.2** |
| **Primary Family Members** | | | | | | | |
| Bipolar | 33.3 | 4.5 | 0 | 0 | 0 | 35.7 | **13.3** |
| Depression | 22.2 | 27.3 | 14.3 | 0 | 20.0 | 14.3 | **20.0** |
| Anxiety | 4.5 | 9.1 | 19.0 | 25.0 | 10.0 | 7.1 | **11.1** |
| Substance | 33.3 | 31.8 | 33.3 | 0 | 20.0 | 35.7 | **24.4** |
| Cognitive | 11.1 | 9.1 | 9.5 | 0 | 0 | 0 | **6.6** |
| Psychosis | 22.2 | 9.1 | 14.3 | 0 | 10.0 | 14.3 | **8.8** |
| Childhood | 0 | 13.6 | 4.7 | 0 | 0 | 0 | **6.6** |
| Unknown | 33.3 | 0 | 4.8 | 25.0 | 20.0 | 14.3 | **8.8** |

**Table 4.** Drug Usage and Comorbidity by Diagnostic Category.

Native Americans in rural settings have significant need for psychiatric care, but have trouble accessing such care. Traditional models of accessing healthcare—often simply what is available locally, in nearby small cities or by travelling to metropolitan areas—have significant limitations. New models of service delivery like telepsychiatry appear to be suitable. Many clinical,

| | Inadequate Treatment | | | Adequate Treatment | | Appropriate Non-Treatment | Total |
|---|---|---|---|---|---|---|---|
| Class | Needed, None given | Needed, dosage low | Needed, time short | Needed, given | % of total | None needed or given | |
| Antidepressants | 11 | 1 | 3 | 15 | 15/30 50.0% | 15 | 45 |
| Mood Stabilizers | 4 | 3 | 3 | 3 | 3/13 23.1% | 32 | 45 |
| Antipsychotics | 3 | 2 | 1 | 2 | 2/8 25.0% | 37 | 45 |
| Total | 18 | 6 | 7 | 20 | 20/41 48.7% | N/A | |

**Table 5.** Adequacy of Medication Care Upon Consultation per Drug Class.

technical, administrative, evaluation, and cultural factors affect telepsychiatric patient care. Research is indicated with regard to help-seeking, diagnosis, treatment, and outcomes of IHS populations, preferably via randomized controlled trials.

A delicate issue in dealing with culture and language of patients is the tension between a goal generalizing an approach or the search for "standard" nuances of specific tribes, with the difficulty of stereotyping groups and making clinical errors (Yellowlees et al 2008, Yellowlees et al 2013). Meeting with members of the community, including the health clinic, in advance is recommended to understand cultural issues. In addition, some nuances are best learned "in vivo" (e.g. during a consultation with "real" patients). Ethnocentrism refers to the attitude that one's own culture is the "correct" one, while the relativist approach compares other cultures to one's own in a less punitive way. Adopting a relativist approach to providing e-mental healthcare to individuals from diverse backgrounds is a minimal, essential step toward culturally appropriate care.

Different cultural and ethnic groups value the role and perspective of the individual differently (Yellowlees et al 2008). Certain cultural groups are highly individualistic, such as many individuals in the United States and in many western European countries. Other cultural groups, such as many Asian societies, value instead the goals and needs of the group/society as a whole. With regard to their mental healthcare, they may not see mental health problems as individual challenges that can be successfully treated, but as shameful or burdensome to themselves or to their families. The value of the individual should be a consideration when planning e-mental health interventions.

Another issue for rural Native Americans is confidentiality in dealing with life's stresses or steps, as well as mental/substance illness/disorders (Yellowlees et al 2008). Our previous work noted that Native Americans had different frameworks for labeling traumas, and in addition, were worried about seeking services due to concern that in small communities that "everyone would know". Certainly trained professionals do their best on these concerns, but the introduction of telemedicine facilitated a more open framework for discussing past events. Providers outside the reservation were seen as neutral parties. Attention was paid, of course, to what was disclosed to the local providers, particularly when one covered for another.

Telepsychiatric consultation may help provide psychiatric services with primary care in Native American communities, which is important because substance abuse/dependence, mental health, and medical treatments are often not integrated and communication between clinicians may be rare (Manson 2000). Patients' comments about their preference for telepsychiatric consultation, because of community stigma and uncertainty about confidentiality, may be significant and require further evaluation. The preliminary high satisfaction rates for patients and staff are encouraging, considering rural and cultural factors that may affect service delivery.

An "effective" program considers clinical, technical, administrative, evaluation, and cultural factors, based on conversations with patients, staff, clinicians, administrators and technicians of this project and according to the literature (Table 6) (Hilty et al 2013; Hilty et al 2004a; Darkins 2001). A developmental model of rural telepsychiatry emphasized stages of needs identification, infrastructure survey, partnership organization, structure configuration, pilot implementation, and solidification (Shore 2005). In particular, cultural factors that affect help-seeking, diagnosis, treatment, and outcomes need to be measured and explored. In the clinical/educational realm, it is important to remember the most complex referrals come first. It is important to be patient with these and the process, in building the relationship with the rural team and using them as opportunities to learn about rural patients' needs, or the "holes" in the rural service delivery system (that can be filled as in the case above).

While technology is certainly reported as being highly beneficial in enhancing mental health outcomes, actual access to information technology is extremely variable and such technologies themselves may also be viewed and understood differently by individuals of different ethnic and cultural backgrounds. The issue of disparate access to technology by individuals of different ethnic and cultural backgrounds reveals that access to information technology differs significantly, depending not only on an individual's race or ethnicity, but also their income, their education level, and their geographical location (Mossberger et al 2006). African American and Hispanic/Latino individuals tend to report more affinity for information technology than whites do, but tended to have lower access to this type of technology, and poorer skills to use it effectively. When poverty and low socioeconomic status were taken into account, only the Hispanic/Latino group in Mossberger and colleagues' study actually had significantly poorer access to technology than the other two groups.

More concerted research on intersecting issues of culture, language, social class, ethnicity, geography, and e-mental health (Yellowlees et al 2008). Scientific and policy recommendations from this discussion include:

| *Clinical/Educational* |
| --- |
| 1. Obtain a telepsychiatric champion and provide adequate training for others with regard to the technology, adapt clinical practice to fit its use, and identifying its limitations. |
| 2. Coordinate timing of consults (i.e., patient is there at the right time, telepsychiatrist has adequate time, and/or referring providers or staff stop in if desired). |
| 3. Adequately train all site coordinators in the technical and procedural aspects of the service, including referral guidelines and transfer of patient medical information to the specialist and back to the referral site. |
| 4. Documentation: appropriate policy and procedures for consent, forwarding pertinent information in advance (e.g., medications, illnesses). |
| 5. Remember, with new services, the most complex of cases often are tried first (i.e., be patient). |
| 6. Integrate telepsychiatric service with spoke on-site care: therapy, substance or cultural. |
| 7. Match the type of service (e.g., consultation to spoke physician, triage, psychological testing, management) to the goal and/or request, as well as standard and reasonable practice (e.g., may be hard to manage from afar, who handles emergencies). |
| *Technical* |
| 8. Use clinically proven technology. |
| 9. For each consult, be certain that the technical quality equipment is appropriately matched to the service and needs of the patient and their condition. |
| 10. Provide regular technical maintenance and prompt trouble-shooting. |
| 11. Have a back-up coordinator at spoke sites for unexpected times the primary coordinator is out. |
| 12. Match the type of technology to the goal and/or service: video for patient evaluation; secure e-mail or telephone for physician-to-physician consultation. |
| *Administrative* |
| 13. Do a site visit to spokes to build relationships and trust. |
| 14. Do a thorough needs assessment in the region that the program is planning to serve |
| 15. Obtain overall and financial support of the program from senior leadership of the organization; ensure telemedicine and outreach is aligned with spoke's overall mission of the organization |
| 16. Develop financial stability after start-up funds with grants and/or contracts. |
| *Evaluation: hub and spoke* |
| 17. Patients' data: sociodemographics, medical and psychiatric diagnoses and satisfaction. |
| 18. Outcomes: disorder-specific (e.g., symptoms), adherence and functional (e.g., SF-12). |
| 19. Services: type preferred and used; adherence; boundary with other system's services; holes. |
| 20. Sites: physicians (e.g., education, skill, performance), staff and clinic system. |
| 21. Costs: patient, hub and spoke. |
| *Culture* |
| 22. Obtain consultation from spoke and/or hub specialist on Indian culture, history and illness, as indicated. |
| 23. Include a section on documentation (e.g., brief note the day of, the dictation) re: cultural and/or spiritual issues. |

**Table 6.** Key Issues in Telepsychiatric Consultation to CA Indian Health Sites.

- What kind of assessment tools, methods, and measures are needed to assess the patients, providers, systems, technology, and other important issues?
- What are the intersections of culture, class, geography, and technology in our current mental health system, and how do these intersections vary across differing racial/ethnic and class subculture groups?

- To what extent can technology be used to increase access to high-quality mental health services, and how will confounding/mediating) variables such as geography, poverty, education, and socioeconomic status prevent effective care?
- Will patients' disorder, racial/ethnic identity, socioeconomic status, and geographic characteristics determine whether e-mental health or face-to-face care is more effective, and should electronic services be used in concert with face-to face services?
- Should policymakers downplay the influence of culture on the use of technology, and pay more attention to factors such as poverty and socioeconomic status when planning the provision of e-mental health services?
- What is the most cost-effective and logistically feasible way to provide language and interpreting support for e-mental health programs (and where…interpreters at which end and who)?
- What new approaches to care, that take into account cultural and ethnic issues, can we create using technologies (e.g. using store-and-forward technologies)?

## Acknowledgements

UC Davis Health System Center for Health and Technology (UCDHS CHT)

California Indian Health Service

California Telemedicine and E-health Center

UC Davis Department of Psychiatry and Behavioral Sciences

Sashi Bandhu, Telemedicine Coordinator, UCDHS CHT

## Author details

Donald M. Hilty[1], Peter M. Yellowlees[1], Nicole Tarui[2], Steven R. Viramontes[3], Margo D. Kerrigan[3], David L. Sprenger[3] and Jay Shore[4]

*Address all correspondence to: dmhilty@ucdavis.edu

1 Telepsychiatric Services, University of California Davis, Sacramento, CA, USA

2 UCLA School of Medicine, USA

3 Indian Health Service, USA

4 University of Colorado Denver American Indian and Alaska Native Programs, USA

## References

[1] A Bill to Reauthorize the Indian Health Care Improvement Act and H.R. 2440, Indian Health Care Improvement Act Amendments of 2003: Joint Hearing Before the Senate Committee on Indian Affairs and the House Resources Committee, Office of Native American and Insular Affairs, 108th Cong. (2003) (statement of Dr. Charles W. Grim, Director, Indian Health Service). See also H.R. 2440, Indian Health Care Improvement Act Amendments of 2003.

[2] AACAP Practice Parameter for Telepsychiatry with Children and AdolescentsJ Am Acad Child Adol Psychiatr, (2007). , 47(12), 1468-1483.

[3] American Academy of Child and Adolescent Psychiatry(2004). AACAP Work Force Data Sheet. Status of Work Force and Prevalence Issues for Child and Adolescent Psychiatrists. See http://www.aacap.org/training/workforce.htm.Last accessed: 1 April 2013.

[4] American Psychiatric AssociationPractice Guideline for the Treatment of Patients with Bipolar Disorder (Revision). Am J Psychiatry, (2002). SS50., 1.

[5] American Psychiatric AssociationPractice Guideline for the Treatment of Patients with Schizophrenia, (2006). See http://www.psych.org/psych_pract/treatg/pg/SchizPG-Complete-Feb04.pdf.Last accessed: 1 April 2013.

[6] Bailey, J, Black, M, & Wilkin, D. Specialist outreach clinics in general practice. BMJ, (1994). , 308, 1083-1086.

[7] Beals, J, Manson, S. M, Whitesell, N. R, Spicer, P, Novins, D. K, & Mitchell, C. M. Prevalence of DSM-IV disorders and attendant help-seeking in 2 Native American reservation populations. Arch Gen Psychiatry, (2005a). , 62, 99-108.

[8] Beals, J, Novins, D. K, Whitesell, N. R, Spicer, P, Mitchell, C. M, & Manson, S. M. Prevalence of mental disorders and utilization of mental health services in two Native American reservation populations: mental health disparities in a national context. Am J Psychiatry, (2005b). , 162, 1723-32.

[9] Beals, J, Piasecki, J, Nelson, S, Jones, M, Keane, E, & Dauphinais, P. Red Shirt R, Sack W, Manson SM. Psychiatric disorder among American Indian adolescents: Prevalence in Northern Plains youth. J Am Academy Child Adol Psychiatry, (1997). , 36, 1252-1259.

[10] Bohn, D. K. Lifetime physical and sexual abuse, substance abuse, depression, and suicide attempts among Native American women. Issues Ment Health Nurs, (2003). , 24, 333-352.

[11] Butler, T. N, & Yellowlees, P. Cost analysis of store-and-forward telepsychiatry as a consultation model for primary care. Telemed J E Health, (2012). , 18(1), 74-77.

[12] Cerda, G. C, Hilty, D. M, Hales, R. E, et al. Use of telemedicine with ethnic groups (letter). Psychiatric Serv, (1999).

[13] Chong, J, & Moreno, F. A. Feasibility and acceptability of clinic-based telepsychiatry for low-income Hispanic primary care patients. Tel e-Health, (2012). , 18(4), 297-304.

[14] Cluver, J. S, Schuyler, D, Frueh, B. C, et al. Remote psychotherapy for terminally ill cancer patients. J Tel Telecare, (2005). , 11, 157-159.

[15] Costello, E. J, Farmer, E. M, Angold, A, Burns, B. J, & Erkanli, A. Psychiatric disorders among American Indian and white youth in Appalachia: The Great Smoky Mountains Study. Am J Public Health, (1997). , 87, 827-832.

[16] Darkins, A. Program management of telemental health care services. J Geriatr Psychiatry Neurol, (2001). , 14, 80-87.

[17] Depression in Primary CareTreatment. Clinical Practice Guideline, Rockville, MD. U.S. Department of Health and Human Services, Public Health Service, Agency for Health Care Policy and Research. AHCPR Publication No. 93-0551, (1993). , 2(5)

[18] Dick, P. T, Filler, R, & Pavan, A. Participant satisfaction and comfort with multidisciplinary pediatric telemedicine consultations. J Pediatric Surg, (1999). , 34, 137-141.

[19] Dixon, M. Access to Care Issues for Native American Consumers. In Dixon M, Roubideaux Y, eds. Promises to Keep: Public Health Policy for Native Americans & Alaska Natives in the 21st Century. Washington DC: American Public Health Association, (2001). , 61-88.

[20] Fortney, J. C, Pyne, J. M, Mouden, S. P, et al. Practice-based versus telemedicine-based collaborative care for depression in rural federally qualified health centers: A pragmatic randomized comparative effectiveness trial. Amer J Psychiatry, (2013). , 1-12.

[21] Geller, J. M, & Muus, K. J. The Role of Rural Primary Care Physicians in the Provision of Mental Health Services. Letter to the Field Frontier Mental Health Services Resources Network. Accessed at www.wiche.edu/mentalhealth/frontier/letter5.html, (2002). (5)

[22] Geller JM: Rural primary care providers' perceptions of their roles in the provision of mental health services: Voices from the plainsJ Rural Health, (1999). , 15(3), 326-334.

[23] Health Data Summaries for California CountiesDepartment of Health Services. State of California, (2000).

[24] Hilty, D. M, Ingraham, R. L, Yang, S. P, et al. Multispecialty phone and email consultation to primary care providers for patients with developmental disabilities in rural California. J Telemed E-Health, (2004b). , 10, 413-421.

[25] Hilty, D. M, Lim, R. F, Koike, A. K, et al. Planning for telepsychiatric consultation: A needs assessment for cultural and language services at rural sites in California. J Rural Mental Health, (2013). Submitted

[26] Hilty, D. M, Marks, S. L, Urness, D, et al. Clinical and educational applications of telepsychiatry: a review. Can J Psychiat, (2004a). , 49(1), 12-23.

[27] Hilty, D. M, Marks, S. L, Wegeland, J. E, et al. A randomized controlled trial of disease management modules, including telepsychiatric care, for depression in rural primary care. Psychiatry, (2007b). , 4(2), 58-65.

[28] Hilty, D. M, Nesbitt, T. S, Kuenneth, T. A, et al. Telepsychiatric consultation to primary care: rural vs. suburban needs, utilization and provider satisfaction. J Rural Health, (2007a). , 23(2), 163-165.

[29] Hilty, D. M, Servis, M. E, Nesbitt, T. S, et al. The use of telemedicine to provide consultation-liaison service to the primary care setting. Psychiatric Annals, (1999). , 29, 421-427.

[30] Hilty, D. M, Yellowlees, P. M, & Cobb, H. C. Models of telepsychiatric consultation-liaison service to rural primary care. Psychosomatics, (2006b). , 47, 152-157.

[31] Hilty, D. M, Yellowlees, P. M, Ferrer, D, et al. The effectiveness of telepsychiatry: A (2013). review. Tel J e-Health, In Press

[32] Hilty, D. M, Yellowlees, P. M, & Nesbitt, T. S. Evolution of telepsychiatry to rural sites: change over time in types of referral and PCP knowledge, skill, and satisfaction. Gen Hosp Psychiatry, (2006). , 28(5), 367-373.

[33] Hollingsworth, J. M, Saint, S, Hayward, R. A, et al. Specialty care and the patient-centered medical home. Med Care, (2011). , 49(1), 4-9.

[34] Katon, W, Von Korff, M, Lin, E, et al. Collaborative management to achieve treatment guidelines. JAMA, (1995). , 273, 1026-1031.

[35] Katon, W, Von Korff, M, Lin, E, et al. Collaborative management to achieve depression treatment guidelines. J Clin Psychiatry, (1997). suppl 1):20-24.

[36] Koike, A. K, Unutzer, J, & Wells, K. B. Improving the care for depression in patients with comorbid medical illness. Am J Psychiatry, (2002). , 159, 1738-1745.

[37] Levine, S. R. Gorman M: Telestroke: The application of telemedicine for stroke. Stroke, (1999). , 30, 464-469.

[38] Lishner, D. M, Richardson, M, Levine, P, et al. Access to primary care among persons with disabilities in rural areas: a review of the literature. Seattle, WA: WAMI Rural Health Research Center, (1995).

[39] Lopez, A. M, Cruz, M, Lazarus, S, et al. Use of American sign language in telepsychiatry consultation. Tel e-Health (2004). , 10(3), 389-391.

[40] Manson, S. Mental health services for Native Americans and Alaska Natives: need, use, and barriers to effective care. Can J Psychiatry, (2000). , 45, 617-626.

[41] Manson, S. M. Long-term care of older American Indians: Challenges in the development of institutional services. In C. Barresi & D. E. Stull (Eds.), Ethnicity and Long-term Care, (1992). New York: Springer., 1992, 130-143.

[42] Manson, S. M. The wounded spirit: A cultural formulation of post-traumatic stress disorder. Culture, Medicine and Psychiatry, (1996a).

[43] Martinez, N. C. Diabetes and minority populations: Focus on Mexican Americans. Nurs Clin North Am, (1993). , 28, 87-95.

[44] Moreno, F. A, Chong, J, Dumbauld, J, et al. Use of standard webcam and internet equipment for telepsychiatry treatment of depression among underserved Hispanics. Psychiatric Serv, (2012). , 63(12), 1213-1217.

[45] Mossberger, K, Tolbert, C. J, & Gilbert, M. Race, place, and information technology. Urban Affairs Rev, (2006). , 41, 583-620.

[46] Mucic, D. Transcultural telepsychiatry and its impact on patient satisfaction. J Tel Telecare, (2010). , 16(5), 237-242.

[47] Murray, C. J. Lopez AD (Eds). "The global burden of disease. A comprehensive assessment of mortality and disability from diseases, injuries, and risk factors in 1990 and projected to 2020". ((1996). Cambridge, MA: Harvard School of Public Health.

[48] National Institutes of HealthOffice of the Director, Office of Behavioral and Social Sciences Research. Strategic Plan for Health Disparities Research, FY 2002.2006. Mar. 28, 2001, www.obssr.od.nih.gov/Activities/HealthDisp.htm.Last accessed: 1 April (2013). See generally Institute of Medicine of the National Academies, Unequal Treatment: Confronting Racial and Ethnic Disparities in Health Care (Washington, DC: National Academies Press, 2002) (hereafter cited as Institute of Medicine, Unequal Treatment).

[49] National Women's Health Information CenterHealth Problems in Native American/ Alaska Native Women. (2005). See http://www.4woman.gov/faq/american_indian.htm.Last accessed: 1 April 2013.

[50] Nelson, S. H, Mccoy, G. F, Stetter, M, & Vanderwagen, W. C. An overview of mental health services for Native Americans and Alaska Natives in the 1990s. Hosp Community Psychiatry, (1992). , 43, 257-261.

[51] Nesbitt, T. S, Dharmar, M, Bell, J, et al. Telehealth at UC Davis-A 20-Year Experience. Tel e-Health, (2013). , 19(5), 1-6.

[52] Nesbitt, T. S, Hilty, D. M, Kuenneth, C. A, & Siefkin, A. Development of a telemedicine program: a review of 1,000 videoconferencing consultations. Western J Med, (2000). , 173, 169-174.

[53] Neufeld, J. D, Bourgeois, J. A, Hilty, D. M, et al. The e-Mental Health Consult Service: providing enhanced primary care mental health services through telemedicine. Psychosomatics, (2007). , 48, 135-141.

[54] Nieves, J, & Stack, K. M. Hispanics and telepsychiatry. Psychiat Serv, (2007). , 58, 877-878.

[55] Office of Technology AssessmentHealth care in rural America (Publication No. OTA-H-434). Washington, DC: US Government Printing Office, (1990).

[56] Office of the General Counsel US. Commission on Civil Rights. Native American Health Care Disparities Briefing, Executive Summary. (2004). Available at: http://www.law.umaryland.edu/marshall/usccr/documents/nativeamerianhealthcare-dis.pdf.Last accessed: 1 April 2013.

[57] Office of the Surgeon General (US); Center for Mental Health Services (US); National Institute of Mental Health (US)Mental Health: Culture, Race, and Ethnicity: A Supplement to Mental Health: A Report of the Surgeon General. Rockville (MD): Substance Abuse and Mental Health Services Administration (US); (2001). Aug. Chapter 4 Mental Health Care for American Indians and Alaska Natives. Available at: http://www.ncbi.nlm.nih.gov/books/NBK44242/.Last accessed: 1 April 2013.

[58] Office of the Surgeon General (US); Center for Mental Health Services (US); National Institute of Mental Health (US)Mental Health: Culture, Race, and Ethnicity: A Supplement to Mental Health: A Report of the Surgeon General. Rockville (MD): Substance Abuse and Mental Health Services Administration (US); (2001). Aug. Chapter 4 Mental Health Care for American Indians and Alaska Natives. Available at: http://www.ncbi.nlm.nih.gov/books/NBK44242/.Last accessed: 1 April 2013.

[59] Pincus, H. Patient-oriented models for linking primary care and mental health care. Gen Hosp Psychiatry, (1987). , 9, 95-101.

[60] Preston, J, Brown, F. W, & Hartley, B. Using telemedicine to Improve health care in distant areas. Hosp Community Psychiatry, (1992). , 43, 25-32.

[61] Regier, D. A, Goldberg, I. D, & Taube, C. A. The de facto US mental health services system. Arch Gen Psychiatry, (1978). , 46, 971-982.

[62] Robin, R. W, Chester, B, Rasmussen, J. K, Jaranson, J. M, & Goldman, D. Prevalence and characteristics of trauma and posttraumatic stress disorder in a southwestern American Indian community. Am J Psychiatry, (1997). , 154, 1582-1588.

[63] Rosenthal, T. C. The medical home: Growing evidence to support a new approach to primary care. J Am Board Fam Med, (2008). , 21(5), 427-440.

[64] Rost, K, Fortney, J, Zhang, M, Smith, J, & Smith, G. R. Treatment of depression in rural Arkansas: policy implications for improving care. J Rural Health, (1999). , 15, 308-315.

[65] Rost, K, Zhang, M, Fortney, J, Smith, J, & Smith, G. R. Rural-urban differences in depression treatment and suicidality. Med Care, (1998). , 36, 1098-1107.

[66] Rural Policy Research InstituteRetrieved July 12, 2001, from http://www.rupri.org/policyres/rnumbers/demopop/demo.html. ((1999). Last accessed: 1 April 2013.

[67] Savin, D, Garry, M, Zuccaro, P, & Novins, D. Telepsychiatry for treating rural Native American youth. J Am Acad Child Adol Psychiatry, (2006). , 45, 484-488.

[68] Shore, J, Kaufmann, L. J, Brooks, E, et al. Review of American Indian veteran telemental health. Telemed J E-Health, (2012a). , 18(2), 87-94.

[69] Shore, J. H, Brooks, E, Anderson, H, et al. Characteristics of telemental health service use by American Indian veterans. Psychiatric Services, (2012b). , 63, 179-181.

[70] Shore, J. H, Brooks, E, Savin, D, Orton, H, Grigsby, J, & Manson, S. Acceptability of telepsychiatry in American Indians. Tel e-Health, (2008). , 14(5), 461-466.

[71] Shore, J. H, & Manson, S. M. A developmental model for rural telepsychiatry. Psychiatric Serv, (2005). , 56, 976-980.

[72] Shore, J. H, & Manson, S. M. Telepsychiatric care of Native American veterans with post traumatic stress disorder: Bridging gaps in geography, organizations and culture. Tel J E-health, (2004b). SS69., 64.

[73] Shore, J. H, & Manson, S. M. The Native American veteran and posttraumatic stress disorder: a telehealth assessment and formulation. Cult Med Psychiatry, (2004a). , 28, 231-43.

[74] Shore, J. H, Savin, D, Orton, H, et al. Diagnostic reliability of telepsychiatry in American Indian veterans. Am J Psychiat (2007). , 164, 115-118.

[75] Shore, J. H, Savin, D. M, Novins, D, & Manson, S. M. Cultural aspects of telepsychiatry. J Telemed Telecare, (2006). , 12, 116-121.

[76] Shore, P. VISN 21 Home Based Telemental Health Pilot Project Program. Veteran's Health Administration. Portland, OR, (2011). Available at:

[77] Simon, G. E, Vonkorff, M, Rutter, C, et al. Randomised trial of monitoring, feedback, and management of care by telephone to improve treatment of depression in primary care. BMJ, (2000). , 320, 550-554.

[78] Spicer, P, Beals, J, Croy, C. D, Mitchell, C. M, Novins, D. K, Moore, L, & Manson, S. M. Re-examining alcohol problems among Native American communities. Alcoholism: Clin Exper Res, (2003). , 27, 1785-1797.

[79] Straker, N, Mostyn, P, & Marshall, C. The use of two-way TV in bringing mental health services to the inner city. Am J Psychiatry, (1976). , 133, 1202-1205.

[80] Strathdee, G. Primary care-psychiatry interaction: a British perspective. Gen Hosp Psychiatry, (1987). , 9, 102-110.

[81] Substance Abuse and Mental Health Services Administration (SAMSHA) Center for Substance Abuse Treatment (CSAT)See http://www.samhsa.gov/centers/csat2002.Last accessed: 1 April (2013).

[82] U. S. Census Bureau. Profile of General Demographic Characteristics: Vol Census 2000 Summary File 1 (SF 1) 100-Percent Data. 2000. Last accessed: 1 April 2013.

[83] U. S. Department of Health and Human Services, Office of the Surgeon General, SAMHSA. Surgeon General's report: Factsheet Native Native Americans, 2004. See http://www.mentalhealth.samhsa.gov/cre/fact4.asp.Last accessed: 1 April 2013.

[84] Unutzer, J, Katon, W, & Callahan, C. M. Williams Jr JW, Hunkeler E, Harpole L, et al. Collaborative care management of late-life depression in the primary care setting. JAMA, (2002)., 288, 2836-2845.

[85] Vernellia Randall Institute of RacismRacial Discrimination in Health Care in the United States as a Violation of the International Convention on the Elimination of All Forms of Racial Discrimination, 14 J. LAW & PUB. POL.Y 45, 57.8 ((2002). Last accessed: 1 April 2013.

[86] Weiner, M, Rossetti, H, & Harrah, K. Videoconference diagnosis and management of Choctaw Indian dementia patients. Alzheim Dement, (2011)., 562-566.

[87] Weinick, R. M, Zuvekas, S. H, & Cohen, J. W. Racial and ethnic differences in access to and use of health care services, 1977 to 1996. Med Care Res Rev, (2000)., 57, 36-54.

[88] Wells, K. B, Unutzer, J, Sherbourne, C, et al. Cost-effectiveness of practice-initiated quality improvement for depression. JAMA, (2001)., 286(11), 1325-1330.

[89] Wittson, C. L, Affleck, D. C, & Johnson, V. Two-way television group therapy. Ment Hosp, (1961)., 12, 22-23.

[90] Ye, J, Shim, R, Lukaszewski, T, Yun, K, et al. Telepsychiatry services for Korean immigrants. Tel e-Health, (2012)., 18(10), 797-802.

[91] Yellowlees, P. M, Hilty, D. M, Marks, S. L, et al. A retrospective analysis of child and adolescent e-mental health. J Am Acad Child Adol Psychiatry, (2008)., 47(1), 1-5.

[92] Yellowlees, P. M, Marks, S, Hilty, D. M, & Shore, J. H. Using e-Health to enable culturally appropriate mental health care in rural areas. J Tel E-Health, (2008)., 486-492.

[93] Yellowlees, P. M, Odor, A, Burke, M. M, et al. A feasibility study of asynchronous telepsychiatry for psychiatric consultations. Psychiatric Serv, (2010)., 61(8), 838-40.

[94] Yellowlees, P. M, Shore, J, & Roberts, L. Practice Guidelines for Videoconferencing-Based Telemental Health, American Telemedicine Association. Tel J e-Health, (2010)., 16, 1074-1089.

# 4

# Telemedicine in Management of Retinoblastoma

Sarah Moran and Michael O' Keefe

## 1. Introduction

Retinoblastoma is a highly malignant tumor of the eye that manifests most often in the first 3 years of life. Early detection is essential to preserve visual function, and decrease mortality from retinoblastoma. Late diagnosis globally results in up to 70% mortality; where optimal therapy is accessible, more than 95% of children are cured.

Telemedicine has many possible applications in ophthalmology, from community screening to the provision of expertise in areas where it is otherwise not available. Broad-based applications of telemedicine could greatly enhance screening efforts for potentially blinding conditions such as diabetic retinopathy, macular degeneration, glaucoma, retinopathy of prematurity as well as retinoblastoma. In this chapter we discuss specifically the application of telemedicine in management of retinoblastoma. Telemedicine can help to bring subspecialty expertise to small or rural communities, as well as to the developing world.

## 2. Retinoblastoma

### 2.1. Epidemiology

Retinoblastoma is the most common intraocular malignancy of childhood.[1] It represents about 4% of all pediatric malignancies, and affects approximately 1 in in 20,000 live births each year.[2] Most studies indicate that the incidence of retinoblastoma among various geographic populations is relatively constant. There is a 95% survival rate in developed countries, however the worldwide survival rate is closer to 50%. This is largely due to earlier detection in developed countries, when the tumor is still confined to the globe. This is in contrast to underdeveloped areas where retinoblastomas are often diagnosed at an advanced stage, when they have already invaded the orbit or brain.

### 2.2. Genetics

Retinoblastoma arises from malignant transformation of primitive retinal cells before final differentiation. It can be inherited as a familial tumor in which the affected child has a positive family history of retinoblastoma or as a non-familial (sporadic tumor) in which the family history is negative. Approximately 94% of newly diagnosed retinoblastoma cases are sporadic, and 6% are familiar.

Retinoblastoma can be classified in 3 ways: familial or non-familial, heritable or non-heritable, unilateral or bilateral, however the 3 classifications are interrelated [3] Bilateral and familial retinoblastomas are caused by a germline tumor and are therefore heritable. Unilateral sporadic retinoblastoma is usually non-heritable, however it is estimated that 10-15% of children with unilateral sporadic retinoblastoma can have a germline mutation.

The retinoblastoma gene is located on the long arm of chromosome 13 (13q14). In order for retinoblastoma to develop, both copies of the gene at the 13q14 locus must be affected. If either the maternal or paternal copy of the gene that is inherited by an individual is defective, then the individual is heterozygous for the mutant allele. Tumor formation requires both alleles to be mutant or inactive- the concept of the "two-hit" hypothesis of Knudson. In familial cases, all the retinal precursor cells contain the initial mutation, and a when a second hit occurs, the cell undergoes malignant transformation. These children develop multifocal and bilateral tumors, and are at higher risk of non-ocular secondary tumors such as pinealoblastomas and osteosarcomas. In contrast, patients with unilateral sporadic retinoblastoma have normal chromosome structure elsewhere in the body and are at no higher risk of secondary tumors. In heritable retinoblastoma, the mutation is transmitted in 50%, but due to incomplete penetrance only 40% of offspring will be affected. If a child has heritable retinoblastoma, the risk to siblings is 2% if the parents are unaffected, and 40% if a parent is affected. In non-heritable cases the risk in each sibling and offspring is about 1%.

Genetic testing using DNA analysis of the patient's tumor can help to identify those with a germline or heritable mutation. Heritable tumors account for approximately 40% of tumors with the remainder being non-hereditary.

### 2.3. Presentation and clinical features

Presentation is usually within the first year of life if the tumor is bilateral or second year of life if the tumor is unilateral. Clinical features vary according to time of presentation. Leukocoria is the most common presenting feature (60%) and may be first noticed in family photographs. (Figure 1.) Strabismus is the next most common form of presentation (20%); therefore dilated fundal examination is mandatory in all cases of childhood strabismus. Retinoblastoma may also present with chronic uveitis, orbital inflammation, secondary glaucoma, or orbital invasion in advanced cases. Metastatic disease before the detection of ocular involvement is rare.

The growth pattern of retinoblastoma can be endophytic, exophytic, and intraretinal. Exophytic tumors grow from the retina outwards into the subretinal space, whereas endophytic tumors grow inward from the retina towards the vitreous cavity. Occasionally the retinoblas-

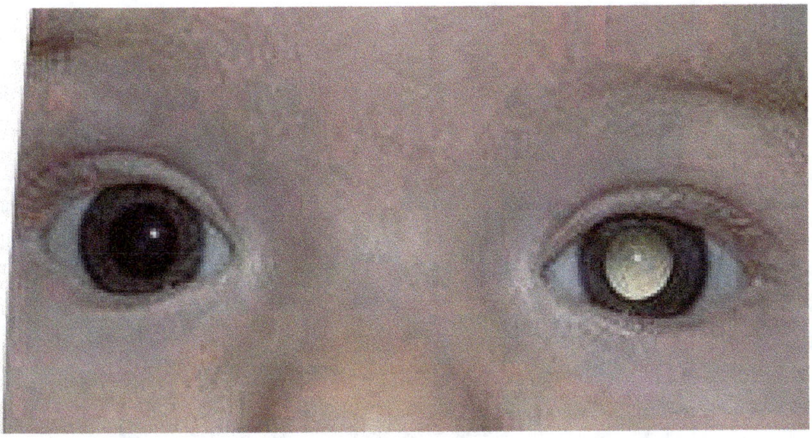

**Figure 1.** Leukocoria in a child with Retinoblastoma

toma can have a diffuse infiltration pattern, which manifests as a relatively flat infiltration of the retina without an obvious tumor mass.

| **Group 1**: Very favorable for maintenance of sight |
|---|
| A. Solitary tumor, smaller than 4 disc diameters (DD), at or behind the equator.<br>B. Multiple tumors, none larger than 4 DD, all at or behind the equator. |
| **Group 2**: Favorable for maintenance of sight |
| A. Solitary tumor, 4 to 10 DD at or behind the equator<br>B. Multiple tumors, 4 to 10 DD behind the equator. |
| **Group 3**: Possible for maintenance of sight |
| A. Any lesion anterior to the equator.<br>B. Solitary tumor, larger than 10DD behind the equator. |
| **Group 4**: Unfavorable for maintenance of sight |
| A. Multiple tumors, some larger than 10 DD.<br>B. Any lesion extending anteriorly to the ora serrata. |
| **Group 5**: Very unfavorable for maintenance of sight |
| A. Massive tumors involving more than one half the retina.<br>B. Vitreous seeding. |
| The system was designed to predict outcome from treatment with external beam radiotherapy (EBRT), used internationally as the primary eye salvage treatment until introduction of chemotherapy in the 1980s. |

**Table 1.** Reese-Ellsworth Classification

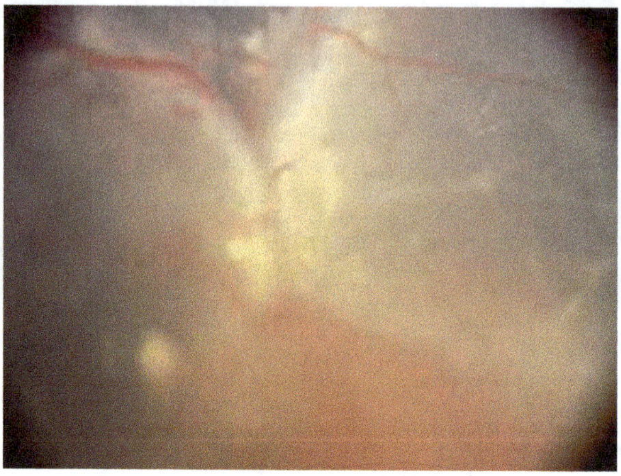

**Figure 2.** Group V Tumor Left Eye on Presentation (December 2011) The eye was subsequently enucleated.

| The International Classification for Intraocular Retinoblastoma is a newer staging system. It divides intraocular retinoblastomas into 5 groups, labeled A-E, based on the chances that the eye can be saved using current treatment options. |
|---|
| **Group A** |
| Small tumors away from foveola and disc<br>•Tumors <3mm confined to retina<br>•Located at least 3mm from foveola and 1.5mm from optic disc |
| **Group B** |
| All other tumors confined to the retina.<br>•Subretinal fluid <3mm from base of tumor |
| **Group C** |
| Local subretinal fluid or vitreous seeding<br>•Subretinal fluid alone >3mm and <6mm from tumor<br>•Vitreous or subretinal seeding <3mm from tumor |
| **Group D** |
| Diffuse subretinal fluid or seeding<br>•Subretinal fluid >6mm from tumor<br>•Vitreous or subretinal seeding >3mm from the tumor |
| **Group E** |
| Presence of 1 or more of following poor prognostic features<br>•More than two-thirds of the globe filled with tumor<br>•Tumor in anterior segment or anterior to vitreous<br>•Tumor in/on ciliary body<br>•Iris neovascularization<br>•Neovascular glaucoma<br>•Opaque media from hemorrhage |

**Table 2.** International Classification of Retinoblastoma

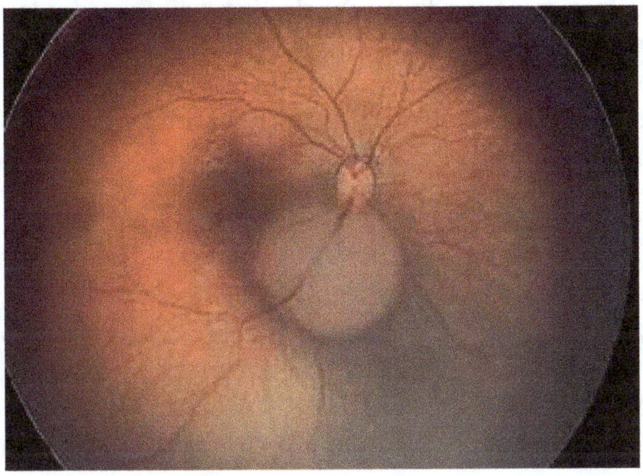

**Figure 3.** Fellow eye of the same patient: Multiple Tumors in Right eye at time of presentation (December 2011)

## 2.4 Differential diagnosis

Approximately 50% of patients diagnosed with possible retinoblastoma prove to have simulating conditions and not retinoblastoma. [4] Differential diagnoses include Persistent Hyperplastic Primary Vitreous, Coats disease, and ROP. It is essential to establish the diagnosis of retinoblastoma prior to commencing treatment.

## 2.5 Diagnosis

Diagnosis is established through a combination of history and physical examination, usually requiring binocular indirect fundoscopy with scleral indentation. This is generally performed under anesthesia to precisely determine the number and location of tumors. An experienced examiner can establish the diagnosis based on the clinical appearance of the tumor. Ancillary diagnostic studies can be helpful if the diagnosis is uncertain. Ultrasonography and computed tomography can demonstrate the mass and detect presence of calcium. Magnetic resonance imaging is of value for assessing the optic nerve, orbit, and brain and evaluating spread outside the globe.

## 3. Management of retinoblastoma

The primary objective in management of retinoblastoma is survival of the child, and secondly the preservation of the globe. After safety of the patient and the globe is established comes the focus on maintaining visual acuity. Treatment is tailored to each individual case, and there are several options. Intraocular retinoblastoma continues to be managed with a wide range of treatment modalities including cryotherapy, laser photocoagulation, transpupillary thermotherapy, brachytherapy, external beam radiation, and enucleation. Newer treatment modalities include intra-vitreal and subconjunctival chemotherapy for advanced tumors, and the recently described technique of ophthalmic artery catheterization with chemotherapy infusion. [5, 6, 7]

The approach to retinoblastoma management has changed significantly over the last 10 years, with a move away from external beam radiation and increased use of focal treatment methods and chemoreduction. It has been well demonstrated that patients with germline tumors are at increased risk of developing secondary cancers if they receive external beam radiation. In recent years, eyes with unilateral retinoblastoma are generally managed with enucleation if the eye is classified as Reese-Ellsworth group V. For those eyes in group I-IV, chemoreduction or focal treatment is used. In bilateral cases, chemoreduction is used in most cases unless there is very asymmetric disease.

### 3.1. Chemoreduction

Chemoreduction is a method of reducing tumor volume to allow for focal therapeutic measures such as cryotherapy or laser photocoagulation. This approach helps to preserve vision and avoid external beam radiotherapy. Tumors may show dramatic response in the first few months of treatment, however they will recur if treatment is not consolidated with local methods. Choice of agents as well as number and frequency of cycles varies between institutions. The main problem with chemoreduction is the recurrence of vitreous or subretinal seeds, which may respond to initial chemoreduction, but later recur.

### 3.2. Periocular chemoreduction

Local periocular chemotherapy can be administered in the subconjunctival or subtenons space. For children with advanced retinoblastoma, systemic chemoreduction with a local periocular boost of subconjunctival or subtenon chemotherapy can be used in advanced tumors. If used alone, recurrence is inevitable, therefore, periocular chemotherapy is combined with systemic chemotherapy for best results. For small volume intraocular retinoblastomas, focal therapy may be potentially curative but can threaten vision if the tumor is adjacent to the macula or optic nerve. In these cases, periocular chemoreduction can be effective whilst avoiding systemic chemotherapy or damaging vision using focal therapies.

### 3.3. Intravitreal chemotherapy

The use of intravitreal chemotherapy was pioneered by Ericson and Rosengren, [8] and has been studied extensively in animal models. It is widely used in Japan but has largely been avoided elsewhere due to concerns regarding tumor seeding. A recent technique has described combining the intravitreal injection with a bleb of subconjunctival chemotherapy to avoid tumor seeding.[9]

### 3.4. Intra-arterial chemotherapy

The concept of intra-arterial chemotherapy for retinoblastoma was introduced more than 50 years ago, when the alkylating agent triethylene melanamine was used via puncture sites in the carotid artery in the side of the eye to be treated.

Most recently, the technique of supraselective intraarterial chemotherapy appears to significantly improve the prognosis for eye preservation (70-80%) of group D eyes. [10, 11] Currently this treatment is employed in retinoblastoma patients as primary treatment for unilateral or bilateral retinoblastoma and as secondary treatment following failure from other treatments. This technique allows selective delivery of chemotherapy to the eye with minimal systemic absorption. The dose delivered to the eye is 10 times that achieved with systemic chemotherapy. This high dose of chemotherapy delivered to the eye accelerates regression of tumor and seeds. The chemotherapy infusion has to be repeated every 3-4 weeks for up to 3-6 injections for complete regression of tumor. Cannulation of the ophthalmic artery is difficult in children particularly in infants less than 6 months and requires surgical expertise and precision. As it is an invasive procedure the risk of neurological complications has to be considered though they are rare.

### 3.5. Focal therapy

Modalities of focal therapy include laser photocoagulation, cry therapy, thermotherapy, and plaque radiotherapy. These are mostly used for small tumors, in particular those which have been already reduced by chemo reduction.

#### *3.5.1. Laser photocoagulation*

Laser photocoagulation is usually employed for small tumors posterior to the equator of the eye.It tends not to be used in conjunction with chemo reduction as its success depends on vascular coagulation and tumor ischemia, which is the opposite case for chemoreduction. It is performed using argon or diode laser, with two rows of photocoagulation surrounding the tumor base. The tumor itelf is avoided as this could lead to vitreous seeding. It is repeated at approximately 1-month intervals for 3 sessions.

#### *3.5.2. Cryotherapy*

Cryotherapy was first introduced by Linkoff in 1967. It causes cell death by destroying circulation during the freeze, via damage to the vascular endothelium and decreased blood flow. This is a useful treatment for equatorial and peripheral small retinoblastomas. The tumor is destroyed with one or two sessions of triple freeze-therapy. It is an important method of tumor consolidation following chemoreduction, and is especially useful for management of recurrent subretinal seeds near the ora serrate

#### *3.5.3. Thermotherapy*

Thermotherapy coupled with chemoreduction is suited for tumors adjacent to the fovea and optic nerve where radiation or laser would possibly induce visual loss. It involves heating the tumor using a diode infrared laser system, and is usually performed in conjunction with chemoreduction.

*3.5.4. Plaque radiotherapy*

This is a form of brachytherapy in which a radioactive implant is placed on the sclera over the base of a retinoblastoma. An average of 2 to 4 days of treatment time is required to deliver the total radiation dose to the tumor. It is useful for tumors less than 8mm thick and 16mm in base. Plaque radiotherapy can be used as a primary or secondary treatment. In the majority of cases it is used as a secondary treatment to salvage a glove after prior failed treatment. The visual outcome varies with tumor size and location as well as side effects such as radiation retinopathy and papillopathy. Overall following 1 application of plaque radiotherapy there is an approximately 80% tumor control rate at 4 years.[13]

### 3.6. External beam radiotherapy

Retinoblastoma is generally a radiosensitive tumor. External bean radiotherapy is a method of delivering whole eye irradiation to treat advanced retinoblastoma, particularly when there is advanced vitreous seeding. Recurrence of retinoblastoma after external beam radiation is a problem that can develop in the first 1 -4 years after treatment. Radiation damage to the retina, optic nerve, and lens can be challenging to manage.

External beam radiation was once employed in a large percentage of patients but has fallen out of favor, largely because external beam radiation has the potential to increase the risk of the development of additional nonocular cancers in survivors of germline retinoblastoma. It is estimated that the risk approximates 1% per year of life.[13] Patients who develop a second cancer and then survive that cancer have an increased risk for the development of nonocular tumors of approximately 2% per year from the time of the second tumor diagnosis. The average latency period between subsequent tumor diagnoses becomes progressively less with each additional cancer that develops. Children radiated during the first year of life are between 2-8 times as likely to develop second cancers as those radiated after the age of 1 year.

Nonetheless external beam radiation remains an excellent method of preserving vision in a child with retinoblastoma, and certain clinical situation demand its use. Unlike focal therapies, external beam radiation can provide an excellent opportunity for useful vision in a macula that is not affected by tumor. It may be considered as a primary option in children with small tumors located within the macula, or for multifocal tumors where focal therapies are ineffective. External beam radiation also continues to be the salvage treatment of choice after focal treatments have failed. For children with advanced extraoculaar or metastatic disease, radiation can also play a role in palliation along with chemotherapy.

### 3.7. Enucleation

Enucleation continues to be a frequently used and important method for managing retinoblastoma If there is advanced disease with no hope for useful vision in the affected eye, or there is concern regarding tumor invasion into the optic nerve, choroid or orbit, then enucleation is appropriate. Also best considered for enucleation, are children with secondary glaucoma, pars plana seeding, or anterior chamber seeding, Over 99% of patients with unilateral retinoblastoma without microscopic or macroscopic extraocular disease are cured by enucleation. The technique of enuclation is to gently remove the eye intact without seeding any malignant cells into the orbit.

## 4. Telemedicine in management of retinoblastoma

### 4.1. Telemedicine

Telemedicine can be defined as the delivery of healthcare and sharing of medical knowledge over distance using telecommunication means. It is used to support health care between participants who are separated from each other.[14] It has the potential to improve the accessibility, quality, and cost of healthcare, and may also contribute to medical education and research. The concept of telemedicine was introduced about 30 years ago through the use of telephones and facsimile machines. However today, telemedicine has advanced, integrating medical and network technology, comprising remote diagnosis, expert consultation, information service, online checkups, and remote communication.

Telemedicine can be broadly divided into two categories: synchronous telemedicine uses telecommunications for real-time interactions between participants (i.e. Videoconferencing), as compared to store-and-forward telemedicine which captures patient data for subsequent interaction with a remote expert (i.e. Digital radiology)

### 4.2. Applications in ophthalmology

The potential benefits of an effective telemedicine system in ophthalmology are many. Telemedicine has a variety of possible applications in ophthalmology, from community screening to the provision of expertise in areas where it is otherwise not available. Broad-based applications of telemedicine could greatly enhance screening efforts for potentially blinding conditions such as diabetic retinopathy, macular degeneration, glaucoma, retinopathy of prematurity and retinoblastoma to name but a few. Telemedicine can bring subspecialty expertise to small or rural communities, as well as to the developing world.

Tele-medicine applications in ophthalmology comprise both clinical and educational processes between the send and receive sites. These can include:

- screening of a disease;
- formulation of a diagnosis and clinical management plan;
- secondary advice and support in clinical management plan;
- peer supervision and support;
- professional development through group discussion, lectures, and tutorials

• research and administration activities.

Typical telemedicine application in retinoblastoma includes the transfer of basic patient information, transfer of high resolution images such as fundal photographs, pathology images, magnetic resonance imaging pictures.

The use of telemedicine in retinoblastoma is not only useful to the specialist managing the condition, but is also of a source of confidence and comfort to parent and families of children with retinoblastoma to know that multiple experts are involved in the care of their child, and their child is receiving the best possible treatment.

### 4.3. Importance of imaging in management of retinoblastoma

The RetCam® wide-angle camera provides wide-field imaging of the retina and anterior segment, including the anterior chamber angle. Some small retinoblastomas, and vitreous seeds, may be better seen on RetCam® images than with indirect ophthalmoscopy. Sequential images are useful to determine if the tumors are growing or regressing. The anterior segment and anterior chamber angle can also be well visualized with the RetCam®. Fluorescein angiography using the RetCam® can assess vascularity, residual tumor activity, and recurrences within laser scars.

### 4.4. Images used in telemedicine for the management of retinoblastoma

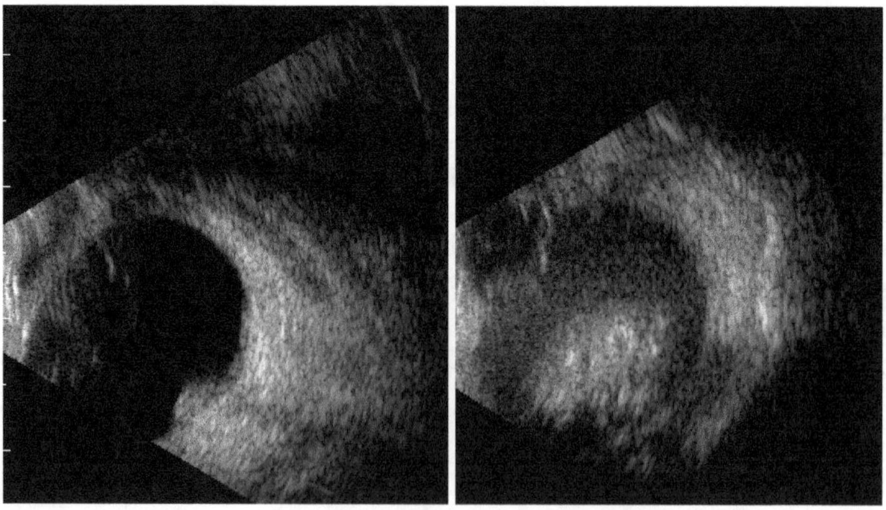

**Figure 4.** B scan ultrasonography of right and left eye of same patient at time of presentation in December 2011 showing multifocal tumors in the right eye, and the left globe filled with large tumor

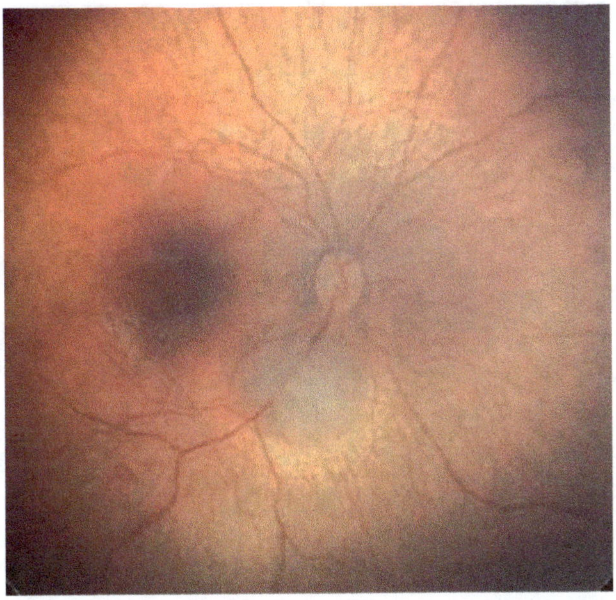

**Figure 5.** Right Fundus following chemoreduction February 2012

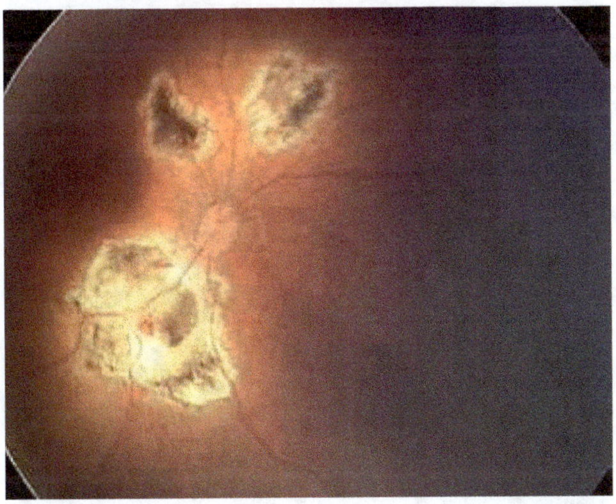

**Figure 6.** May 2012: Images of the right eye during treatment with chemoreduction and focal therapy with laser photocoagulation

#### *4.4.1. Diagnosis*

Telemedicine is invaluable when the diagnosis of retinoblastoma is in doubt. Diagnosis is generally established by the classic appearance of the retinal tumors by an experienced examiner. The sooner the diagnosis is established the sooner the appropriate treatment can be implemented and the better the prognosis.

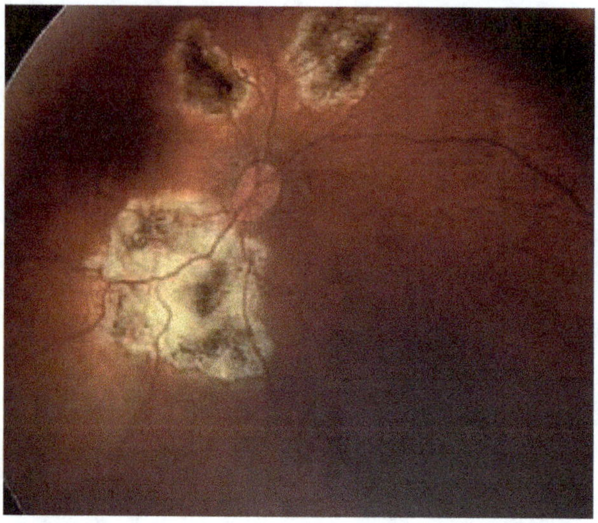

**Figure 7.** June 2012: Image from examination under anesthesia following chemoreduction and focal laser consolidation

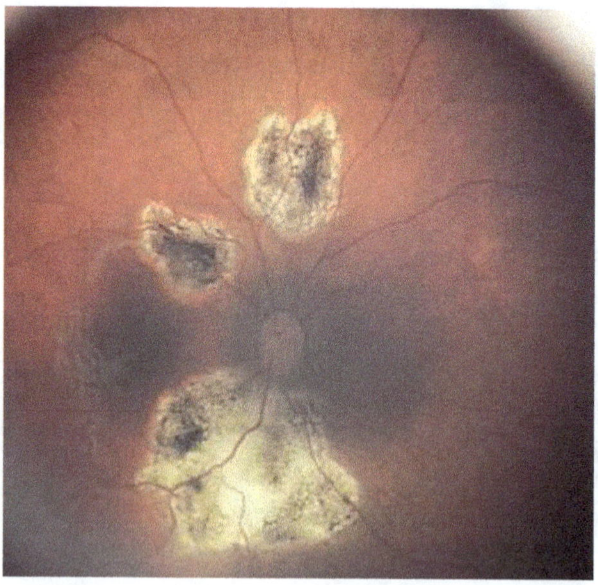

**Figure 8.** August 2012. Fundal image from right eye following chemoreduction and focal laser photocoagulation

In our experience in the Children's University Hospital in Dublin, all new cases of retinoblastoma are discussed using an internet consultation service where fundus images, clinical history, and proposed treatment are reviewed with a leading expert in retinoblastoma in the Hospital for Sick Kids in Toronto, Canada. The diagnosis is confirmed, and a treatment plan is agreed upon. This ensures standards of retinoblastoma management are of the highest

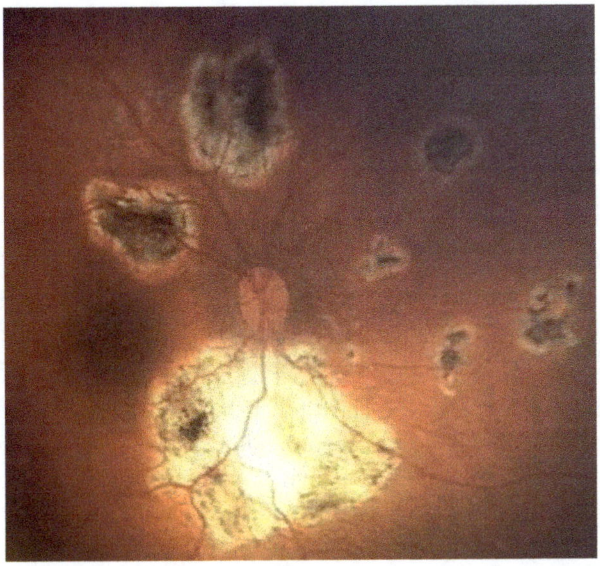

**Figure 9.** September 2012.Fundal image from right eye taken during examination under anesthesia showing multiple treated areas and inactive tumor

quality, and the most up-to-date treatments are employed. Selected cases may be further discussed via videoconferencing and electronic mail.

### 4.5. Treatment planning

As discussed earlier there are multiple treatment modalities available to treat retinoblastoma. Treatment plans tailored to specific cases can be formulated between experts in different countries by sharing medical knowledge and experiences. Remote experts can closely monitor the progress of patients by sharing fundus images and other clinical information. In difficult cases, or cases requiring enucleation it is especially useful to have the second opinion of an objective expert to ensure the best possible care is delivered.

### 4.6. Cost effectiveness

The relatively small numbers of retinoblastoma patients worldwide means that ophthalmologists and oncologists in developing countries are unlikely to have the experience to treat without expert advice. As this is a curable disease, efforts toward early diagnosis and treatment are not only worthwhile, but cost effective. In countries with limited resources especially, telemedicine provides invaluable support and advice. For example, a telemedicine programme for retinoblastoma has been implemented in Jordan and has improved treatment and survival for children in that country. The RetCam allows for real-time teleconferencing.

There are strong arguments for tackling long term conditions to improve quality of life, while being mindful of the need to contain costs. In particular, there is considerable interest in the potential of telemedicine to generate cost effectiveness gains and even to yield cost savings, while maintaining or improving patient outcomes. Evidence on the cost-effectiveness of telehealth is accumulating; systematic reviewers have judged it as promising for managing respiratory and cardiac disease and diabetes. Although evidence of the effect of telemedicine on retinoblastoma cost effectiveness remains scarce, it is promising.

### 4.7. Medico-legal aspects

#### *4.7.1. Protocols for telemedicine*

To avoid medico-legal pitfalls, comprehensive policies should be in place to ensure that patients receive the maximum benefit.

The limits of a telemedicine should be clarified. It is important to identify and outline the responsibilities of everyone in who is involved in telemedicine interactions to ensure seamless patient management. The credentials and insurance coverage of all licensed practitioners involved in telemedicine applications should be clear. Failure to verify the credentials of a consulting specialist could lead to claims of negligent referral if there is an adverse outcome.

The accepted "standard of care" for telemedicine in the relevant area should be identified. The process for assuring confidentiality of patient information should be outlined including: security and retention protections for electronic communication; protocols for identifying people at distant locations; confidentiality agreements for third-parties; compliance with confidentiality, and patient informed consent.

It is necessary also to outline standards for image acquisition, resolution bandwidth, transmission, storage resolution, method and time, retrieval, and manipulation, and to have backup procedures in place in case of equipment failure, weather interference, or other emergency.

## 5. Summary

Retinoblastoma is the most common intraocular cancer of childhood; it continues to be a challenge both diagnostically and therapeutically. Telemedicine has a large role to play in the diagnosis and management of this retinoblastoma. In our experience, telemedicine enables invaluable expert collaboration to ensure the best outcomes for patients with retinoblastoma. Telemedicine has many potential applications in retinoblastoma management, both in the developing and developed world.

## Author details

Sarah MoranMichael O' Keefe

Mater Private Hospital, Dublin, Ireland

## References

[1] Shields JA, Shields CL. Management and prognosis of Retinoblastoma. In: Intraocular Tumors: A text and Atlas. Philadelphia, Pa: WB Saunders; 1992.

[2] Devesa SS. The incidence of retinoblastoma. Am J Ophthalmol. 1975;80:263-265.

[3] Shields CL, Shields JA. Genetics of Retinoblastoma. In :Tasman WS, Jaeger E,eds. Duane's foundations of Clinical Ophthalmology. 3rd ed. Philadelphia, Pa: Lippincott Williams and Wilkins;2002.

[4] Shields JA, Parsons HM, Shields CL, et al. Lesions simulating retinoblastoma. J Pediatr Ophthalmol Strabismus. 1991;28:338-340.

[5] Aziz HA, Boutrid G, Murray TG, et al. Supraselective injection of intra-arterial melphalan as the primary treatment for late presentation of unilateral multifocal stage Vb retinoblastoma. Retina 2010;30:S63-5

[6] Abramson DH, Dunkel IJ, Brodie SE, et al. A phase I/II study of direct intraarterial ophthalmic artery) chemotherapy with melphalan fro intraocular retinoblastoma initial results. Ophthalmology 2008;115:1398-404

[7] Shields CL, Ramasubramanian A, Rosenwasser R, et al. Supraselective catheterization of the ophthalmic artery for intrarterial chemotherapy for retinoblastoma. Retina 2009;29:1207-9

[8] Ericson LA, Rosengren BH. Present therapeutic resources in retinoblastoma. Acta Ophhalmol 1961;39:569-76

[9] Smith SJ, Pulido JS, Salomao DR et al. Combined intravitreal and subconjunctival carboplatin for retinoblastoma with vitreous seeds. Br J Ophthalmol 2012;96:1073-1077

[10] Shields CL, Bianciotto CG, Jabbour P, et al. Intra-arterial chemotherapy fro retinoblastoma: Report No.q, Control of retinal tumors, subretinal seeds, and vitreous seeds. Arch Ophthalmol 2011;129:!399-406

[11] Munier FL, Beck-Popovic M, Balmer A, et al. Occurrence of sectoral choroidal occlusive vasculopathy and retinal arteriolar embolization following supraselective ophthalmic artery chemotherapy for advanced intraocular retinoblastoma. Retina 2011;31:566-73

[12] Shields CL, Shields JA, Cater J et al. Plaque radiotherapy in the management of retinoblastoma:long-term tumor control and treatment complication in 208 tumors. Ophthalmology. 2001;108:2116-2121

[13] Abramson DG, Ellsworth RM. The surgical management of retinoblastoma. Ophthalmic Surg 1980;11(8):596-8

[14] Field MJ. Telemedicine: a guide to assessing telecommunication in healthcare. J Digit Imaging. 1997;10 (3 Supp;1):28

5

# Teleophthalmology: Eye Care in the Community

Daniel Dragnev, Usman Mahmood,
Chris Williams and Manoj Kulshrestha

## 1. Introduction

The difficulties of sustaining care in hospitals are forcing health economies to deliver health care closer to the home in the community. The increased use of Vasoactive Endothelial Growth Factor (VEGF) antagonists to treat patients with wet age related macular degeneration has exponentially increased the need for additional clinic and treatment capacity. New National Institute of Clinical Excellence (NICE) guidelines for glaucoma (2009) have increased the number of referrals into secondary care. This chapter will explore how additional capacity may be created using digital imaging transfer techniques, to allow patients to be seen in virtual clinics, which may be located in either primary or secondary care.

The learning goal of this chapter is better understanding of novel ophthalmic technology for retinal disease management and glaucoma assessment deployed in the digital health environment. This is a topic of considerable significance in retinal care given the explosion of relevant clinical imaging technology and the huge burden of certain retinal disease (age related macular degeneration, retinal vein occlusion and diabetic retinopathy) on National Health Service (NHS) services and which is set to expand even more with further new and welcome treatments for these conditions. It is also of importance in view of the increased glaucoma referrals into secondary care in the light of recent NICE guidance, increasing the need for more advanced imaging techniques in the diagnosis and investigation of these patients. Glaucoma patients are now more commonly undergoing Optical Coherence Tomography (OCT) scanning of the optic disc, or advanced disc imaging for follow up purposes and diagnosis.

Smarter ways of working, using new technology, are required to cope with this clinical need and organisational burden. The need includes better use of IT infrastructure; innovation in primary care to secondary care referral management and enhanced productivity in secondary care. The development of "Virtual Clinics" using this technology will be discussed.

Some clinical IT/imaging driven solutions to such challenges will be explored in this and with emphasis on retinal/glaucoma care pathways and treatment of eye emergencies.

Tele ophthalmology is a visual specialty with a long history. Therefore, the development of image and video transmission through a telephone line makes it possible to transfer ophthalmologic images over long distances. Li H (1999) reported a modern application in the late 1980s: NASA developed a real time transmission system of retinal images acquired using a portable video funduscope. Shimmra et. al (1998) used a conventional telephone system to transmit slit lamp images of the eye and evaluate the feasibility of real-time video and audio transmission. Yoshida A (1998) used video conferencing systems to transmit full-motion colour images between a university and hospital.

Using those early systems, an expert remote presenter who is trained in the use of the ophthalmic peripherals, hardware, and software can capture still and moving images of the eyes can transmit them to ophthalmologists. The current status of teleophthalmology applications has been limited to specific purposes such as doctor-to-doctor consultation, research and clinical trial collaboration, and distance learning for medical professionals. The purpose of this chapter is to demonstrate how refinement of this technology has successfully led to the clinical application of teleophthalmology systems for the benefit of patients.

Barsela and Glovinsky examined the feasibility of a low-bandwidth, Internet-based teleophthalmology system for consultation in an ophthalmic emergency room. Forty-nine patients were seen in the eye casualty by a resident and ocular images were taken using a slit-lamp connected to a video camera and transmitted to a senior ophthalmologist by email. A telephone was used for real-time audio communication of each case. Each case was re-examined by the same senior ophthalmologist the following day. Each case was assigned a feasibility score (0-100%), which was defined as the contribution made by the transmitted images in presenting clinical details which could not have been described verbally.

High feasibility scores from 85 to 90% were found for the following images: ocular surface, anterior chamber, anterior chamber angle, pupils, lens, optic nerve and macula. Images of vitreous and peripheral retina received low feasibility scores (mean score 65%). There was 100% agreement between the diagnosis made during consultation and the examination made by the consultant ophthalmologist later on. This illustrates the feasibility of teleophthalmoogy consultations in the emergency room. It has also proven to overcome the barriers and improve quality, access and affordability in eye care in South India, (John S et al 2012) in teleophthalmology mobile units in the community, a topic which will be discussed in more detail in section 3.

### 1.1. Eye care using wireless smart phone technology

Tele-ophthalmology is taking an increasing role in the provision of primary emergency services. Digital images, slit lamp video conferencing and transfer of fundus images allow the provision of substantial clinical care. Most urgent ophthalmic diagnosis may be made and treatment prescribed remotely. Decisions to transfer patients urgently can also be made. For instance the difference between acute iritis and acute angle closure glaucoma can be established with slit lamp videos after telephone input of history. Urgent corneal conditions such as microbial keratitis, herpetic eye disease, etc can be initially managed urgently via elinks of photographs and videos. Images of optic discs can help in the diagnosis of papilloedema in an emergency setting. Images may now be transmitted to pads, phones and blackberry devices, so diagnosis and treatment may be made remotely.

The initial cost of investing in tele-ophthalmology in an emergency department is returned favourably by the savings in on call hours. This strategy is being employed at various rural centres across Australia, Wales and Canada. In Australia, most rural emergency departments now have tele links with one on call ophthalmologist covering several areas at once.

It has been shown to be feasible to apply satellite based tele-ophthalmology for making a presumptive diagnosis and planning further management of adnexal and orbital diseases based on live interaction and digital still images of the patients taken by a digital video slit lamp in rural areas of Tamil Nadu as demonstrated by Verma et al (2009). It has been demonstrated to be reliable in the assessment of ocular trauma as researched by Simon et al (2003).

In Sweden and Australia, General Practitioners have used these digital slit lamps in rural settings to gain experience in management of primary care emergencies and are supervised in the removal of corneal foreign bodies by the technology as shown by Hall et al (2005). A general ophthalmologist, Camara et al (2000) has used teleophthalmology to link up with an orbital surgeon to assist in the removal of a lateral orbital tumour.

Nurse Practitioners can be well trained to take anterior segment photographs on the slit lamp. (Kulshrestha MK, Williams C, Lewis D, Axford A (2010) A pilot trial of tele-ophthalmology services in North Wales. J Telemed Telecare;16:196-197).

Smart phones have been used in ophthalmology emergency departments to document visual acuity and examination findings. They have been used in dermatology and radiology to transfer images, but there is limited published use documented for image transfer in ophthalmology. The Foto-Ed Study by Lamirel et al (2012) compared the quality of images of non-mydriatic fundus images on a phone vs a computer screen, showing no loss of resolution of the image.

Smart phones, such as the iphone, therefore present a unique opportunity for a role in teleophthalmology. They have a high resolution "retinal" screen with 326dpi resolution located between two glossy panels of aluminosilicate glass (the same glass used in the windshields of helicopters and high speed trains). It has 78% of the pixels of a larger tablet or pad in a far smaller screen size. The resolution is therefore optimised to the way the human eye sees things at the normal distance from the eyes.

We therefore explored the use of the smart phone to take photos of the digitally captured image and transfer these to the Consultant Ophthalmologist in charge of the Tywyn Eye Clinic in North Wales through MMS smart phone text.

Smart phone technology has already been used in emergencies in the Norway's Arctic Svalbard archipelago where British students were recently attacked by a polar bear (www.myfox8.com/

news/wghp-story-deadly-polar-bear-attack-norway). Images were sent through a phone to University Hospital Tromsoe for immediate advice on first aid to be obtained.

We used smart phone technology to transfer a digital image taken on a slit lamp of the anterior segment of the eye in rural North Wales to a Consultant Ophthalmologist in the local District General Hospital, over 1 hour away by ambulance transfer to gain an instant, rapid opinion on diagnosis. This reduced unnecessary travelling down to Swansea, over 3.5 hours away. Eye Emergencies have been shown to be treated in rural areas by Nurse Practitioners obtaining advice directly from a Consultant Ophthalmologist through high resolution images of the eye seen on a smart phone.

Larger pads and tablets may also be used to send macular Optical coherence tomography images to a Consultant Ophthalmologist wirelessly using appropriate apps to carry out Virtual Clinics, run by Nurse Practitioners or Opticians, so that treatment decisions may be made remotely if the ophthalmologist is working many miles away from the rural centre.

## 1.2. Smart phone images used for diagnosis and treatment of eye emergencies in rural North Wales

### *1.2.1. Brief outline of problem*

Tywyn, Gywnedd, North Wales at the Tywyn War Memorial Cottage Hospital, is a rural outreach clinic in the Betsi Cadwaladr University Health board. One hundred and twenty four eye emergencies are seen at this unit by Nurse Practitioners in casualty per year. Twenty four of these emergencies have needed referral per year to a Consultant Ophthalmologist on call at Bronglais Hospital, Aberystwyth for assessment. Bronglais Hospital is in the neighbouring Hywel Dda Health Board.

Nurse Practitioners have already undergone training in use of the Topcon SL D7 slit lamp to take photos of the anterior segment of the eye and send these images to Bronglais casualty for assessment through a Polycom Telemedicine monitor

Last year, Consultant Ophthalmologists in Hywel Dda Health Board were taken out of the on call rota and no longer carried out on call duties. Nurse Practitioners in Tywyn would therefore have to send eye emergencies to Swansea for assessment, which is 3 hours away.

The Nurse Practitioner is well trained to take anterior segment photographs on the slit lamp. We therefore explored the use of the smart phone to take photos of the digitally captured image and transfer these to the Consultant Ophthalmologist in charge of the Tywyn Eye Clinic through MMS texting.

### *1.2.2. Assessment of problem and analysis of its causes*

Twenty four patients with eye emergencies would need to be transferred to Swansea per year, involving 144 hours of travelling time per year or 1526 kg of $CO_2$ pollution per year, to gain a Consultant Ophthalmologist opinion.

The Trust Telemedicine Board and the Caldicott Guardian were consulted to discuss in detail issues in regard to transfer of images through smart phones to a Consultant Ophthalmologist to obtain an expert opinion and avoid hospital transfer

*1.2.3. Strategy for change*

A pilot in the use of smart phone technology to transfer digital images was discussed in the Telemedicine Board. The Caldicott Guardian stated that in an emergency transfer of an image for an expert opinion could be justified on clinical need. None of the anterior segment photos would show an identifiable face, and no patient identifiable information would be on the image. After the emergency decision and treatment were carried out the images were to be deleted from the Smart phones by the Nurse Practitioner and the Consultant.

Patients presenting to casualty with an eye emergency which the Nurse Practitioner on call deemed to need a Consultant opinion were asked and given the option of transfer to Swansea or for an image of the anterior segment of the eye to be sent to the Consultant Ophthalmologist in charge of the Tywyn Eye Clinic.

The experience/success of the pilot was to be fed back to the Telemedicine group for further discussion/improvements.

*1.2.4. Measurement of improvement*

Over a 12 month period from September 2011– August 2012, there were 12 eye casualties who needed assessment by digital transfer of images through the smart phone to the Consultant. The Consultant gave help on history/investigation/diagnosis and treatment

These patients were then assessed in Tywyn clinic at an appropriate time interval, the diagnosis confirmed and the outcome on symptoms/visual acuities assessed.

*1.2.5. Effects of changes*

We used smart phone technology to transfer a digital image taken on a slit lamp of the anterior segment of the eye to a Consultant Ophthalmologist to gain an instant, rapid opinion on diagnosis. This reduced unnecessary travelling down to Swansea, with a total of 84 hours or 2800 miles saved over 12 months for patients and hospital transport. Twelve patients had their eye findings correctly diagnosed through the smart phone image by an expert and appropriate treatment was given rapidly with excellent visual outcomes in all cases

This had allowed eye emergencies to be seen in Tywyn, despite changes in the on call arrangements. Patients can still gain an expert opinion through use of digital photography, and gain rapid treatment by instruction to a trained Nurse Practitioner. This has been useful for patients who present with anterior segment disorders of the eye, but is not as useful for disorders of the posterior segment of the eye. These patients would need assessment of their symptoms and are referred for urgent assessment in the local clinic.

The main problem encountered in the change was the issue of confidentiality. The Caldicott Guardian deemed that the clinical need was greater in these instances, and once the decision was made, the images were to be deleted form both Smart phones

*1.2.6. Lessons Learnt*

Smart Phone technology has been shown to be useful in the assessment and treatment of eye emergencies. All patients showed improvements in visual acuity ranging from 1 line to 7 lines, and complete resolution of symptoms due to prompt diagnosis and therapy.

A Consultant opinion was gained quickly in all 12 cases. The costs of patient and hospital transport were saved. There is a role for the use of smart tablets in digital image transfer to provide a larger image, and these could also be used for transfer of retinal optical coherence tomography images in a macular clinic. There is the potential for use of smart phone images in dermatological emergencies

Eye Emergencies can be effectively treated in rural areas by Nurse Practitioners obtaining advice directly from a Consultant through high resolution images of the eye seen on a smart phone.

### 1.3. Smart phone adapters for slit lamps

It is possible to take slit lamp photos by placing the lens of a smart phone against the slit lamp lens; however, the use of an adapter will allows higher quality photographs. This may help to facilitate teleophthalmology for nurse practitioners and optometrists in the primary care setting.

The Keeler Portable Slit Lamp iPhone 4 image adapter has been reported to be compatible with the Haag-Streit 900 BM (older series) and Topcon SL-3F slit lamps. The adapter is not compatible with Topcon SL-D7, Mentor. When using the Keeler adapter, a moderate amount of force has to be applied to attach the adapter to most Haag-Streit slit lamp oculars (the diameter of my slit lamp's ocular is 30 mm and it requires a moderate amount of force to attach).

## 2. Eye care in the optometry setting using community based optical coherence tomography and virtual glaucoma clinics

Current treatment for age related macular disease requires patients to be monitored closely ( usually on a monthly basis ) for recurrence of the disease. This disease affects elderly people, who may be unable to drive due to loss of visual acuity below driving standards. In rural areas, where there is a greater travel burden ( for example in rural Wales ) there is a major challenge for people to keep up with their appointments. Elderly people are increasingly reliant on relatives, neighbours and carers to transport them to clinics, and in many cases ambulance transfer is needed for routine clinic appointments. This causes additional stress and inconvenience for these patients. It increases the chance of further health problems as for example increased rate of falls. This costs either the health authorities and/ or the patients for organising and supplying this transport. More CO2 gases are released in the atmosphere from the increased pollution.

The solution for all these issues is to deliver healthcare closer to the home in the community. This can be achieved with community based OCT machines, together with (non- ) mydriatic fundus cameras. In areas with not very dense population or in countries, where the purchase of enough equipment is an issue, this equipment can be integrated into special mobile vans. Mobile vans can visit different areas with a pre- determined schedule, and are the topic of discussion of the next section in this chapter.

The information obtained with this equipment is sufficient for a trained ophthalmologist to assign appropriate treatment or follow up, using modern telemedicine equipment, even if he or she is thousands of miles away. This allows remote diagnosis and management of patients.

Glaucoma is a chronic disease, in which in the majority of cases lifetime follow up is required. This puts a large strain on the ophthalmology clinics. For most of the patients with stable glaucoma follow up in a virtual clinic is possible.

Trained opticians or nurses can check visual acuity, IOP ( Goldman application ), perform visual acuity test, nerve fibre layer scans (OCT, GDX, HRT ) and record fundus photos with a (non)- mydriatic camera. All these tests can be done in the community and after that the information can be digitally transferred to a regional ophthalmology centre, where it can be interpreted by ophthalmologists. In this way patients are not going to have travel long distances. The ophthalmologists will be able to increase the capacity of their clinics. They will have all the required information for changing treatment and assigning follow up appointments. Prioritisation of patients who need to be seen for a face to face consultation can be made from the information.

### 2.1. Optometry and teleophthalmology

In the UK there are currently 2.3 ophthalmologists per 100 000 population, as described by Kulshrestha and Kelly (2011). This is the lowest pro rata than any other European Union country (www.uems.net). In the UK, optometrists play an important role in managing patients with eye complaints. Most of the patients seen in the Hospital Eye Service (HES) are referred by them either directly or through the patient's general practitioner (GP) (Bell and O'Brien 1997). For example more than 90 % of all suspected cases of primary open angle glaucoma are referred to the HES by optometrists according to Harrison and Wild et al (1988). The National Health Service (NHS) hospitals in the United Kingdom are a part of the public system. Optometry practices are private and have a dual role: they carry sight tests and dispense spectacles and contact lenses. The sight tests are reimbursed by the NHS.

The Hospital Eye Services (HES) in the UK are usually overloaded with patients and have waiting times of several months for new patients. There are also waiting times for follow up appointments. This means that for many patients allocated 6 months follow up appointments, the appointment may be delayed by a number of months. This is called slippage, and slippage has increased in recent years due to the introduction of new NICE guidance for glaucoma, which has increased referrals into HES from primary care. In addition, increased workload from the Vasoactive Endothelial Growth Factor antagonist treatment of wet age related macular disease has overloaded the service due to the demands of monthly OCT scanning and injections. This service is now affecting appointments in general ophthalmology clinics where glaucoma patients are seen.

With an aging population (baby-boomers are currently retiring) and financial strain on the NHS hospital services, new technological and organizational solutions are in need of implementation to solve the capacity problems brought about by an increased demand on services. Involving optometrists as part of a team is one potential solution. To ensure that quality is guaranteed, this can be done under the direct supervision of the consultant ophthalmologist (or other trained HES trained staff) with the help of an IT teleophthalmology connection between them. In addition to assisting the Hospital Eye Service by using the human, technological and the space capacity available at the optometry practices in urban areas, teleophthalmology provides invaluable benefits in rural areas. The availability of ophthalmology services at the community reduces the need of transport (cost and carbon emissions) and reduces the inconvenience (need of accompanying relative/ absence from work).

For example in the Hywel Dda Health Board, patients from Wales have to travel sometimes more than 1 hour in each direction for a HES appointment. Ophthalmology patients are usually elderly, some with impaired eyesight and not fit to drive. Even if they are fit to drive they usually need somebody accompanying them, because of the need for pupillary dilation. Very often the general health of these patients is impaired as well which makes the journeys even more unpleasant and add to the psychological burden on the patient. Many of the ophthalmology conditions are chronic and need multiple follow up appointments (sometimes monthly visits) or on a lifelong basis (for example glaucoma). Waiting times for optometric appointments are usually a few days and these practices are situated in the community.

The teleophthalmology connection between HES and optometry practices can be significantly helpful in managing patients with 1) Glaucoma 2) Macular diseases 3) Emergency eye conditions.

### 2.2. Teleophthalmology in glaucoma patients

Management of patients with glaucoma and ocular hypertension is a significant part of the everyday workload in the glaucoma clinics. The North London Eye study and other population based surveys estimate that patients with ocular hypertension or primary open angle glaucoma (POAG) will increase by one third by 2021, as demonstrated by Morley and Murdoch (2006). According to Lockwood et al (2010) the positive predictive rate in the diagnosis of glaucoma and ocular hypertension was 0.37 before the National Institute of Clinical Excellence (NICE) guidelines published in April 2009 and has dropped to 0.2 after that. There are several glaucoma refinement schemes such as the Manchester, and Carmarthenshire Refinement Scheme, which rely on a specially trained optometrist to reduce the number of false positive glaucoma referrals and increase the positive predictive rate of HES referrals as described by Hensen et al (2003) and Devarajan et al (2011).In these schemes specially trained optometrists take the decision on which patients are to be referred to HES and which have to be discharged.

Teleophthalmology provides us with the opportunity for these patients to be reviewed directly by the consultant and the HES staff who are already trained to do this by using virtual glaucoma clinics. At the Portsmouth-based glaucoma refinement scheme (Trickha et al 2012) designated refinement scheme optometrist examined the patients followed by a standard Humphrey 24-2 visual field (SITA fast) (Carl Zeiss Meditec,Dublin, CA, USA), applanation tonometry assessment of IOP (Goldmann model; Haag-Streit, Bern, Switzerland), and a digital disc photograph (Topcon, Tokyo, Japan). All the information is processed digitally to a named consultant, who takes the decision at a specially designated virtual glaucoma clinic, whether the patient needs an appointment at the HES or can be discharged and followed up in the community by a community optometrist. In this project only 11 % of the referrals to the virtual clinic needed an appointment in the HES and the other 89% did not need it. The positive predictive rate of the refinement scheme was 0.78 compared to 0.37 for the unrefined one.

In addition to refining patient referrals, teleophthalmology can be used for glaucoma patients follow up in the community. In a study performed by Bunduchi et al. (2010) in Scotland, stable glaucoma patients were followed up in the community by a designated optometrist.They had visual acuities, visual fields test, intraocular pressure measurement and fundus photograph of the eye done at a local optometrist sometimes many miles away from the HES. All the information was transferred via secure electronic information exchange system to the hospital where the information was assessed by the consultant or trained hospital staff at a virtual glaucoma clinic. In the virtual glaucoma clinic more patients can be assessed compared to a standard glaucoma clinic. In this way more slots were available for the unstable glaucoma patients. This can reduce the waiting time for follow up appointments and reduce the necessity for the patients to travel long distances usually every 6 months with all the associated drawbacks.

Teleophthalmology provides the opportunity of setting up an efficient glaucoma referral refinement and follow up system under the care of consultant ophthalmologist. In this way patients can receive quality specialised hospital services in their local community without the need for travel. This can lead to savings for the NHS and the patient, as it can increase the capacity of the existing glaucoma services.

### 2.3. Teleophthalmology and macular diseases

The optical coherence tomography (OCT) is the gold standard for diagnosis and follow up of many macular diseases. Many community optometry practices have OCT machines currently. In a study performed by Kelly at al. (2011) fundus photos and OCT scans were transferred by secure file transfer email (National Health Service or NHS mail) to the hospital ophthalmologist. The images transferred via email are with superior quality compared to the standard method of communication (faxing) and are much faster than posting of hard copies or using a CD. In 96 % of cases in this study analysis of the referrals and a working diagnosis/care pathway was provided by the ophthalmologist to the optometrist within the next calendar day. In the cases where ophthalmic examination was required patients were referred through the GP. In some cases on the basis of information provided by the optometrist urgent ophthalmology appointments were scheduled.

In the last few years wet age related macular degeneration (AMD) and the intravitreal anti-VEGF injection treatment has put unprecedented strain on the ophthalmology services worldwide. Even when the patients do not need treatment they have to be followed up on monthly basis, because of the possibility of recurrence. Stable wet AMD patients can be followed up locally with their community optometrist. Optometrists can examine the patients; take OCT scans and fundus photos and all this information can be transferred digitally via secure connection to the eye clinic. Consultants or other trained staff at the HES virtual AMD clinic can assess the information and manage the patients appropriately. In this way the current capacity of the eye clinics can be increased.

### 2.4. Teleophthalmology and urgent ophthalmology referrals

Many of the patients with eye complaints present initially at the optometrists practices. Sometimes the cases can be solved just with the advice of the ophthalmologist. The percentage of these cases can be increased significantly by using the opportunities of teleophthalmology. In this way unnecessary appointments at the HES and travel can be avoided. If emergency phone calls from the optometrists are accompanied by anterior segment photo or fundus photo the hospital ophthalmologist will receive much more information and can take immediate decision in most of the cases, whether to see the patient as an emergency or even to give appropriate management plan to the optometrist.

Most of the referral to the HES, even if they come from the GP are seen prior by their optometrists. If most of the referrals are accompanied by digital information received at the hospital the prioritisation consultant can more easily detect urgent cases, so they can receive sooner appointment.

Optometrists have the expertise to manage ophthalmology patients and with the help of teleophthalmology technology these skills can be expanded. The variety of patients managed in the community setting under the direct teleophthalmology supervision of a hospital consultant can be increased. In this way more resources at the hospitals can be spared for more challenging cases. On the other hand patients can receive high quality hospital service at their local community.

## 3. Eye care in mobile vans in urban and rural populations for macular disease and diabetic retinopathy

As the wet macular service continues to exponentially multiply the capacity issues in performing OCT scans (instrumental in the management of this condition) are becoming a limiting factor in this service. The use of transport mobile vans that perform these scans with technicians and nurses is now becoming a more viable option.

Mobile van units have been used successfully to deliver eye service in the community in York, Exeter and Wales. In Wales there is the National Diabetic Retinopathy Screening Service, where vans are used throughout the country to take fundus photos of diabetics. Images are then transferred to a grading centre in Cardiff. In Exeter there is a mobile glaucoma service which has been developed to provide additional clinic capacity, run by Glaucoma Nurse Practitioners. In York there is a Box Van where patients are seen to have OCT scanning and lucentis injections in the van.

### 3.1. Diabetic retinopathy screening service for Wales

In Wales all diabetic patients undergo annual screening in local community hospitals or GP surgeries depending on the rural location. Digital fundus imaging is carried out with dilated pupils. The photographs are saved onto laptops with strict security access codes. Images are stored in data centres in North Wales, (Canaervon), Mid and South West Wales (Carmarthen) and Trefforest near Cardiff at Fairway Court which is the main centre to which all images are sent for data backup. These centres are linked through a DAWN$_2$METRO VPN. Graders at Trefforest carry out primary and secondary retinal screening.

Any patients with sight threatening diabetic retinopathy are referred to their local eye clinic by a fax or letter referral depending on the urgency and the patients are seen appropriately in specialised diabetic eye clinics within the hospital eye service. Patients with background diabetic retinopathy or no retinopathy at all have annual follow up screening assessments. This has proved to be a world class, efficient and well coordinated screening service for all diabetics in Wales. Consultant Ophthalmologists throughout Wales have regular group meetings to discuss how the service is to be delivered and improved, and provide regular training for all the Graders at Trefforest. In addition, it has standardised ophthalmic care for diabetics throughout the whole country. Consultants may view images at the local Screening Centre. There are now developments in place to allow the images to be digitally transferred to individual clinics from the main centre, so Consultants can visualise them in the clinic setting

### 3.2. Exeter mobile glaucoma service

This service was set up to screening for new referrals and follow up care of stable patients according to NICE standards The Royal Devon & Exeter Hospital Wonford have a dedicated Mobile Eye Unit which goes out across the community which screens new referrals and provides follow up care of stable patients. It is Nurse led, the Specialist Glaucoma Nurses carrying out investigations in the mobile unit including:

- Visual field assessments,
- visual acuity,
- Goldman tonometry,
- gonioscopy,
- Pupil assessment,
- Pachymetry,
- Heidelberg Retinal Tomography,

- Digital fundus photography
- Optic nerve head assessments

The Specialist Nurses also drive the mobile units around the area

The Nurse Practitioners work closely with the consultants and other members of the health service such as Opticians and GPs to provide screening and follow-up care for glaucoma patients. Glaucoma Practitioners undergo MSc Glaucoma modules in assessment and management of Glaucoma and non medical independent prescribing qualifications.

Glaucoma Imaging Technicians provide technical support for Glaucoma Practitioners in carrying out Glaucoma screening and follow-up clinics. They record patients' visual acuities, carry out Humphrey visual field assessments, perform digital stereoscopic optic disc photography, retinal topography scans and optical coherence tomography images of the optic disc

### 3.3. York mobile service

AMD is the leading cause of blindness in the UK, and predominantly affects those aged 55 and over. It currently affects an estimated 500,000 people in the UK and approximately 26,000 new cases of the more severe wet form are reported each year. This includes over 10,000 people across the North and East of Yorkshire.

Eye patients based in East Yorkshire are now able to reap the benefits of a newly launched Mobile Community Eye Care Centre based at Bridlington and District Hospitals. Previously over 140, mostly elderly, patients from the Bridlington, Scarborough and Whitby area had to make a round trip of 80 miles or more to receive treatment at York Hospital once a month. This meant that a clinic visit which should not take longer than two hours could sometimes take a whole day.

Designed as a dedicated service for local people with wet Age-related Macular Degeneration (AMD), the new clinic has slashed patient travelling times by over half, also relieving local health services of some of the capacity issues currently being faced.

The York Mobile Unit is a large Box van in which there is a waiting area, visual acuity assessment, OCT scanning and injection facilities.

The mobile clinic has saved the local NHS money in transport costs, as patients will be able to receive treatment closer to home. On average, 50 patients required hospital transport to their AMD clinic appointments over a 3 month period previously.

Incorporation of" Iris software" into the van has enabled the development of an electronic patient record in the mobile unit and has the potential to transmit image data wirelessly to a smart phone or tablet, allowing remote teleophthalmology assessment of images to take place. The unique thing about iris is that it uses the cloud to store data so can be accessed more easily in peripheral locations than Stand alone systems. It's is connected via the National Health Service n3 secure network via a password that is sent to the users mobile phone on logging in. It is a paperless system that mails a summary to the General Practitioner direct.

### 3.4. Setting up a mobile ophthalmology service: Rural Wales

The aim of the Project is to improve the quality and convenience of care for Ophthalmology patients by providing clinical reviews in the community by setting up a mobile assessment service with the capability of performing OCTs, automated visual fields, and slit-lamp based clinical examinations. This mobile assessment service will assist in overcoming current clinic capacity issues experienced by the general ophthalmology service (especially the wet AMD and glaucoma service) within the Hywel Dda Health Board Ophthalmology Department and reduce the requirement for extra out-of-hours / weekend clinics. The Mobile Ophthalmic Review Service (The Review Van) will be used in varying locations for patients to visit and receive their follow up wet AMD assessments (OCT scan and fundoscopy), and glaucoma assessments (optic disc imaging via the OCT machine, visual field analysis, and intraocular pressure check). Two possible models may be used. 1. Decisions can be made immediately in the van by an appropriate doctor or nurse practitioner. 2. The images can be transferred to the Department of Ophthalmology to be reviewed by clinicians at Hywel Dda Health Board. The mobile unit could be used to monitor other ophthalmic conditions such as pre-op and post-op cataracts, diabetic macular oedema (DMO), retinal vein occlusion (RVO) etc.

In West Wales, there are a number of community hospitals in rural areas, where elderly people find it difficult to access care. We are in the process of piloting an OCT Scan Van which will provide local OCT scanning for macular patients undergoing lucentis therapy. This will reduce the travel burden for these elderly patients who would otherwise have to access this care at District General Hospitals which are more than 1 hour away. It will also provide OCT scanning of the Optic Disc for Glaucoma patients. Some of the local community hospitals have injection facilities/theatres which could be used at a later stage to provide a one stop service. There will also be the option of providing an Injection van for carrying out Lucentis injections at certain community locations at a later stage.

Hywel Dda Health Board is the operational name of Hywel Dda Local Health Board.

Hywel Dda Local Health Board provides healthcare services to a total population of around 372,320 throughout Carmarthenshire (178,119), Pembrokeshire (116,001), and Ceredigion (78,200). It provides Acute, Primary, Community, Mental Health and Learning Disabilities services via General and Community Hospitals, Health Centres, GP's, Dentists, Pharmacists, Optometrists and other sites. The Headquarters is at Merlin's Court, Winch Lane, Haverfordwest.

The map below provides a visual overview of the wide area covered by Hywel Dda Health Board.

The map shows the site of the 4 general hospitals (white circles 1-4) within Hywel Dda Health Board. For geographic reasons the ophthalmology service for Hywel Dda has historically developed as 2 separate departments each with its own separate group of staff. The wet AMD and glaucoma services that the Hywel Dda Health Board Mobile Outreach Joint Working Project Group applies to are delivered by the department serving Carmarthenshire and Pembrokeshire (and some patients from Ceredigion) serving a total population of approxi-

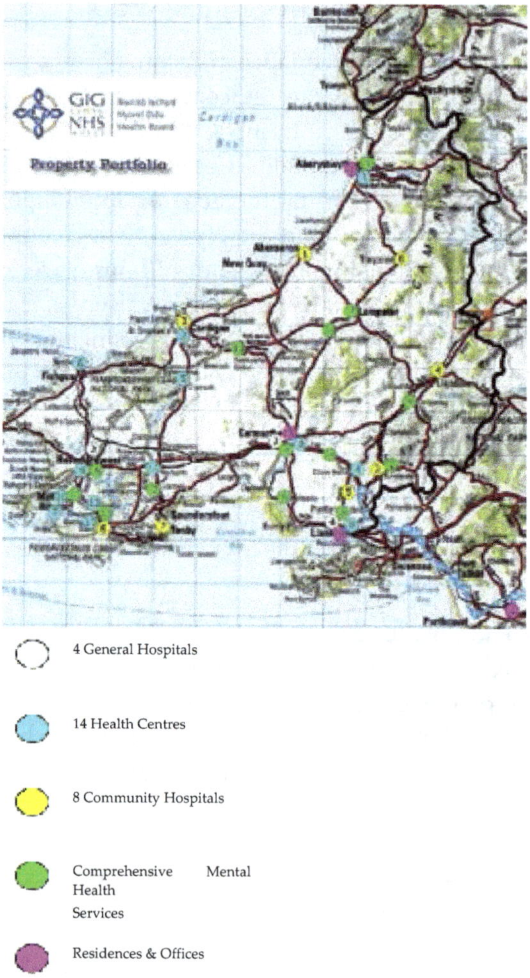


**Figure 1.** Map of Wales with locations of Hospitals served by Hywel Dda Health Board

mately 300,000. The intravitreal service for this area currently operates out of Amman Valley Hospital (yellow circle 2). The day surgery unit at this community hospital accepts patients for its intravitreal service from the catchment areas of 3 general hospitals: Withybush Hospital (WBH) in Haverfordwest (white circle 3), West Wales General Hospital (WWGH) in Carmarthen (white circle 2), Prince Phillip Hospital (PPH) in Llanelli (white circle 4). Thus Amman Valley Hospital provides a wet AMD service for Carmarthenshire, Pembrokeshire and parts of Ceredigion which covers a population of approximately 300,000 drawing patients from a wide geographical area.

The AA route finder shows that a return journey from Haverfordwest to Amman Valley Hospital is 110 miles taking 2 hours and 50 minutes, from Fishguard it is 140 miles with an estimated return travel time of 3.5 hours. Only a proportion of this journey has a dual carriageway, patients often have longer travel times than this, especially when using hospital transport. A public transport journey is complicated, exceptionally long, and not practical for patients, and is never undertaken. The above example (the catchment area for Withybush Hospital in Haverfordwest) applies to approximately one third of the departmental catchment area (serving 116,000 people). There are currently 460 wet AMD patients in this service for regular follow up and treatment, approximately 1/3 of this population each lives in the catchment area of PPH (Llanelli), WWGH (Carmarthen), Withybush (Haverfordwest, Pembrokeshire). This represents a significant travel burden on patients and their relatives, especially for the patients from Pembrokeshire. Costs of travel are met by patients and family (75% of journeys), and Hywel Dda Health Board via the Welsh Ambulance Service (25% of journeys).

An audit of 26 recent clinics (June, July 2011) has shown that the number of patients injected per clinic has fallen from 75-80% in 2009, to 50% currently (due to the increased proportion of stable wet age related macular disease patients as the macular service service has matured). This has resulted in an inefficient use of the injection facilities available, and unnecessary travel for the 50% of patients who do not receive injections. Not all 'non-injection' decisions can be predicted, but many can, especially those patients who have been recently dry for 4 months or more.

The Ophthalmology service is currently operating beyond capacity and the expected increase in patient numbers would mean the service would be further stretched. An increased time interval between intravitreal treatments has been proven to reduce visual outcomes. The service currently requires a combination of extra Saturday clinics or volunteers to cross-cover for colleagues when they take annual leave from the service. The current guidelines from the Royal College of Ophthalmologists on the standard of care for the management of wet AMD is that initial treatment be given within two weeks of presentation and that patients be followed up four weekly. The current average follow up time at Hywel Dda Health Board is 5 weeks for patients with active wet AMD, longer for those patients who have been 'dry' for successive visits, as long as extra clinics and cross-cover can be arranged. The extra out-of-hours clinics and volunteer based cross-cover is no longer sustainable.

New treatment modalities have recently been approved for Diabetic Macular Oedema (DMO)and Retinal Vein Occlusion (RVO). These developments will increase the burden on theintravitreal service over and above the burden from the wet AMD service. The wet AMDservice continues to accumulate patients at a rate of 11-14 new patients per month, thiscontinues to far exceed the number of discharges from the service despite now entering its 4th year. Experience from around the UK is showing only a 5% discharge at year one, only 25% at year two, the predicted service plateau at end of year three has not materialised.

Within the Department of Ophthalmology, the medical retina service has been a priority due its immediate capacity needs. However, the service cannot keep up with the demand, and the new treatment modalities now available for DMO and RVO will impact this service further. This growth in demand for intravitreal treatments has had a major impact on the ability and capacity to deliver the general ophthalmic service, especially the glaucoma and cataract services.

The glaucoma service for this department currently operates out of the 3 main district general hospitals described above (WBH, WWGH and PPH – white circles 3, 2 and 4 respectively). The extra capacity demands placed on the Ophthalmology department following the development of the new wet age related macular disease service in 2008 has resulted in a lack of building space and staff to cope with the increased demands placed on the glaucoma service via recent NICE guidelines and the new National (NHS Wales) Glaucoma pathway. The glaucoma service cannot currently meet these guidelines predominantly due to capacity issues, created by recent intravitreal service development

Delivering a health system focused on care closer to home will require support from the population of Carmarthenshire, Ceredigion and Pembrokeshire, as well as stakeholders. The key driver for change is the opportunity to improve the quality and the safety of health services. This project fits perfectly with the stated aims of the Health Board by moving wet age related macular disease consultations from a day surgery unit hospital environment into the community, and nearer to the home of the patient. As stated above there is a considerable travel burden for one third of the intravitreal population, and in comparison to a non-rural region there is still a significant travel burden for the other two thirds of the population. The costs for 25% of journeys are met by the Health Board; costs for 75% of journeys are met by patients and their families. The table below provides a snapshot of the travel burden.

| Catchment area | Approx proportion of population (Total 300,000) | Minimum return journey time* | Frequently quoted return journey time | Return mileage from district general hospital to intravitreal centre (AVH, Glanamman) |
|---|---|---|---|---|
| WBH, Pembrokeshire | 33% | 2 hrs 50mins | 4 hrs WBH<br>5 hrs Fishguard | 110 miles |
| WWGH, Carmarthen | 33% | 80 mins | 80 mins | 52 miles |
| PPH, Llanelli | 33% | 60 mins | 60 mins | 31 miles |

*AA route finder quote

NB: Carmarthen to AVH is the only journey which is predominantly dual carriageway, the other 2

**Table 1.** journeys are predominantly single carriageway roads

- The Health Board has limited buildings and infrastructure to grow and develop the Ophthalmology service. This has significant implications for the intravitreal service (wet age related macular disease, Diabetic macular oedema and retinal vein occlusion), and the Glaucoma service, both of which have NICE guidelines and new NHS Wales pathways to adhere to. The Glaucoma service does not have the required buildings / space to expand into in any of the above 3 district general hospitals (WBH, WWGH, PPH – white circles 3, 2, 4 above).

- There are demands on the Ophthalmology service to follow up patients at regular intervals which cannot be achieved with current staff / service logistics / capacity.
- Adherence to National Institute of Clinical Excellence guidelines (for both wet age related macular disease and glaucoma) and the new NHS Wales 'Focus on Ophthalmology' Pathways (for both wet age related macular diseases and glaucoma) cannot be guaranteed with current demands and activities

The proposed project is to set up a mobile assessment unit (review van) complete with an OCT machine, visual field machine and slit-lamp to follow-up recently 'dry' macular disease patients nearer to their home rather than in Amman Valley Hospital; plus follow-up glaucoma patients at an approved interval near to or at their local district general hospital thereby:

- Reducing the number of unused injection slots in the Amman Valley Hospital (AVH) theatre
- Reducing considerably the travel time burden on patients and their family to AVH
- Reducing considerably the travel cost burden on the Health Board, patients and their families
- Reducing the time interval between reviews in wet age related macular disease, thus facilitating improved visual outcomes due prompt recognition of the requirement for further intravitreal therapy.
- Reduce the time interval between glaucoma follow-up reviews to that required by NICE guidelines and NHS Wales 'Focus on Ophthalmology' Pathways, thus facilitating enhanced visual outcomes.

The 'Review Van' will be used in varying locations for patients to visit and receive their follow up macular and glaucoma assessments. 2 models are available:

- Data (intraocular pressure and images for glaucoma, images for macular assessment) can be transferred to the Department of Ophthalmology at Hywel Dda Health Board to be reviewed by clinicians, or
- The assessments can be reviewed in real-time by a doctor or nurse practitioner present within the van

For macular disease, the first locations for the mobile unit to provide follow up appointments have been identified in Pembrokeshire. There is an aspiration to achieve further locations within twelve months in/near Carmarthen and Llanelli.

For glaucoma, WWGH Carmarthen has been identified as the primary area of interest due to acute constraints of available building space and staff. There is an aspiration to pilot the review van for glaucoma reviews in WBH and PPH (both also have constraints on available building space and staff).

There is also the potential for the review and monitoring of other patients that require OCT scanning and slit-lamp review as part of their regular monitoring eg diabetic macular oedema, retinal vein occlusion, pre and post-op cataract assessments.

By moving a proportion of the wet AMD service and glaucoma service out of the main unit it is proposed that there will be more capacity to meet the current and immediate future demands for intravitreal therapies. It is proposed that after 3-4 months of 'dry' status patients could be seen in the review van for follow up.

The lucentis service at Aberystwyth caters for the population of Ceredigion (90,000), South Gwynedd (50,000 of a total of 130,000 for Gwynedd county and Powys (120,000). Some patients in Powys are managed by the medical retina teams of Shrewsbury and Hereford.

All patients undergo OCT scanning at North Road Eye Clinic, and lucentis injection at Bronglais Hospital at a separate booked appointment. Currently up to 20-25 patients are booked for lucentis injection from North Road onto one injection list at Bronglais Hospital as a two stop service.

Patients are seen at local community clinics of Tywyn (South Gywnedd), Machynlleth (North Powys), Llanidloes (North Powys), Newtown (Mid Powys), Aberaeron (South Ceredigion) and Cardigan (South Ceredigion). All patients from these community clinics therefore have to travel twice per month when undergoing review of lucentis therapy for OCT scanning at North Road and subsequent injection at Bronglais. Provision of local Optical Coherence Tomography scanning in the van in the community will allow this travel burden to be halved.

Patients from Aberaeron, Machynlleth are within 30 minutes of Aberystwyth and can therefore continue to have their injections in Bronglais. Patients from South Gwynedd and Mid Powys may have to travel in excess of 1 hour to access the theatre facilities in Aberystwyth. This travelling time can be up to 1.5 or 2 hours in snowy winter conditions, where the roads are full of traffic from holiday makers from the Midlands in the summer or in rare instances where there has been a road traffic accident

This group of patients can potentially have injections in theatre facilities within Tywyn for South Gwynedd patients and Llandrindod Wells Hospital for Mid Powys patients. Cardigan patients are over 1 hour from Aberystwyth, and they may have the travel burden reduced by having both the OCT scan and injection facilities to be made available in two separate vans. It would be possible therefore, for certain sited to have a one stop service (Tywyn, Llandrindod Wells, Cardigan) and some to remain as a two stop (Aberaeron, Machynlleth) depending on the facilities available on each site.

There remains scope to reduce the travel burden on patients from Powys who currently are scanned in Shrewsbury or Hereford to have local OCT scanning and/or injections in the community at Welsh Community Hospitals in the future to reduce their travel burden. This may be incorporated into the project once the project has been established within Hywel Dda Health Board.

In order to set this develop this project, an Ophthalmic Mobile Unit team was set up to discuss development of a business case with regular meetings monthly for a year. The Project is now about to hit the road, and has had a successful demonstration using the Mobile van for optical coherence tomography scanning

## 4. Eye care to the paediatric population

### 4.1. Medico legal issues

The diagnosis of non-accidental injuries in children and babies frequently requires the presence of retinal haemorrhages. Court conviction depends on the testimony of the ophthalmologist who has to rely only on clinical notes as evidence. Having retcam video and photographs carry huge weight age in such proceedings.

### 4.2. Retinopathy of prematurity

Babies born prematurely or underweight are at risk of developing a devastating proliferative retinopathy of prematurity (RoP) that can be blinding. It remains a major cause of visual loss worldwide and there is approximately 50 000 babies annual rate of global blindness from RoP. This is potentially a treatable condition and therefore requires thorough and extensive screening. Unfortunately screening is dependant on the presence of highly skilled paediatric ophthalmologists. Most babies with RoP are in developing countries where there is a lack of properly trained paediatric ophthalmologists. Having a device that can photograph the fundus appearance and then either email or share these pictures with a central resource where trained ophthalmologists can grade them will obviously save sights. The answer has been in the use of the retcam, which can photograph and even video the fundi of such babies. The retcam images are now increasingly replacing the indentation indirect approach of fundoscopy.

Another source of problems is intra and inter grader variability. To overcome this issue software are in the process of development for "Automated Quantification of Retinal Vessel Morphology". Human input is still required, but the aim of development is to make screening entirely computerized.

### 4.3. Retcam images

Retcam images are similarly used for screening of premature or low birth weight babies for Retinopathy of Prematurity (ROP) using ophthalmoscopy and image-based telemedicine examinations. The number of premature infants is increasing throughout the world, and a larger percentage of them are surviving. A Telemedicine examination from images obtained from a Retcam may be more reproducible than if you see an infant's retina only briefly during ophthalmoscopy. These are manufactured by Spectrum and Clarity Medical systems. There is a rationale that image-based examination may be better because findings are documented photographically, rather than an indirect ophthalmoscopic examination, which may also be more uncomfortable for the baby. In many other ophthalmic diseases, definitions are based on standard images, so this has implications for the way we might deliver the best care to patients in the future.

The Retcam does require contact with the cornea and will therefore require training. It uses pupillary illumination to take digital photos of the fundus and skilled screeners may grade these images in a central location that can be remote from the neonatal unit. Where a shortage of trained paediatric ophthalmologists is stretching the services of ROP screening, this mode of teleophthalmology is not only valuable, but is in fact the only solution to maintaining a credible service. Other paediatric ophthalmic pathology can also be excluded via the retcam. An example is the presence of retinoblastomas[4] in an eye with a white reflex, allowing decisions to be made on urgency of referrals. Photographs of shaken babies for diagnostic and medico legal purposes can also be taken via a Retcam and the images subsequently transferred for opinion.

Advantages of the Retcam include its portability and manoeuvrability in constrained areas such as on the Neonatal Intensive Unit and outpatients. It is easily transportable between hospitals and clinics, and allows transfer of images to any networked system. It allows timely remote evaluation of patient images and provides advanced image analysis and comparison capability of previous images with retcam review software.

In 2008 at Nayayana Nethralaya Postgraduate Institute of Ophthalmology, Bangalore, India, a tele ROP service was initiated using a nonphysician screening model as described by Vinekar A (2008). This was entitled KIDROP (Karanataka Internet Assisted Diagnosis of ROP). The Retcam Shuttle (clarity MSI) and a portable laser indirect ophthalmoscope were transported by a clinical team to 23 Neonatal Intensive Care Units in 7 districts around Bangalore city.

The images are exported from a laptop using a portable wireless data card which allows internet access. The images are uploaded onto a secure server using an n indigenously designed software (i2i Telesolutions;Bangalore, India), which are backed up at 2 geographic sites. A remotely situated expert will login read and report the image live.

Since 2009, images have been visualised on a smart phone remotely using a specially designed application for the device. The reports created on the smart phone are in PDF, and on submission to the expert, they enter the server through the GSM cellular network and are accessible to the technician in any remote rural area.

## 5. Conclusion

Governments are now focusing on delivering care closer to the patient's home. With the ever increasing number of patients we need to see in our clinics, these clinically driven IT solutions may allow patients to have investigations carried out either in their local community hospitals, primary care setting or in mobile ophthalmic units. The various solutions discussed in this chapter using wireless technology to set up virtual clinics will:

- Increase productivity of healthcare professionals
- Strengthen referral patterns
- Effectively educate hospital staff, clinicians and the community

- Extend patient care and expertise to remote areas
- Improve patient care with mobility solutions

We would envisage that this will help to reduce slippage on patient appointments, distribute the workload to the community staff and help to increase capacity. This will help to reduce also the travel burden on patients traveling to the main centre every month for some patients. This becomes increasingly more difficult for elderly patients with time, and saves them many hours of a long trip, with reduced need for hospital transport, or patients own transport costs in many instances. There is also reduced pollution directly arising from reduced travel needs.

## Author details

Daniel Dragnev[1], Usman Mahmood[1], Chris Williams[2] and Manoj Kulshrestha[1]

1 Hywel Dda Health Board, UK

2 Betsi Cadwaldr University Health Board, UK

## References

[1] Bar-sela, S. M, & Glovinsky, Y. (2007). A feasibility study of an Internet-based telemedicine system for consultation in an ophthalmic emergency room J Telemed Telecare., 13(3), 119-24.

[2] Bell, R. D, & Brien, O. C. Accuracy of referral to a glaucoma clinic. Ophthal Physiol Opt (1997)., 17, 7-11.

[3] Bunduchi, R, Smart, A, Charles, K, & Mckee, L. and Azuara-Blanco A Boundary spanning process innovation: The role of institutional pressures in shaping process innovation across public and private sectors

[4] Blomdahl, S, Calissendorff, B, & Jacobsson, U. (2002). Patient-focused urban tele-ophthalmology services. J Telemed Telecare. 8;Suppl , 2, 43-4.

[5] Camara, J. G, Zabala, R. R, Henson, R. D, & Senft, S. H. (2000). Teleophthalmology: the use of real-time telementoring to re move an orbital tumor.*Ophthalmology*. Aug;, 107(8), 1468-71.

[6] Devarajan, N, Williams, G. S, Hopes, M, Sullivan, O, & Jones, D. D.The Carmarthenshire Glaucoma Referral Refinement Scheme,a safe and efficient screening service. Eye (2011)., 25(1), 43-49.

[7] Glaucoma Diagnosis and management of chronic open angle glaucoma and ocular hypertension NICE clinical guideline 85 Developed by the National Collaborating Centre for Acute Care Issue date: April 2009

[8] Kelly, S. P, Wallwork, I, & Haider, D. Qureshi K Epub ((2011). Teleophthalmology with optical coherence tomography imaging in community optometry. Evaluation of a quality improvement for macular patients. *Clin Ophthalmol.* 2011;, 5, 1673-8.

[9] Kulshrestha, M, Kelly, S, & Mahmood, U. (2011). Teleophthalmology in Practice, Telemedicine Techniques and Applications, Georgi Graschew and Stefan Rakowsky (Ed.). In Tech , 19, 393-412.

[10] Kulshrestha, M. K, Williams, C, Lewis, D, & Axford, A. (2010). A pilot trial of teleophthalmology services in North Wales. *J Telemed Telecare* , 16, 196-197.

[11] Hall, G, Hennessy, M, Barton, J, & Coroneo, M. (2005). Teleophthalmology-assisted corneal foreign body removal in a rural hospital. Telemed J E Health. Feb;, 11(1), 79-83.

[12] Harrison, R. J, Wild, J. M, & Hobley, A. J. Referral patterns to an ophthalmic outpatient clinic by general practitioners and ophthalmic opticians and the role of these professionals in screening for ocular disease. BMJ (1988). , 297, 1162-1167.

[13] Henson, D. B, Spencer, A. F, Harper, R, & Cadman, E. J. Community refinement of glaucoma referrals. Eye (2003). , 17, 21-26.

[14] John, S, Sengupta, S, Reddy, S. J, Prabhu, P, Kirubanandan, K, & Badrinath, S. S. (2012). The Sankara Nethralaya mobile teleophthalmology model for comprehensive eye care delivery in rural India Telemed J E Health. Jun;, 18(5), 382-7.

[15] Lamirel, C, Bruce, B, Wright, D, Newman, N, & Biousse, V. (2012). Nonmydriatic Digital Ocular Fundus Photography on the Smart Phone 3G: The FOTO-ED Study *Arch Ophthalmol* , 130(7), 939-940.

[16] Li H Telemedicine and ophthalmology (1999*) Survey of Ophthalmology* 44:1999;61-72.

[17] Lockwood, A. J, Kirwan, J. F, & Ashleigh, Z. Optometrists referrals for glaucoma assessment: a prospective survey of clinical data and outcomes. Eye (2010). , 24(9), 1515-1519.

[18] Morley AMSMurdoch I. The future of glaucoma clinics.BJO (2006). , 90, 640-645.

[19] Shimmura, S, Shinozaki, N, Fukagawa, K, Shimazaki, I, & Tsubota, K. (1998). Realtime telemedicine in the clinical assessment of the ocularsurface. American Journal of Ophthalmology 125; , 388-390.

[20] Simon, D. P, Thach, A. B, & Bower, K. S. (2003). Teleophthalmology in the evaluation of ocular trauma. Mil Med. Mar:168(3);, 205-11.

[21] Trikha, S, Macgregor, C, Jeffery, M, & Kirwan, J. (2012). The Portsmouth-based glaucoma refinement scheme: a role for virtual clinics in the future?. Eye. Jul 6.;10:1038

[22] Verma, M, Raman, R, & Mohan, R. (2009). Application of tele-ophthalmology in remote diagnosis and management of adnexal and orbital diseases. Indian J Ophthalmol. Sep-Oct; , 57(5), 381-384.

[23] Vinekar, A. (2008). The ROP Challenge in rural India:preliminary report of a telemedicine screening model. In:International experience with photographic imaging for paediatric and adult eye disease. Retina Physician ;suppl , 9-10.

[24] wwwmyfox8.com/news/wghp-story-deadly-polar-bear-attack-norway

[25] www.uems.net

[26] Yogesan, K, Cuypers, M, Barry, C. J, Constable, I. J, & Jitskaia, L. (2000). Tele-ophthalmology screening for retinal and anterior segment diseases.*J Telemed Telecare*. 6; Suppl 1:S, 96-8.

[27] Yoshida, A. (1998). The importance of informed consent in the field of ophthalmology," [Hokkaido igaku zasshi] The Hokkaido Journal of Medical Science;, 73

6

# Quality of Life in Telemedicine-Based Interventions for Type-2 Diabetes Patients: The TECNOB Project

Stefania Corti, Gian Mauro Manzoni,
Giada Pietrabissa and Gianluca Castelnuovo

## 1. Introduction

Worldwide, diabetes has become an overwhelming problem due to the increase of overweightness and obesity. As estimated by WHO in 2011 [1], 346 million people globally suffer from diabetes and there is an approximate 3,4 million mortality rate from the consequences of DMT. WHO predicts that diabetes related deaths will double by 2030. Throughout the course of time, diabetes damages the heart, blood vessels, eyes, kidneys, and nerves. Indeed, 50% of people with diabetes die due to cardiovascular disease (primarily heart disease and stroke). Reduced blood flow and neuropathic pain can increases the chances of complications such as ulcers and even limb amputations. Diabetic retinopathy represents a significant cause of blindness, as a consequence of damage to blood vessels in the retina. 2% of diabetics become blind after 15 years. Diabetes can result in neuropathy, whose common symptoms are tingling, pain, numbness, or weakness both in feet and hands. Diabetes is the seventh leading cause of death in the US [2]. These complications are very important determinants of quality of life. Low QoL may, in turn, affect metabolic control by reducing regimen adherence. Treatment of diabetes involves lowering blood glucose and the levels of other known risk factors that could damage blood vessels. Lifestyle measures, such as the control of body weight, physical activity, a healthy diet and avoidance of tobacco use, have been shown to be effective in preventing the onset of type 2 diabetes.

In addition, estimated global healthcare expenditures to treat and prevent diabetes and its complications total at least $376 billion in 2010. By 2030, this number is projected to exceed some USD490 billion. Expressed in International Dollars (ID), which correct for differences in purchasing power, estimated global expenditures on diabetes was ID418 billion in 2010, and it will be at least ID561 billion in 2030. An estimated average of USD703 (ID878) per person will be spent on diabetes in 2010 globally [3]. Besides excess healthcare expenditure, diabetes also imposes large economic burdens in the form of lost productivity and foregone economic growth. The American Diabetes Association estimated that the US economy lost USD58 billion, equivalent to about half of the direct healthcare expenditure on diabetes in 2007, as a result of lost earnings due to lost work days, restricted activity days, lower productivity at work, mortality and permanent disability caused by diabetes [4]. The largest economic burden, therefore, is the monetary value associated with disability and loss of life as a result of the disease itself and its related complications. This economic burden, however, can be reduced by implementing many inexpensive, easy-to-use interventions, most of which are cost-effective or cost-saving. Advancement in treatment for diabetes have resulted in reduced lengths of hospital stay and, in some cases, the avoidance of hospital visits, so the demand for home care services has increased [5]. Health-care providers can deliver home care services by visiting the patient at home or by using information and communication technology, also known as telehealth or telemedicine.

## 2. Quality of life in diabetic population

In the past two decades, research has increasingly highlighted quality of life (QoL) as an important health outcome in diabetes, if not the 'ultimate goal' of treatment [6, 7]. In recent years, there has been a burgeoning interest in quality of life issues, and especially in health-related quality of life, fueled by several factors, including a growing body of evidence concerning the potent effect of psychosocial factors on physical health outcomes, and dramatic changes in the organization and delivery of health care. People with diabetes often feel challenged by their disease and its day-to-day management demands. And these demands are substantial. Patients must deal with their diabetes all day, every day, making countless decisions in an often futile effort to approximate the non-diabetic metabolic state. Diabetes therapy, such as taking insulin, can substantially affect quality of life either positively, by reducing symptoms of high blood sugar, for instance, or negatively, by increasing symptoms of low blood sugar, for example. The psychosocial toll of living with diabetes is often a heavy one, and this toll can often, in turn, affect self-care behaviour and, ultimately, long-term glycaemic control, the risk of developing long-term complications, and quality of life. Psychological adjustment to chronic disease embraces emotional, cognitive and behavioural dimensions. Several adaptation tasks need to be accomplished, such as negative and positive affective self-regulation, daily functioning contingent to treatment needs and the reformulation of beliefs and expectancies about health and disease, self and others, life and death. It is a complex dynamic process for someone with a chronic disease [8-10]. The daily psychological stress of living with a chronic disease in a world with professional and interpersonal challenges and specific diabetes-related psychological distress, associated with repetitive intrusive treatment regimens or disabling chronic complications are two correlated sources of stress in people with DMT2 [11-13]. There is good evidence that psychosocial issues are critical to good diabetes care [14, 15]. Psychosocial factors often determine self-management behaviours, and psychosocial variables (such as depression) are often stronger predictors of medical outcomes such as hospitalization and mortality than are physiologic and metabolic measures (such as the presence of complications, BMI and HbA1c)[16]. Greater attention is now being devoted to evaluating the quality of health care and the economic value associated with new interventions. Managed care organizations have stimulated a growing effort to determine whether the costs associated with new or existing therapies and educational interventions are justified within fairly short time frames, often less than 3 years. Quality of life is a multidimensional construct comprising the individual's subjective perception of physical, emotional and social well-being, including both a cognitive component (e.g. satisfaction) and an emotional component (e.g. happiness)[17]. In addition to overall or global quality of life there are many specific sub-domains (e.g. health, job, family, friends, community, etc.). Some research on the impact of health on quality of life has examined the impact of domain-specific satisfaction on global life satisfaction. There has been substantial research on the effect of objective health status on overall life satisfaction or on a global measure of health-related quality of life. Yet, while the objective dimension of health status (as assessed by physicians' reports of symptoms or the presence of complications, for instance) is important, the patient's subjective perceptions of health translate the objective facts of his or her health status into an actual quality of life experience. This view is generally endorsed by researchers in this field [18-20] who point out that since expectations regarding health and the ability to cope with limitations and disability can greatly affect a person's perception of health and satisfaction with life, two people with the same objective health status may have a very different quality of life [21]. There is also general consensus that various domains of functioning and well-being can each contribute independently to global quality of life, thus making multidimensional measurement of quality of life necessary [19]. Simply asking one question, such as 'please rate your overall health-related quality of life on a scale from 0 to 100', may provide a useful global assessment, but it does not identify the underlying dimensions which contribute to the overall or health-specific quality of life [21]. Thus, almost all quality of life research involving people with diabetes employs multidimensional assessment of quality of life and typically assesses several dimensions, including physical, psychological, and social functioning and well-being.

Two broad approaches to health-related quality of life measurement have emerged – generic and disease-specific. The generic approach involves the use of measures applicable across health and illness groups. The most widely used generic measure of quality of life in studies of people with diabetes is the Medical Outcomes Study (MOS) Short-Form General Health Survey [22], in its several forms (SF-36, SF-20, SF-12). The MOS instrument includes physical, social and role functioning scales to capture behavioural dysfunction caused by health problems. Measures of mental health, perceptions of overall health, and pain intensity reflect more subjective components of health and general well-being. The authors of this measure claim that these six health concepts are comprehensive in terms of those aspects of health considered most important to patients [23]. These instruments have been translated into many languages, and used in these forms in studies which include people with diabetes. The Rand Quality of Well-Being Self-Administered (QWB-SA) survey [24] is similar to the SF-36 in its aim to comprehensively assess health-related well-being or quality of life. It contains scales designed to measure acute and chronic emotional and physical symptoms, mobility, and physical activity. Other instruments used at least occasionally to assess general health status in people with diabetes include the

Sickness Impact Profile [25] and the Nottingham Health Profile [26]. Generic measures like the SF-36 are most useful for comparing quality of life in people with different diseases and the quality of life in people who have no diseases with the quality of life in people who have a disease. Some generic measures, such as the Quality of Well-Being Scale [24], generate a single utility index of overall quality of life. This index usually ranges from 0 to 100 and these values can be used to adjust for years of life by degree of health experience to yield a measure of 'quality-adjusted life years'. Such a measure can be used to assess cost-effectiveness and cost benefits across various interventions and illnesses. Many generic measures of emotional status have been employed in studies which include people with diabetes. These include the Well-Being Questionnaire [27], the Profile of Mood States [28], the Symptom Checklist (SCL-90R) [29], the Mini-Mental Status Exam [30]. Depression in people with diabetes has been studied using the following scales: the Beck Depression Inventory [31] and the Zung Self-Rating Depression Scale [32]. Anxiety in people with diabetes has been studied using the following scales: the Beck Anxiety Inventory [33], and the Zung Self-Rating Anxiety Scale [34]. Both depression and anxiety in people with diabetes have been studied using the Hospital Anxiety and Depression Scale [35]. Illness-specific quality of life measures can focus on the specific problems posed by an individual illness. For example, even a well-designed generic quality of life scale will not address certain aspects of life with diabetes such as hypoglycaemia, insulin injections, self-monitoring of blood glucose (SMBG), and dietary restrictions, which may be critical to an individual's health-related quality of life. Generic measures may not be specific enough to detect effects in some areas of functioning among some people with diabetes. For example, generic measures of mental health may not identify fear of complications as an important contributing factor. More and more, researchers have added disease-specific assessments to generic ones, to increase the ability of their measures to identify the factors most relevant to the health-related quality of life of people with a specific disease. Some [18] have even advocated a 3-level approach for clinical trials, incorporating generic and disease-specific measures and, finally, situation-specific questions that apply to the specific condition (neuropathy, for example) or intervention being investigated.

As shown in literature, individuals with DMT2 are known to have lower health-related quality of life (HRQOL) and more depressive symptomatology than those without diabetes [36-39]. The comorbidity of depression in patients with type 2 diabetes mellitus has been observed in several studies [40, 41]. Anderson [41] summarized 20 cross-sectional reports and found that the odds of depression in the diabetic group was twice that of the nondiabetic comparison group. In a population-based study of adults with and without DMT2, investigators found EQ-5D index scores and visual analogue scores were significantly lower for respondents with DMT2 and those with 3–5 risk factors for DMT2 than for those with 0–2 risk factors [42]. In a longitudinal analysis of EQ-5D data collected in 2004 and 2009 among SHIELD (Study to Help Improve Early Evaluation and management of risk factors Leading to Diabetes) respondents with DMT2, found their health status declined significantly, indicating that burden of disease has a long-term detrimental impact on the QoL of individuals living with DMT2 [43]. The high prevalence of depressive symptoms among people with diabetes can be explained by two scenarios: that depression may occur as a consequence of having diabetes or a risk factor for the onset of DMT2. The first prospective study where this association was suggested emerged from the work of Eaton and collaborators in 1996 [44]. Afterwards, several prospective studies provided further solid evidence of this fact, even when controlling for usual T2DM risk factors, such as BMI, sedentary lifestyle or family diabetes [45-49]. Two meta-analyses based on 9 [50] and 13 [48]) prospective studies, reported an increase of 37% risk of depressed adults or a global risk increase of 1.6 (CI 95% 1.37–1.88) which led to T2DM later on. In recent study by Pan [51], conduced on a total of more than 55'000 US women with a 10 years' follow-up, was shown that depression and diabetes are closely related to each other, and this reciprocal association depends on the severity or span of these conditions

Depressive symptoms and diabetes-specific distress correlate with each other, although only specific distress displays more links with behavioural markers, such as self-management. treatment adherence, exercise and glycaemic control [52-55]. Psychological adjustment to type 2 diabetes explains 48% of the variance in diabetes-specific distress [56]. Nevertheless, diabetes distress remains the most prevalent long-lasting factor associated with hyperglycaemia in DMT2 [53]. Predictors of diabetes stress are related to chronic complications, negative life events, chronic stress in daily life, setbacks in diet and exercise management and previous history of depression. Also, depressive symptoms emerge mostly when more intrusive kinds of treatment begin, such as insulin use [51, 57] or if some complications in late diabetes arise [58, 59]. Furthermore, it has been shown that diabetic patients with severe depressive symptoms adhere less well to diet and medication regimes than patients with less severe or no depressive symptoms [60-63]. In particular, depressed mood in diabetic patients might lead to pessimism regarding perceived benefits and lowered self-efficacy, and could result in poor self-care and compliance [64]. The diabetes patient who has low adherence to their diabetes management, lipid, or blood pressure medication as a result of depression is placed at greater risk for both micro- and macrovascular comorbid events and retinopathy [65, 66]. Finally, the course of depression is also more chronic and severe in people with diabetes [67].

## 3. Telemedicine

One of the most promising methods for the management of chronic illness and, in particular, diabetes and its consequences is represented by the use of Information and Communication Technology (ITC) tools [68]. Telemedicine includes timely transmission and remote interpretation of patient data for follow-up and preventative interventions. The main purpose of this approach is to facilitate a productive interaction between the patient and the health care provider in order to achieve improved treatment results and lower treatment costs. The five components of a sound telemedicine system include:

1. a process for accurate data collection in digital format,
2. an electronic medical record for data incorporation and remote transmission,
3. a set of protocols for distant data analysis,
4. a variety of communication tools to permit effective dialogue between patients and health care providers, and
5. a system for automatically flagging and providing feedback for outlier data [69].

Telemedicine interventions can be communicated from handheld hardware devices to a remote Web server. Hardware for transmission may include

1. cell phones [70],
2. handheld personal digital assistant devices or diaries [71], and
3. portable/laptop computers or desk computers [72].

Data may be transmitted in the form of

1. voice messages over the phone,
2. text messages (short message services) over wireless networks to Web interfaces,
3. email messages over the internet, or
4. live streaming audio or video over the internet.

Data are then incorporated into the patient's electronic medical record, analyzed, flagged if necessary, and responded to by way of automatic or personalized treatment recommendations, which are transmitted into the patient's computer, cell phone, or other handheld device.

Telemedicine is an automated support tool for patients with diabetes to facilitate better decisions by patients and health care providers. Although some of the most widely implemented applications of telemedicine have been designed to support recording and interpretation of serial blood glucose measurements by patients with diabetes, systems have been developed to organize a broadest variety of uploaded objective and subjective data of interest to managing diabetes [73], including patient-collected physiological data, such as

1. blood glucose levels, continuous glucose levels, and blood pressure;
2. laboratory data, such as haemoglobin A1c (A1C) or lipid levels;
3. behavioural information, such as dietary intake and exercise patterns;
4. medication dosages, allergies, and other history;
5. subjective symptoms of hypoglycaemia or other complaints;
6. pertinent event data, such as emergency room visits, hospitalizations, scheduled ophthalmology visits, vaccines, and missed clinic appointments; and
7. images of retinal photos, wounds, or other structures. The pattern of information can be analyzed with decision support software.

A physician can contact the patient either on a scheduled regular response basis if the situation is safe or on an automatic immediate as-needed basis in the event of a high-risk dangerous event [74]. Images of retinal examinations [75] or foot wounds [76] can be transmitted from a general practitioner's office to a specialist consultant at a remote central location.

Telemedicine programs can impact various aspects of patient care, including informational, clinical, behavioural, structural, and economic [77, 78]. The informational impact is a better quality of information than handwritten records, which may be incomplete or inadvertently forgotten at home on appointment days. The clinical impact is a more frequent communication of information and instructions, which can lead to improved outcomes with lower A1C levels or fewer adverse sequelae. The behavioural impact is more frequent therapy adjustments and reminders, leading to greater patient education and empowerment. The structural impact is usually time-saving for patients who might need to come in to the physician's office for fewer visits; however, the physician workload of reviewing messages and updated data on a regular basis may actually increase.

In a recent review and meta-analysis [79], carried out to determine the effects of telemedicine and teleconsultation regarding clinical, behavioural, and care coordination outcomes of diabetes care compared to usual care, twenty-six studies related to home telehealth for diabetes are included. Results show that, overall, home telehealth interventions were found to be effective in improving glycaemic control (HbA1c) for diabetic persons. Patients in telemedicine group are encouraged to self-monitor blood glucose levels as a part of their disease management programme. The home telehealth interventions help to reduce the number of patients who are hospitalized, number of hospitalizations and bed days of care. However, nonuniform outcomes on the effects of DMT control on quality of life are shown. In fact, in literature, QoL in diabetes is measured by a broad range of validated instruments (the World Health Organization Quality of Life-Bref, World Health Organization–Diabetes Treatment Satisfaction Questionnaire, SF-12, SF-36, Diabetes Quality of Life, Depression Scale CES-D, Problem Areas in Diabetes Scale, Visual Analog Scale, Zung Self-Rating Depression Scale, Depression Short-CARE, Diabetes Distress Scale and Health-Related Quality of Life). Despite these reported methodological issues, telemedicine interventions in DMT control show an increase in contact between health care provider and patient, health care perceived as more supportive according to patients, more effective communication, increased metabolic data transmission, availability and completeness of data among health carers, and improved communication both with health carers and peers [80].

A telemedicine program can be judged as successful if it meets four criteria by being (1) sound, (2) effective, (3) cost-effective, and (4) practical [69]. A sound telemedicine technology facilitates accurate collection of data, accurate input of data, verification of data accuracy, and a process to correct incorrect data. A sound technology will include time stamping of input data to avoid back filling, forward filling, or other data manipulation. An effective technology allows for the determination of process outcome measures, clinical outcome measures, and patient satisfaction. First, the effectiveness of automated telemedicine systems can be measured to assess the adoption of process outcomes, such as timely foot screenings, retinal evaluations, vaccine administrations, and measurement of laboratory tests. These tests include A1C, glucose, lipids for all patients with diabetes, and other laboratory analyses for selected diabetes patients, including serum creatinine levels in users of metformin, liver tests in users of statins, serum potassium in hypertensive patients on selected blood pressure medications, and serum fructosamine in some patients with hemoglobinopathies. Second, the effectiveness of telemedicine programs can be assessed on the basis of improvements in objective clinical outcomes, such as A1C levels, number of hypoglycaemic events, glycaemic variability according to a predefined formula, or emergency room visits for diabetes-related events. Finally, patient satisfaction can also be used to measure the effectiveness of a telemedicine program. User experience can be quantified by using surveys to measure patient satisfaction, classifying patient feedback in response to provider instructions, and determining the amount of system use by patients [81]. A cost-effective telemedicine technology, compared to usual care, will provide benefits for a cost that is either less expensive than current care ('cost-saving intervention') or a cost-per-benefit ratio, which is within a range that society is already willing to pay for other widely used services. This amount is typically in the range of a cost of up to $50,000 per each quality adjusted life year gained [82]. At last, a practical telemedicine program will overcome technical and structural problems that have hindered the adoption of many new medical programs. Such problems have included (a) a lack of connectivity between stand-alone diabetes telemedicine systems and hospital electronic medical record systems, (b) inadequate decision support software, and (c) inadequate data encryption and security systems to fully ensure patient privacy. Based on these four criteria for a successful telemedicine program, telemedicine has been demonstrated to be substantial, possibly effective, and somewhat practical, but has not been demonstrated to be cost-effective. Research on telemedicine programs that has been published has typically described short-term projects of up to 12 months. Although most studies of telemedicine programs for type 2 diabetes mellitus have demonstrated improved A1C outcomes [83], such programs in type 1 diabetes have not consistently demonstrated improved A1C levels [84]. One on the largest telemedicine studies conducted was the Informatics for Diabetes Education and Telemedicine project [85]. This study compared the outcomes of a combined Web and streaming video telemedicine system against base therapy without a telemedicine system in 1665 Medicare patients. Telemedicine subjects experienced an improvement in glycaemia control, blood pressure levels, and total and low-density lipoprotein cholesterol levels at 1 year of follow-up. The long-term costs and benefits of telemedicine programs are unknown [84]. Cost-effectiveness data are very sparse, however, because there has been very little work in the way of realistic economic modeling or empiric data analysis in the field of diabetes telemedicine [86]. Patients and providers will need to demonstrate continued ongoing compliance and favourable medical and economic results before these programs will be funded on a widespread basis for long-term care. Telemedicine systems are hindered by technical and structural problems that are being corrected gradually and will likely be solved in the near future.

## 4. Technology for obesity project

In order to determine which features of telemedicine and internet-based interventions are critical in a cost-effective approach, TECNOB project has been developed. TECNOB (TECh-Nology for OBesity) Project is a comprehensive two-phase stepped down program enhanced by telemedicine for the medium-term treatment of obese and diabetic people seeking intervention for weight loss [87, 88]. Its core features are the hospital-based intensive treatment (1-month), that consists of diet therapy, physical training and psychological counselling, and the continuity of care at home using new information and communication technologies (ICT) such as internet and mobile cell phones. The effectiveness of the TECNOB program compared with usual care (hospital-based treatment only) will be evaluated in a randomized controlled trial (RCT) with a 12- month follow-up. The primary outcome is weight in kilograms. Secondary outcome measures are energy expenditure measured using an electronic armband, glycated haemoglobin, binge eating, self-efficacy in eating and weight control, body satisfaction, healthy habit formation, disordered eating-related behaviours and cognitions, psychopathological symptoms and weight-related quality of life (The Self-Report Habit Index – SRHI[89], Weight Efficacy Life Style Questionnaire – WELSQ [90], Body Uneasiness Test – BUT [91], Binge Eating Scale – BES [92, 93], Eating Disorder Inventory EDI-2 [94], Symptom Check List - SCL-90 [95], Impact of Weight on Quality of Life-Lite - IWQOL-Lite [96], The Outcome Questionnaire - OQ 45.2 [97]). According to the Consensus Statement on the Worldwide Standardization of the Haemoglobin A1C Measurement [98], the haemoglobin A1C (A1C) assay has become the gold-standard in measurement of chronic glycaemia for over two decades. Anchored in the knowledge that elevated A1C values increase the likelihood of the micro-vascular complications of diabetes (and perhaps macro-vascular complications as well), the assay has become the cornerstone for the assessment of diabetes care. In this study, we adopt the measurement method (concentration of only one molecular species of glycated A1C) and results reporting (mmol/mol and derived NGSP %) developed by the International Federation of Clinical Chemistry and Laboratory Medicine (IFCC)

In this paper only weight and disordered eating-related behaviours and cognitions (EDI- 2) data were analyzed and reported. Weight was assessed with the participant in lightweight clothing with shoes removed on a balance beam scale. The EDI-2 is a widely used, standardized, self-report measure of psychological symptoms commonly associated with anorexia nervosa, bulimia nervosa and other eating disorders. The EDI-2 does not yield a specific diagnosis of eating disorder. It is aimed at the measurement of psychological traits or symptom clusters presumed to have relevance to understanding and treatment of eating disorders. The EDI-2 consists of 11 subscales derived from 91 items. Three of the subscales were designed to assess attitudes and behaviours concerning eating, weight and shape (Drive for Thinness, Bulimia, Body Dissatisfaction) and the remaining eight ones tapped more general constructs or psychological traits clinically relevant to eating disorders (Ineffectiveness, Perfection, Interpersonal Distrust, Interoceptive Awareness, Maturity Fears, Asceticism, Impulse Regulation and Social Insecurity) [94, 99].

During the in-patient phase, participants attend an intensive four-week hospital-based and medically-managed program for weight reduction and rehabilitation. All patients are placed on a hypocaloric nutritionally balanced diet tailored to the individual after consultation with a dietician (energy intake around 80% of the basal energy expenditure estimated according to the Harris-Benedict equation and a macronutrient composition of 16% proteins, 25% fat and 59% carbohydrates). Furthermore, they receivegeneral well-being. The authors of this measure nutritional counselling provided by a dietician, brief psychological counselling provided by a clinical psychologist and physical activity training provided by a physiotherapist. Nutritional rehabilitation program's aim to improve and promote change in eating habits and consists of both individual sessions (dietary assessment, evaluation of nutrient intake and adequacy, nutritional status, anthropometric, eating patterns, history of being overweight, readiness to adopt change) and group sessions (45 minutes each twice a week) including: information on obesity and related health risks, setting of realistic goals for weight loss, healthy eating in general, general nutrition and core food groups, weight management and behaviour change strategies for preventing relapse). Psychological counselling is provided once a week both individually and in group setting. Individual sessions, lasting 45 minutes each, are mainly based on the cognitive-behavioural approach described by Cooper and Fairburn [100] and emphasize the techniques of self- monitoring, goal setting, time management, prompting and cueing, problem solving, cognitive restructuring, stress management and relapse prevention. Group sessions (small groups of 5/6 persons), lasting 1 hour each, focus on issues such as motivation to change, assertiveness, self-esteem, self-efficacy and coping. Developing a sense of autonomy and competence are the primary purposes of the in-hospital interventions. Patients are afforded the skills and tools for change and are supported in assigning positive values to healthy behaviours and also in aligning them with personal values and lifestyle patterns. Physical activity takes place once a day except for weekends and consists of group programs (20 individuals) based on postural gymnastics, aerobic activity and walks in the open. Patients with specific orthopaedic complications carry out individual activities planned by physiotherapists and articulated in programs of physical therapy, assisted passive and active mobilization and isokinetic exercise. In the last week of hospitalization, just before discharge from the hospital, participants allocated to the TECNOB program are instructed for the outpatient phase. Firstly, they receive a multisensory armband (SenseWear® Pro3 Armband) [101], an electronic tool that enables automated monitoring of total energy expenditure (calories burned), active energy expenditure, physical activity duration and levels (METs). Patients are instructed to wear this device on the back of the upper arm and to record data for 36 hours every two weeks in a free-living context. The Armband holds up to 12 days of continuous data which the outpatients are instructed to download into their personal computer and to transmit online to a web-site specifically designed for data storing. Outpatients are also told that they can review their progress using the SenseWear® 6.1 Software which analyzes and organizes data into graphs and reports. Secondly, participants are instructed to use the TECNOB webplatform, an interactive web-site developed by TELBIOS S.P.A. (http://www.telbios.it). The TECNOB web-platform supports several functions and delivers many utilities, such as questionnaires, an animated food record diary, an agenda and a videoconference virtual room. In the "questionnaires" section, patients submit data concerning weight and glycated hemoglobin. In the "food record diary" participants submit actual food intake day by day through the selection of food images from a comprehensive visual database provided by METEDA S.P.A. (http://www.meteda.it). The same procedure is also possible through a software called METADIETA (Meteda s.p.a.) previously installed on the outpatients' mobile phones before discharge. Through the mobile phones outpatients maintain the contact with the dietitian who regularly sends them SMS containing syntax codes that METADIETA, the software previously installed into the outpatients' mobile phones, used in order to visually display the food choices (frequency and portions) outpatients have to adhere according to dietary prescriptions. In this way, outpatients can keep a food record diary allowing comparisons between current eating and the recommended hypocaloric diet along the whole duration of the program. The"agenda" allows the patients to remember the videoconference appointments with the clinicians and the days when to fill in the questionnaires. Moreover, the patients can use the "memo" space to note down any important event occurred to him/her in the previous week/month. The clinical psychologist has thus the opportunity to discuss with the outpatients about the significant events reported in the "memo" space during the videoconference sessions and cognitively reconstruct dysfunctional appraisals in functional ways. Finally, outpatients are instructed to use the videoconference tool. Thanks to this medium, they receive nutritional and cognitive-behavioural telecounselling with the dietitian and the clinical psychologist who attended the patients inside the hospital. In particular, just after discharge, participants have 6 videoconference contacts with both clinicians along 3 months. From the 3rd to the 6th month sessions are scheduled every 30 days and then even more spaced up to an interval of 60 days. During telesessions, clinicians (psychologist and dietitian) test the outpatients' progress, their mood, the maintenance of the"good alimentary and physical activity habits", the loss/increase of weight and ask about critical moments, especially those ones reported on the "memo"web-space. In particular, telesessions with the clinical psychologist aim to consolidate strategies and abilities acquired during the in-patient phase, to improve self-esteem and self-efficacy, to support motivation, to prevent relapse and to provide problem-solving and crisis counselling. On the other hand, a dietician assesses adherence and compliance to dietary therapy with a special focus on normal eating behaviour, sufficient fluid intake, hunger and fullness regulation, appropriate eating/etiquette (pace and timing of meals), slow rate of eating, and addresses critical points such as plateau in weight loss or lack of readiness to improve dietary habits. In addition to videoconferences, outpatients can further contact clinicians by e-mail. Indeed, each patient is given the possibility to join his clinician beyond the established videoconference contacts in case of urgency or emergency. According to the e-message's content, clinicians choose the most appropriate format for delivering feedback among e-mail or telephone. In order to avoid excessive dependence and to contain costs, a maximum number of 1 not scheduled contact a week is established a priority. Great relevance is given to the clinicians-patient relationship as an important medium and vehicle of change. After discharge, outpatients begin to experience the autonomy and competence to change they develop during the in-patient phase and inevitably face resistances and barriers. Thanks to videoconferences, outpatients are supported by the clinicians who attended them during the in-hospital phase in exploring resistances and barriers they experience and in finding functional pathways to cope. Furthermore, outpatients are helped to experience mastery in terms of the health behaviour change that needs to be engaged.

## 5. Conclusion

Some preliminary results are now available. As indicated in a recent paper [87], at present 72 obese patients with type 2 diabetes have been recruited and randomly allocated to the

TECNOB program (n=37) or to a control condition (n=39). However, only 34 participants have completed at least the 3-month follow-up and have been included in this ad interim analysis. 21 out of them have reached also the 6-month follow-up and 13 have achieved the end of the program. The first ad interim analysis of the data from the TECNOB study has not revealed any significant difference between the TECNOB program and a control condition in weight change at 3, 6 and 12 months. Within-group analysis showed significant reductions of initial weight at all time-points but not at 12-month follow-up. The median percentage of initial weight loss for the whole sample was -5,1 kg (-6,6 to-3,7) at discharge from the hospital. Completers analysis of data collected at 6 and 12 months showed that participants regained back part of the weight loss and the difference between weight at baseline and at 12-month follow-up was no more statistically significant.

Differences in eating-related behaviours and cognitions (EDI-2) were also examined. At baseline, the control group showed higher scores in many EDI-2 scales, i.e. Drive for Thinness, Ineffectiveness, Interoceptive awareness, Impulse regulation and Social Insecurity, compared with the TECNOB group. Notably, these groups included selected participants (those patients that have come through at least the 3-month follow-up) and such statistically significant differences were not found when the original groups were compared. Control group showed higher scores also in Interpersonal distrust at 12 months. However, this result has to be seen with caution because of the few patients (n=12) who have achieved the end of the program at present.

Remarkably, sample sizes at 6 and 12 months are small (n=21 and n=12 respectively) due to the ongoing status of the study and these results may be unreliable. These ad interim findings did not support the effectiveness of the TECNOB protocol over a control condition. Notably, this kind of data analysis (ad interim analysis) is underpowered and results obtained may not be reliable, in particular at 6 and 12 months. However, we gained a significant insight into an important component of the study design, i.e. the hospital-based program. The effect that such uncontrolled factor has on weight loss was very high and probably overwhelmed the effect of the TECNOB intervention. Hence, much statistical power is necessary to enhance the chance to detect the effect of the TECNOB program: the hospital-based program has a very high effect in the first months after discharge but such effect may reduce in the long term. A 12-month follow-up is probably sufficient to detect the TECNOB effect over and above the weakened effect of the hospital base program. Study and information collection is an on-going process and complete results, in particular about glycated haemoglobin and QoL indices, will be published in the next years.

## Acknowledgements

This chapter is related to the TECNOB Project (Technology for Obesity Project) supported by the "Compagnia di San Paolo" private foundation. Our technological partners are TELBIOS (http://www.telbios.it) and METEDA (http://www.meteda.it).

## Author details

Stefania Corti[1,2], Gian Mauro Manzoni[1,3], Giada Pietrabissa[1,3] and Gianluca Castelnuovo[1,3]

1 Istituto Auxologico Italiano IRCCS, Psychology Reseach Laboratory, Ospedale San Giuseppe, Verbania, Italy

2 Department of Psychology, University of Bergamo, Italy

3 Department of Psychology, Catholic University of Milan, Italy

## References

[1] Organization WH. Diabetes. 2011 [cited Fact sheet N°312 27 August 2012]; Available from: http://www.who.int/mediacentre/factsheets/fs312/en/index.html.

[2] Prevention CfDCa. Diabetes. 2012 [cited 2012 28 August 2012]; Available from: http://www.cdc.gov/nchs/fastats/diabetes.htm.

[3] Federation ID. The Economic Impacts of Diabetes 2009 [cited 2012 28 August]; Available from: http://www.idf.org/diabetesatlas/economic-impacts-diabetes.

[4] Economic costs of diabetes in the U.S. In 2007. Diabetes Care. 2008 Mar;31(3):596-615.

[5] Irish C. Home health care: helping to prevent and treat diabetes. Caring. 2011 Jul; 30(7):28-32.

[6] Rubin RR, Peyrot M. Quality of life and diabetes. Diabetes Metab Res Rev. 1999 May-Jun;15(3):205-18.

[7] Speight J, Reaney MD, Barnard KD. Not all roads lead to Rome—a review of quality of life measurement in adults with diabetes. Diabetic Medicine. 2009;26(4):315-27.

[8] de Ridder D, Geenen R, Kuijer R, van Middendorp H. Psychological adjustment to chronic disease. Lancet. 2008 Jul 19;372(9634):246-55.

[9] Sharpe L, Curran L. Understanding the process of adjustment to illness. Soc Sci Med. 2006 Mar;62(5):1153-66.

[10] Stanton AL, Revenson TA, Tennen H. Health psychology: psychological adjustment to chronic disease. Annu Rev Psychol. 2007;58:565-92.

[11] Fisher L, Chesla CA, Mullan JT, Skaff MM, Kanter RA. Contributors to depression in Latino and European-American patients with type 2 diabetes. Diabetes Care. 2001 Oct;24(10):1751-7.

[12] Fisher L, Mullan JT, Arean P, Glasgow RE, Hessler D, Masharani U. Diabetes distress but not clinical depression or depressive symptoms is associated with glycemic con-

trol in both cross-sectional and longitudinal analyses. Diabetes Care. 2010 Jan;33(1): 23-8.

[13] Fisher L, Mullan JT, Skaff MM, Glasgow RE, Arean P, Hessler D. Predicting diabetes distress in patients with Type 2 diabetes: a longitudinal study. Diabet Med. 2009 Jun; 26(6):622-7.

[14] Fisher EBJ, Arfken CL, Heins J, Houston C, Jeffe D, Sykes R. Acceptance of diabetes in adults. In: DS G, editor. Handbook of Health Behavior Research. New York: Plenum Publishing Corp; 1996.

[15] Glasgow RE, Osteen VL. Evaluating diabetes education. Are we measuring the most important outcomes? Diabetes Care. 1992 Oct;15(10):1423-32.

[16] Rosenthal MJ, Fajardo M, Gilmore S, Morley JE, Naliboff BD. Hospitalization and mortality of diabetes in older adults. A 3-year prospective study. Diabetes Care. 1998 Feb;21(2):231-5.

[17] Campbell A, Converse PE, Rodgers WL. The Quality of American Life. New York: Russell Sage; 1976.

[18] Jacobson AM. Quality of Life in Patients With Diabetes Mellitus. Semin Clin Neuropsychiatry. 1997 Jan;2(1):82-93.

[19] Rose M, Burkert U, Scholler G, Schirop T, Danzer G, Klapp BF. Determinants of the quality of life of patients with diabetes under intensified insulin therapy. Diabetes Care. 1998 Nov;21(11):1876-85.

[20] Testa MA, Simonson DC. Health economic benefits and quality of life during improved glycemic control in patients with type 2 diabetes mellitus: a randomized, controlled, double-blind trial. JAMA. 1998 Nov 4;280(17):1490-6.

[21] Testa MA, Simonson DC. Assesment of quality-of-life outcomes. N Engl J Med. 1996 Mar 28;334(13):835-40.

[22] Stewart AL, Greenfield S, Hays RD, Wells K, Rogers WH, Berry SD, et al. Functional status and well-being of patients with chronic conditions. Results from the Medical Outcomes Study. JAMA. 1989 Aug 18;262(7):907-13.

[23] Ware JH, Sherbourne CD. The MOS 36-Item Short Form Health Survey (SF-36). I: Coneptual framework and item selection. Med Care. 1992;30:473-83.

[24] Bush JM, Kaplan RM. Health-related quality of life measurement. Health Psychology. 1982;1:61-80.

[25] Bergner M, Bobbitt R, Carter W, Gilson B. The Siskness Impact Profile: development and final revision of a health status measure. Med Care. 1981;19:787-805.

[26] Hunt SM, McKenna SP, McEwen J, Williams J, Papp E. The Nottingham Health Profile: subjective health status and medical consultations. Soc Sci Med A. 1981 May;15(3 Pt 1):221-9.

[27] Bradley C, Lewis KS. Measures of psychological well-being and treatment satisfaction developed from the responses of people with tablet-treated diabetes. Diabet Med. 1990;7:445-51.

[28] McNair DM, Lorr M, Droppelman LF. Manual of the Profile of Mood States. San Diego: Educational and Industrial Testing Service; 1971.

[29] Derogatis LR, Rickels K, Rock AF. The SCL-90 and the MMPI: a step in the validation of a new self-report scale. Br J Psychiatry. 1976 Mar;128:280-9.

[30] Folstein MF, Folstein SE, McHugh PR. "Mini-mental state". A practical method for grading the cognitive state of patients for the clinician. J Psychiatr Res. 1975 Nov; 12(3):189-98.

[31] Beck AT, Beamesderfer A. Assessment of depression: the depression inventory. Mod Probl Pharmacopsychiatry. 1974;7(0):151-69.

[32] Zung WW, Richards CB, Short MJ. Self-rating depression scale in an outpatient clinic. Further validation of the SDS. Arch Gen Psychiatry. 1965 Dec;13(6):508-15.

[33] Steer R, Beck A. The Beck Anxiety Inventory. In: Zalaquette CP, Wood RJ, editors. Evaluating Stress: a Book of Resources. Lanham, Maryland: Scarecrow Press; 1997. p. 23-40.

[34] Zung WWK. Assessment of anxiety disorders: qualitative and quantitative approaches. In: Fann WE, editor. Phenomenology and the Treatment of Anxiety. New York: SP Medical and Scientific; 1978. p. 1-17.

[35] Zigmond AS, Snaith RP. The hospital anxiety and depression scale. Acta Psychiatr Scand. 1983 Jun;67(6):361-70.

[36] Grandy S, Chapman RH, Fox KM. Quality of life and depression of people living with type 2 diabetes mellitus and those at low and high risk for type 2 diabetes: findings from the Study to Help Improve Early evaluation and management of risk factors Leading to Diabetes (SHIELD). Int J Clin Pract. 2008 Apr;62(4):562-8.

[37] Luscombe FA. Health-related quality of life measurement in type 2 diabetes. Value Health. 2000 Nov-Dec;3 Suppl 1:15-28.

[38] Watkins K, Connell CM. Measurement of health-related QOL in diabetes mellitus. Pharmacoeconomics. 2004;22(17):1109-26.

[39] Egede LE, Ellis C. The effects of depression on diabetes knowledge, diabetes self-management, and perceived control in indigent patients with type 2 diabetes. Diabetes Technol Ther. 2008 Jun;10(3):213-9.

[40] Ali S, Stone MA, Peters JL, Davies MJ, Khunti K. The prevalence of co-morbid depression in adults with Type 2 diabetes: a systematic review and meta-analysis. Diabet Med. 2006 Nov;23(11):1165-73.

[41] Anderson RJ, Freedland KE, Clouse RE, Lustman PJ. The prevalence of comorbid depression in adults with diabetes: a meta-analysis. Diabetes Care. 2001 Jun;24(6): 1069-78.

[42] Grandy S, Fox KM. EQ-5D visual analog scale and utility index values in individuals with diabetes and at risk for diabetes: Findings from the Study to Help Improve Early evaluation and management of risk factors Leading to Diabetes (SHIELD). Health Qual Life Outcomes. 2008;6:18.

[43] Grandy S, Fox KM. Change in health status (EQ-5D) over 5 years among individuals with and without type 2 diabetes mellitus in the SHIELD longitudinal study. Health Qual Life Outcomes. 2012 Aug 21;10(1):99.

[44] Eaton WW, Armenian H, Gallo J, Pratt L, Ford DE. Depression and risk for onset of type II diabetes. A prospective population-based study. Diabetes Care. 1996 Oct; 19(10):1097-102.

[45] Kawakami N, Takatsuka N, Shimizu H, Ishibashi H. Depressive symptoms and occurrence of type 2 diabetes among Japanese men. Diabetes Care. 1999 Jul;22(7): 1071-6.

[46] Carnethon MR, Kinder LS, Fair JM, Stafford RS, Fortmann SP. Symptoms of depression as a risk factor for incident diabetes: findings from the National Health and Nutrition Examination Epidemiologic Follow-up Study, 1971-1992. Am J Epidemiol. 2003 Sep 1;158(5):416-23.

[47] Arroyo C, Hu FB, Ryan LM, Kawachi I, Colditz GA, Speizer FE, et al. Depressive symptoms and risk of type 2 diabetes in women. Diabetes Care. 2004 Jan;27(1): 129-33.

[48] Mezuk B, Eaton WW, Albrecht S, Golden SH. Depression and type 2 diabetes over the lifespan: a meta-analysis. Diabetes Care. 2008 Dec;31(12):2383-90.

[49] Demakakos P, Pierce MB, Hardy R. Depressive symptoms and risk of type 2 diabetes in a national sample of middle-aged and older adults: the English longitudinal study of aging. Diabetes Care. 2010 Apr;33(4):792-7.

[50] Knol MJ, Twisk JW, Beekman AT, Heine RJ, Snoek FJ, Pouwer F. Depression as a risk factor for the onset of type 2 diabetes mellitus. A meta-analysis. Diabetologia. 2006 May;49(5):837-45.

[51] Pan A, Lucas M, Sun Q, van Dam RM, Franco OH, Manson JE, et al. Bidirectional association between depression and type 2 diabetes mellitus in women. Arch Intern Med. 2010 Nov 22;170(21):1884-91.

[52] Delahanty LM, Grant RW, Wittenberg E, Bosch JL, Wexler DJ, Cagliero E, et al. Association of diabetes-related emotional distress with diabetes treatment in primary care patients with Type 2 diabetes. Diabet Med. 2007 Jan;24(1):48-54.

[53] Fisher L, Skaff MM, Mullan JT, Arean P, Glasgow R, Masharani U. A longitudinal study of affective and anxiety disorders, depressive affect and diabetes distress in adults with Type 2 diabetes. Diabet Med. 2008 Sep;25(9):1096-101.

[54] Nakahara R, Yoshiuchi K, Kumano H, Hara Y, Suematsu H, Kuboki T. Prospective study on influence of psychosocial factors on glycemic control in Japanese patients with type 2 diabetes. Psychosomatics. 2006 May-Jun;47(3):240-6.

[55] Nichols GA, Hillier TA, Javor K, Brown JB. Predictors of glycemic control in insulin-using adults with type 2 diabetes. Diabetes Care. 2000 Mar;23(3):273-7.

[56] Welch GW, Jacobson AM, Polonsky WH. The Problem Areas in Diabetes Scale. An evaluation of its clinical utility. Diabetes Care. 1997 May;20(5):760-6.

[57] Golden SH, Lazo M, Carnethon M, Bertoni AG, Schreiner PJ, Diez Roux AV, et al. Examining a bidirectional association between depressive symptoms and diabetes. JAMA. 2008 Jun 18;299(23):2751-9.

[58] Brown LC, Majumdar SR, Newman SC, Johnson JA. Type 2 diabetes does not increase risk of depression. CMAJ. 2006 Jul 4;175(1):42-6.

[59] Engum A, Mykletun A, Midthjell K, Holen A, Dahl AA. Depression and diabetes: a large population-based study of sociodemographic, lifestyle, and clinical factors associated with depression in type 1 and type 2 diabetes. Diabetes Care. 2005 Aug; 28(8):1904-9.

[60] Rush WA, Whitebird RR, Rush MR, Solberg LI, O'Connor PJ. Depression in patients with diabetes: does it impact clinical goals? J Am Board Fam Med. 2008 Sep-Oct; 21(5):392-7.

[61] Gonzalez JS, Safren SA, Cagliero E, Wexler DJ, Delahanty L, Wittenberg E, et al. Depression, self-care, and medication adherence in type 2 diabetes: relationships across the full range of symptom severity. Diabetes Care. 2007 Sep;30(9):2222-7.

[62] DiMatteo MR, Lepper HS, Croghan TW. Depression is a risk factor for noncompliance with medical treatment: meta-analysis of the effects of anxiety and depression on patient adherence. Arch Intern Med. 2000 Jul 24;160(14):2101-7.

[63] Lin EH, Katon W, Von Korff M, Rutter C, Simon GE, Oliver M, et al. Relationship of depression and diabetes self-care, medication adherence, and preventive care. Diabetes Care. 2004 Sep;27(9):2154-60.

[64] Doherty Y, James P, Roberts S. Stage of Change Couselling. In: Snoek FJ, Skinner TC, editors. Psychology in Diabetes Care. West Sussex, United Kingdom: John Wiley & Sons; 2000. p. 112-3.

[65] Kronish IM, Rieckmann N, Halm EA, Shimbo D, Vorchheimer D, Haas DC, et al. Persistent depression affects adherence to secondary prevention behaviors after acute coronary syndromes. J Gen Intern Med. 2006 Nov;21(11):1178-83.

[66] de Groot M, Anderson R, Freedland KE, Clouse RE, Lustman PJ. Association of depression and diabetes complications: a meta-analysis. Psychosom Med. 2001 Jul-Aug; 63(4):619-30.

[67] Pibernik-Okanovic M, Begic D, Peros K, Szabo S, Metelko Z. Psychosocial factors contributing to persistent depressive symptoms in type 2 diabetic patients: a Croatian survey from the European Depression in Diabetes Research Consortium. J Diabetes Complications. 2008 Jul-Aug;22(4):246-53.

[68] Association TAT, editor. Abstracts2012; San Jose, CA: Telemedicine and E-Health.

[69] Klonoff DC. Using telemedicine to improve outcomes in diabetes--an emerging technology. J Diabetes Sci Technol. 2009 Jul;3(4):624-8.

[70] Adkins JW, Storch EA, Lewin AB, Williams L, Silverstein JH, Malasanos T, et al. Home-based behavioral health intervention: Use of a telehealth model to address poor adherence to type-1 diabetes medical regimens. Telemed J E Health. 2006 Jun; 12(3):370-2.

[71] Garcia-Saez G, Hernando ME, Martinez-Sarriegui I, Rigla M, Torralba V, Brugues E, et al. Architecture of a wireless Personal Assistant for telemedical diabetes care. Int J Med Inform. 2009 Jun;78(6):391-403.

[72] Boren SA, Puchbauer AM, Williams F. Computerized prompting and feedback of diabetes care: a review of the literature. J Diabetes Sci Technol. 2009 Jul;3(4):944-50.

[73] Schnipper JL, Linder JA, Palchuk MB, Einbinder JS, Li Q, Postilnik A, et al. "Smart Forms" in an Electronic Medical Record: documentation-based clinical decision support to improve disease management. J Am Med Inform Assoc. 2008 Jul-Aug;15(4): 513-23.

[74] Watson AJ, Kvedar JC, Rahman B, Pelletier AC, Salber G, Grant RW. Diabetes connected health: a pilot study of a patient- and provider-shared glucose monitoring web application. J Diabetes Sci Technol. 2009 Mar;3(2):345-52.

[75] Cuadros J, Bresnick G. EyePACS: an adaptable telemedicine system for diabetic retinopathy screening. J Diabetes Sci Technol. 2009 May;3(3):509-16.

[76] Clemensen J, Larsen SB, Kirkevold M, Ejskjaer N. Treatment of diabetic foot ulcers in the home: video consultations as an alternative to outpatient hospital care. Int J Telemed Appl. 2008:132890.

[77] Jaana M, Pare G. Home telemonitoring of patients with diabetes: a systematic assessment of observed effects. J Eval Clin Pract. 2007 Apr;13(2):242-53.

[78] Pare G, Jaana M, Sicotte C. Systematic review of home telemonitoring for chronic diseases: the evidence base. J Am Med Inform Assoc. 2007 May-Jun;14(3):269-77.

[79] Polisena J, Tran K, Cimon K, Hutton B, McGill S, Palmer K. Home telehealth for diabetes management: a systematic review and meta-analysis. Diabetes Obes Metab. 2009 Oct;11(10):913-30.

[80] Sharma U, Reed J, Doyle C, Bell D. Challenges in evaluating telehealth through RCT-the problem of randomization. Stud Health Technol Inform. 2012;180:323-7.

[81] Dalton JE. Web-based care for adults with type 2 diabetes. Can J Diet Pract Res. 2008 Winter;69(4):185-91.

[82] Klonoff DC, Schwartz DM. An economic analysis of interventions for diabetes. Diabetes Care. 2000 Mar;23(3):390-404.

[83] Krishna S, Boren SA. Diabetes self-management care via cell phone: a systematic review. J Diabetes Sci Technol. 2008 May;2(3):509-17.

[84] Azar M, Gabbay R. Web-based management of diabetes through glucose uploads: has the time come for telemedicine? Diabetes Res Clin Pract. 2009 Jan;83(1):9-17.

[85] Shea S, Weinstock RS, Starren J, Teresi J, Palmas W, Field L, et al. A randomized trial comparing telemedicine case management with usual care in older, ethnically diverse, medically underserved patients with diabetes mellitus. J Am Med Inform Assoc. 2006 Jan-Feb;13(1):40-51.

[86] Barnett TE, Chumbler NR, Vogel WB, Beyth RJ, Ryan P, Figueroa S. The cost-utility of a care coordination/home telehealth programme for veterans with diabetes. J Telemed Telecare. 2007;13(6):318-21.

[87] Castelnuovo G, Manzoni GM, Cuzziol P, Cesa GL, Corti S, Tuzzi C, et al. TECNOB Study: Ad Interim Results of a Randomized Controlled Trial of a Multidisciplinary Telecare Intervention for Obese Patients with Type-2 Diabetes. Clin Pract Epidemiol Ment Health. 2011;7:44-50.

[88] Castelnuovo G, Manzoni GM, Cuzziol P, Cesa GL, Tuzzi C, Villa V, et al. TECNOB: study design of a randomized controlled trial of a multidisciplinary telecare intervention for obese patients with type-2 diabetes. BMC Public Health. 2010;10:204.

[89] Verplanken B, Orbell S. Reflections on Past Behavior: A Self-Report Index of Habit Strength1. Journal of Applied Social Psychology. 2003;33(6):1313-30.

[90] Castelnuovo G, Gaggioli A, Mantovani F, Riva G. From psychotherapy to e-therapy: the integration of traditional techniques and new communication tools in clinical settings. Cyberpsychol Behav. 2003 Aug;6(4):375-82.

[91] Cuzzolaro M, Vetrone G, Marano GF, Battacchi MW. BUT: una nuova scala per la valutazione del disagio relativo all'immagine del corpo in adolescenza. Psichiatria dell'infanzia e dell'adolescenza. 1999.

[92] Gormally J, Black S, Daston S, Rardin D. The assessment of binge eating severity among obese persons. Addict Behav. 1982;7(1):47-55.

[93] Di Bernardo M, Barciulli E, Ricca V, Mannucci E, Moretti S, Cabras PL, et al. Validazione della versione italiana della Binge Eating Scale in pazienti obesi. Minerva Psichiatrica. 1998;39:125-30.

[94] Garner DM. EDI-2. Eating Disorder Inventory-2. Professional Manual. Odessa, FL1991.

[95] Derogatis LR, Lipman RS, Covi L. SCL-90: an outpatient psychiatric rating scale--preliminary report. Psychopharmacol Bull. 1973 Jan;9(1):13-28.

[96] Kolotkin RL, Crosby RD, Kosloski KD, Williams GR. Development of a brief measure to assess quality of life in obesity. Obes Res. 2001 Feb;9(2):102-11.

[97] Kolotkin RL, Crosby RD, Williams GR. Health-related quality of life varies among obese subgroups. Obes Res. 2002 Aug;10(8):748-56.

[98] Consensus statement on the worldwide standardization of the hemoglobin A1C measurement: the American Diabetes Association, European Association for the Study of Diabetes, International Federation of Clinical Chemistry and Laboratory Medicine, and the International Diabetes Federation. Diabetes Care. 2007 Sep;30(9): 2399-400.

[99] Conti L. Repertorio delle scale di valutazione in psichiatria. E. SE, editor. Florence, Italy2002.

[100] Fairburn CG. Cognitive Behavior Therapy and Eating Disorders. 1 ed: Guilford Press; 2008.

[101] BodyMedia. [cited 2010 31 August]; Available from: http://www.bodymedia.com/Products/Learn-More/What-is-BodyMedia-FIT.

Section 2

# Telemedicine: Present and the Future

7

# The Telemedicine Service Maturity Model: A Framework for the Measurement and Improvement of Telemedicine Services

Liezl van Dyk and Cornelius S.L. Schutte

## 1. Introduction

General consensus exists that information and communication technology has the potential to enhance health systems applications and many good examples of such applications exist all over the world. Unfortunately, with respect to eHealth and telemedicine, there are also examples of disillusionment and scepticism. Many studies acknowledge the importance and challenge of finding models suitable for use in the facilitation, evaluation, and measurement of the success rate of eHealth and telemedicine projects. These measures are vital for facilitating the success, sustainability and optimisation of telemedicine services [1 -4].

### 1.1. Purpose

The purpose of this chapter is to present the *TeleMedicine Service Maturity Model* (TMSMM), a maturity model, including a capability statements that can be used to measure and manage the maturity of any telemedicine process.

### 1.2. Why a maturity model?

In many respects, telemedicine projects have experienced similar problems to those of the US military projects, implemented during the 1980's. These projects, involving software contractors, ran over-budget and were completed far later than planned, if at all. In order to address this, the US Defense Software Engineering Institute (SEI) developed a process maturity framework to aid in the capability evaluation of the software contractors, to be used as part of the contract awarding process [9]. This model, which was orginally based on Crosby's Quality Management Maturity Grid [5], became the Capability Maturity Model (CMM) and later the

Capability Maturity Model Integration (CMMI). The CMM and CMMI also serve as compliance standards [6, 7].

The CMM was the inspiration for the development of dozens of other maturity models which were developed and applied in various domains and contexts. With a maturity model the maturity (i.e. competency, capability, level of sophistication) of a selected domain is assessed based on a more or less comprehensive set of criteria. [6]. Maturity models, firstly, provide a way of measuring the status quo by means of maturity level indicators. Secondly, they facilitate an improvement process that best suits the enterprise, while remaining within the prescribed best practice parameters of the particular domain [8].

Most definitions of maturity combine an evolutionary or experiential element with the adoption of 'good' (or appropriate) practice [9]. It is proposed that a telemedicine service maturity model will address the need for a framework that can be used to measure and grow the maturity of existing and prospective telemedicine services. This model should be useful for self-assessment and well as benchmarking to guide a telemedicine service or project towards the identification and adoption of best practices.

### 1.3. Maturity models within the context of health systems

As result of a meta-analysis of maturity models Fraser et. al. [9] divided maturity models into three groups.

- CMM-like models
- Hybrids and Likert-like questionnaires
- Maturity grids

This categorization appealed to a number of authors to follow [10, 11] and is also of significance to this study:

#### *1.3.1. CMM-like models*

CMM-like models [9] are based upon a more formal architecture, specifying a number of goals and key practices to reach a predefined level of sophistication [11]. Many CMM-like models follow a standard format, are internationally recognized and are also use for certification purposes. Within the context of health systems, the British National Health System Infrastructure Maturity Model (NIMM) is possibly the only maturity model that fits this description.

#### *1.3.2. Hybrids and likert-like scales*

Hybrids and Likert-like questionnaires are comparable with maturity grids, but the focus is more inclined on scoring specific statements of "good practice" and not on describing the overall levels of maturity [11].

Technology readiness, system readiness and organizational readiness instruments are typical examples of this type of maturity assessment [10]. A few readiness instruments are already developed and in use within the context of telemedicine and ehealth. Jennett *et al.* [12] specifically refers to eHealth readiness when arguing that time, money and energy can be saved if the *status quo* of an eHealth/telemedicine system context is determined before implementation.

Legare *et al.* [13] identified six different assessment tools which use likert scale questionnaires to measure e-readiness within a certain health context: The first of these tools were developed in 1996. The *Organizational Information Technology/ Systems Innovation Readiness Scale* supports, within the context of telehealth, the evaluation, diagnosis and treatment selection for different steps in patient care. The second, third and fourth tools mentioned by [13] followed on each other and are focussed on home-based telehealth applications. Specifically the most recent two tools, namely the *eHealth Readiness Assessment Toolset for Healthcare Institutions in Developing Countries* [3] and a generic telehealth readiness assessment tool [12], was considered during the development of the TMSMM.

### *1.3.3. Maturity grid*

Maturity grids are typically descriptive frameworks, used for self-assessment purposes. With a maturity grid a number of levels of maturity are described in a simple, textual manner, normally not exceeding a few pages of text [9, 10].

In contrast to CMM-like models, the purpose of maturity grids is not to provide a means of certification. Companies often follow a number of approaches in parallel and maturity grid assessment may be used as a stand-alone assessment, or as a subset of a broader improvement initiative [10, 11]. Furthermore, a typical maturity grid allows for the visualization of maturity levels, which is not necessarily the case for CMM-like models.

According to the classification presented in this section, the Telemedicine Service Maturity Model (TMSMM) presented in this chapter is considered to be a maturity grid.

Most of the maturity models developed within the context of health systems fit this description. Examples of these include, the Quintegra Maturity Model for Electronic Healthcare [14], the Healthcare Information Management Systems Society (HIMSS) Maturity Model for Electronic Medical Records, the Health Industry Insights Maturity Model for Information Systems and Technology (IST) development in hospitals [15], as well as the Picture Archiving Communication Systems (PACS) maturity model [16].

None of the frameworks mentioned in this section are an „off-the-shelf" answer to the need for a framework to guide in the implementation and management of telemedicine services. However, all of the models mentioned in this section provided input to the development of a new maturity model, which is presented in this chapter.

## 2. Methodology

The scientific approach in the development of the TMSMM (refer to Figure 1), resembles the procedure suggested in [17]. This procedure takes into account the iterative nature of the maturity model development process, as well as the need to combine theoretical and empirical research as recommended by other respected scholars of maturity models [6, 9, 18, 19].

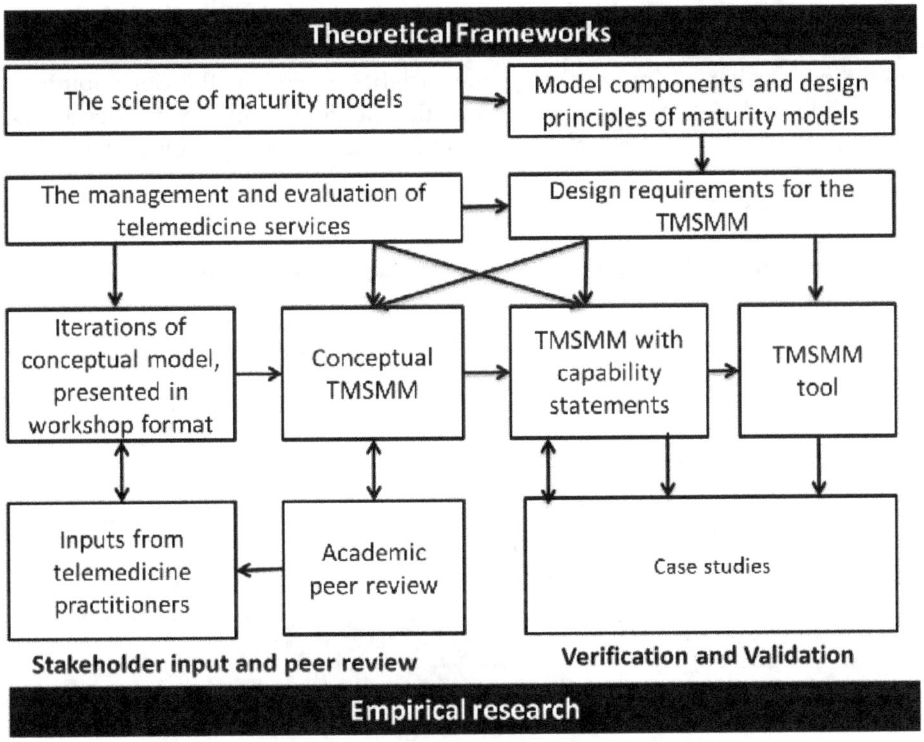


**Figure 1.** Scientific approach to the development of the TMSMM

The conceptual telemedicine service maturity model (TMSMM) was developed by following an iterative process involving telemedicine practitioners from five different South African provincial departments of health (DoH). The involvement of these stakeholders in the process, ensured the contribution of their domain knowledge for solution creation and in turn, contributed to the validity of the model. As a consequence, greater user acceptance was achieved [20].

Between June 2011 and December 2011, a series of workshops was held throughout South Africa. Representatives included healthcare workers (e.g. specialists, radiologists, radiographers and nurses), as well as persons responsible for the development, implementation and maintenance of hospital information and communication technology (ICT).

The first day of these workshops was aimed at educating representatives about current state-of-the-art telemedicine. The second day of each workshop was an interactive session in which groups of delegates engaged with the maturity model. At the end of each session, workshop delegates were asked to reflect upon and provide feedback on the effectiveness of the maturity model in terms of its characteristics. This feedback, together with the thoughts of other researchers from the literature, was used to revise key design features, as well as the maturity model itself [21-23].

Upon finalization of the conceptual model, a top-down approach was followed to develop the descriptive model [6]: An overarching maturity scale was defined, after which domain-specific maturity scales were developed in alignment with these. A first iteration of TMSMM descriptors was defined, using as inputs firstly, the insights gained in the development of the conceptual model and secondly, frameworks and theories for the management and evaluation of telemedicine services. The descriptors were refined, based on stakeholder input.

## 3. The Telemedicine Service Maturity Model (TMSMM)

The conceptual TMSMM is shown in Figure 2, which also provides a framework for the remainder of this chapter.

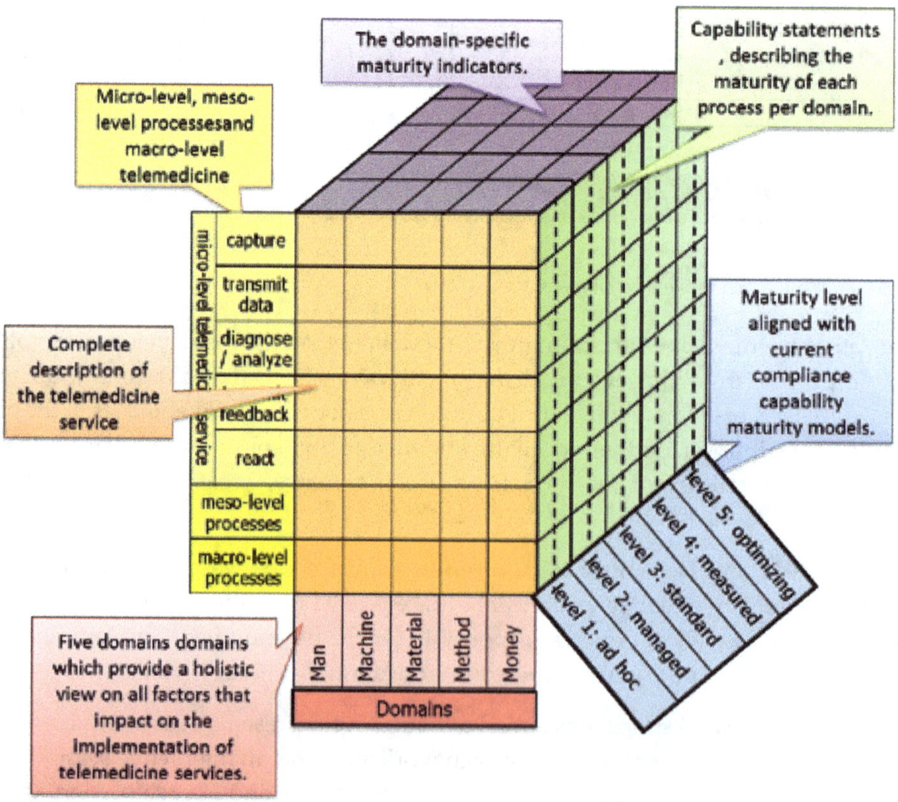


**Figure 2.** Conceptual model of the TMSMM

## 3.1. Design of the TMSMM

The TMSMM is designed along three dimensions. The intercept of each pair of these dimensions form a matrix, each with a specific significance and function.

### *3.1.1. Three dimensions*

Firstly, five domains are defined (*domain* dimension), which provides a holistic view on all factors that impact on the implementation of telemedicine services. Secondly, the *telemedicine service* dimension represents five micro-level processes, one meso-level, and one macro-level process per domain. The third dimension is the *maturity scale*, which provides yardsticks for maturity measurement. The three primary colours are deliberately selected to represent each of these three dimensions. Each of the three dimensions are briefly described in section 3.2 (*telemedicine service*, yellow), section 3.3 (*domain*, red) and 3.5 (*maturity scale*, blue).

### *3.1.2. Three matrices*

The orange matrix (refer to section 3.4) is the intercept of the *telemedicine service* dimension (yellow) and the *domain* dimension (red) and provides a framework, according to which, all aspects of the telemedicine under consideration are described. The domain-specific maturity indicators are outlined on the purple matrix (refer to section 3.6). This is the intercept of *domain* dimension (red) and the *maturiy scale* dimension (blue). The maturiy capability statements (green) in section 4 shows the maturity scale (blue) descriptors per telemedicine service process (yellow) for each respective domain.

## 3.2. The telemedicine service dimension

Telemedicine is per definition the delivery of healthcare service (*medicine*) over a distance (*tele*). This dimension includes all micro-level, meso-level and macro-level processes required to make this happen.

### *3.2.1. Micro-level telemedicine service*

The micro-level telemedicine service is broken up into five generic processes, which are applicable to any telemedicine service. All five of these processes need to be effective for the telemedicine service to be successful. (1) Patient data is captured, (2) transmitted to where the (3) data is analysed and converted into useful information (diagnosis). This useful information is then (4) transmitted back so that it can be (5) acted upon.

### *3.2.2. Meso-level and macro-level telemedicine services*

The systems engineering mindset dictates that complex systems (such as a health system), should be viewed as systems of systems. The meso- and macro-level telemedicine systems are systems which are situated higher up the health systems hierarchy. It does not exclusively relate to the telemedicine service, but it has a significant impact on the success of the telemedicine service. Hence, the maturity of these systems must be evaluated in conjunction with the maturity of the micro-level telemedicine process.

### 3.3. The domain dimension (red)

References are often made to the so-called „alphabet soup" of the business world, for example the 4Ps of marketing, the 5Ps of strategy, the 4Ps of healthcare, the 5Ss of lean manufacturing, the 4Ms, 5Ms, 6Ms and 7Ms of manufacturing, and the list continues. The value of these models (representations of the real world) lies in its simplicity and re-usablity. Furthermore, the fact that these concept groupings are applied repetitively and to a variety of contexts is indicative of its validity and generalizability.

The TMSMM must be simple in structure and language, so that it can be understood and used by a range of stakeholders. Therefore, the domains were named and organized in a way similar to other „alphabet-soup" frameworks. After each iteration of the development of the TMSMM the domains were adjusted, based on new insights gained. The final set of domains resembles the 5Ms for manufacturing, namely „man", „machine", „material", „method" and „money".

At first glance it may seem inappropriote to apply the 5Ms of manufacturing to the domains of the TMSMM. However, the generic description for a manufacturing process is well aligned with the telemedicine service: The telemedicine service entails the sourcing and acquisition of raw material (raw patient data and information) at the right place, the right time, and according to the right specification. This information is then reworked into a useful product (a diagnosis, treatment prescription etc.) which only has value if it reaches the customer (patient) at the right place, the right time, and according to the right specification.

### 3.4. Framework for the description of the telemedicine service

Figure 3 (orange matrix) provides a framework for the description of the telemedicine service, since it provides *domain* (red) -indicators for each of the micro-, meso- and macro-*level telemedicine service* processes (yellow).

| | Micro-Level Telemedicine Processes | | Higher Level Telemedicine Processes | |
|---|---|---|---|---|
| | Capture, Diagnose/ Analyse, React processes | Data Transmission processes | Meso-level processes | Macro-level processes |
| **Man** | patient/ doctor/ nurse etc. | patient/ doctor/ nurse etc. | user community | the society benefiting from this service |
| **Machine** | telemedicine device/ mobile phone ect. | internet service, mobile phone network etc. | service system | national ICT infrastructure |
| **Material** | EHR data/ images/ video ect. | EHR-type data/ images/ video | EHR mgmt within context of the sevice | national EHR mgmt |
| **Method** | work procedure | service levels | change management within service context | national policies, strategies and ethics guidelines |
| **Money** | operational and maintenance costs | cost of transmission service | business model | health economics |

**Figure 3.** Micro-, meso-, and macro-level telemedicine processes

### 3.5. The maturity scale

The maturity scale of the TMSMM is based on the generic level indicators of the capability maturity model (CMM). This is done for two reasons: Firstly, most of the existing maturity models use a maturity scale, which is either identical to, or strongly resembles the CMM-scale. This is indicative of the usefulness and validity of this scale. Secondly, it opens up the possibility that the TMSMM, which is categorized as a descriptive maturity grid, is used in conjunction with comparative CMM-like maturity models, for example those developed for project management and innovation management.

The generic levels are described below:

- **Level 1**:Ad hoc - The service is unpredictable, experimental, and poorly controlled
- **Level 2**:Managed - The service is characterised by projects and is manageable
- **Level 3**:Standard - The service is defined/confirmed as a standard business process
- **Level 4**:Quantitatively managed - The service is quantitatively measured and controlled
- **Level 5**:Optimising - Deliberate focus on continuous improvement

### 3.6. Domain-specific maturity indicators

Domain specific maturity indicators for the micro-level as well as meso- and macro-level telemedicine service processes are shown in Figure 4 and Figure 5 respectively. Each of these rows serves as heading for each of the respective maturity grids, which are presented in the next section.

## 4. Maturity capability statements for the micro-level processes of each domain

If the three-dimensional concept model (Figure 2) is sliced up along the domain dimension, fifteen sets of maturity capability statements (green) are created, three for each domain. The three sets per domain are with respect to the micro-level, meso-level and macro-level processes. This section presents the complete sets of maturity capability statements with respect to micro-level processes. Each of the five rows of Figure 4 represents the heading for each of the five respective sets of maturity capability statements presented in this section.

### 4.1. Users (*Man*-domain)

The capability statements for the micro-level services within context of the *man*-domain is shown in Figure 6.

Telemedicine services have a wide range of users. Depending on how the service is set up, the telemedicine process can include patients as well as healthcare workers, such as medical specialists, nurses, radiologists, midwifes, primary care practitioners and counsellors, amongst

| Micro-level Telemedicine Service | | Level 0 | Level 1 | Level 2 | Level 3 | Level 4 | Level 5 |
|---|---|---|---|---|---|---|---|
| | | *no* | *ad hoc* | *managed* | *standard* | *measured* | *optimising* |
| man | users | no-one | entrepeneur | champion | everyone | workforce | professional |
| machine | devices / appli-cations | nothing | prototype | pilot | standard and (technically) interoperable | monitored | maintenance and upgrades |
| material | electroni c health records | no EHR | uncertain quality | consitent quality | quality standards | quality control | quality improvement |
| method | work procedures | no process | ad hoc | consistent execution | work standards | performance control | continuous improvement |
| money | costs | no funds | R and D / entrepeneur | consitent, but temporary | consitent and permanent | accountability | cost optimisation |
| Meso- and Macro Level Telemedicine Processes | | Level 1 | Level 1 | Level 2 | Level 3 | Level 4 | Level 5 |
| | | *ad hoc* | *ad hoc* | *managed* | *standard* | *measured* | *optimising* |
| man | user community | no community | resistance | acceptable | norm | evidence based medicine | change to community |
| machine | ICT infra-structure | none | insufficient | managed | standard and scalable | monitored | continuous improvement |
| material | EHR mgmt | no EHRs | no EHR mgmt system | consistent EHR mgmt | standard and (semantically) interoperable | business intelligence | business analytics |
| method | change manage-ment | not existing | not existing | defined | institu-tionalized | monitoring and evaluation | optimising |
| money | financial sustain-ability | research and development | research and development | dependent on seed funding | sustainable | cost metrics | value optimisation |

**Figure 4.** Micro-level domain-specific maturity indicators

| Micro-level Telemedicine Service | | Level 0 | Level 1 | Level 2 | Level 3 | Level 4 | Level 5 |
|---|---|---|---|---|---|---|---|
| | | *no* | *ad hoc* | *managed* | *standard* | *measured* | *optimising* |
| man | users | no-one | entrepeneur | champion | everyone | workforce | professional |
| machine | devices / appli-cations | nothing | prototype | pilot | standard and (technically) interoperable | monitored | maintenance and upgrades |
| material | electronic health records | no EHR | uncertain quality | consitent quality | quality standards | quality control | quality improvement |
| method | work procedures | no process | ad hoc | consistent execution | work standards | performance control | continuous improvement |
| money | costs | no funds | R and D / entrepeneur | consitent, but temporary | consitent and permanent | accountability | cost optimisation |

**Figure 5.** Macro-level domain-specific maturity indicators

others. On the the left hand side of examples are given of users (orange) for each of the steps within the micro-level telemedicine service. These examples are derived from a meta-analysis of telemedicine projects on which reports were published between 2007 and 2010 in the International Journal for Telemedicine and Telecare [24].

| users | | | Capture, Diagnose/ Analyse, React processes | Data Transmission processes |
|---|---|---|---|---|
| | | | patient/ doctor/ nurse etc. | patient/ doctor/ nurse etc. |
| Level 0 | no | no-one | ... is non-existing / not part of the system anymore. | ... is non-existing / not part of the system anymore. |
| Level 1 | ad hoc | entrepeneur | ... should possibly be able to do this. | ... should possibly be able to do this. |
| | | | ... has done it before. | ... has done it before. |
| Level 2 | managed | champion | ... has done it before and is willing to do this as default action. | ... has done it before and is willing to do this as default action. |
| | | | ... is willing and mandated to do this as default action. | ... is willing and mandated to do this as default action. |
| Level 3 | standard | everyone | ... is mandated and expected to do this as default action. | ... is mandated and expected to do this as default action. |
| | | | ... is mandated and compelled to do this as default action. | ... is mandated and compelled to do this as default action. |
| Level 4 | measured | workforce | ... is monitored if/ how he does this. | ... is monitored if/ how he does this. |
| | | | ... is monitored and appraised on if/how he does this. | ... is monitored and appraised on if/how he does this. |
| Level 5 | optimising | professional | ... has the support to improve his performance in doing this. | ... has the support to improve his performance in doing this. |
| | | | ... contributesthe training and development of peers towards doing this. | ... contributesthe training and development of peers towards doing this. |

**Figure 6.** Maturity capability statements for the micro-level processes of the "Man" domain

Patients are always the beneficiaries of telemedicine services and are often categorised as users. In home-based telemedicine services, it is common that patients are equipped with appropriate technology enabling them to collect and transmit their healthcare data themselves. On the other hand, patients are not necessarily a user of the system. For example, a nurse can use a telemedicine service to deliver appropriate care to a patient. In this case the nurse would be catagorised as the user of the telemedicine service and not the patient. By the same token, the role of ICT technologists is imperative for the operation of a telemedicine service, but the ICT technologist is not necessarily a user of the system.

Many authors, for example, [25] and [26], agree that the involvement of a so-called champion is one of the contributing factors to the successful implementation of telemedicine services. A champion is a user from the community who takes the role of innovator and advocate. Both level 2 and level 3 imply that the user is appropriately trained and motivated to execute the task consistently and on an ongoing basis. A maturity level of 2 is assigned when this process is driven by a champion. A maturity level of 3 is allocated if every user is trained and motivated to execute the task consistently and on an ongoing basis.

Another determinant for the successful implementation of telemedicine, is the integration of the telemedicine service with other business processes of the hospital or health system [1, 27].

For example, when the users are human resources of the hospital or health system, integration with the human resource business process is expected. The maturity level for the user-domain is scored at level 4 (quantitatively managed) if worker performance metrics exist for each of the steps of the telemedicine process and if data is effectively included in performance management and in the work appraisal process. A maturity level of 5 indicates a deliberate attempt towards continuous professional development with respect to the use of the micro-level telemedicine service.

## 4.2. Devices and software applications (*Machine*-domain)

The maturity capability statements for the micro-level *machine* domain is shown in Figure 7.

| devices / appli-cations | | | Capture, Diagnose/ Analyse, React processes | Data Transmission processes |
|---|---|---|---|---|
| | | | telemedicine device/ mobile phone ect. | internet service, mobile phone network etc. |
| Level 0 | no | nothing | ... is non-existing (not the same as not available) | ... is non-existing (not the same as not available) |
| Level 1 | ad hoc | prototype | ... is used on ad hoc/ experimental basis | ... is assumed to be available. |
| | | | ... meets design requirements | ... is confirmed to be available. |
| Level 2 | managed | pilot | ... is effective | ... transmits data effectively. |
| | | | ... is reliable and available | ... transmits data repeatably. |
| Level 3 | standard | standard and (technically) interoperable | ... was procured/ developed/ considered according to system design standards. | ... was considered in the design of the service. |
| | | | ... 's interoperability is considered in the system's standards design. | ... 's interoperability is considered in the system's standards design. |
| Level 4 | measured | monitored | ... is developed and operated according to specifications of regulatory bodies. | ...'s reliability and availability can be measured. |
| | | | ... is continuously monitored to determine adherance to specifications of regulatory bodies. | ...'s reliability and availability are monitored. |
| Level 5 | optimising | maintenance and upgrades | ... is continuously upgraded to specifications of regulatory bodies and standards organizations. | : Deviations from acceptable levels of availability and reliability is continuously addressed. |
| | | | ... is continuously upgraded to specifications of regulatory bodies and standards organizations. | ... 's capability, reliability and availability is continuously improved. |

**Figure 7.** Maturity capability statements for the micro-level processes of the "Machine" domain

Examples of devices and applications (orange) for each of the steps of the micro-level telemedicine service (yellow) are given. These examples are derived from a meta-analysis of telemedicine projects on which reports were published between 2007 and 2010 in the International Journal for Telemedicine and Telecare [24].

Admittedly, technology is developing at a rapid pace and it is likely that the current list of most used telemedicine devices and software looks somewhat different to those identified in this study. This does not influence the relevance of the TMSMM, since it is technology-independent. The purpose of the TMSMM is not to measure the complexity of technological advancement of the devices and software. Telemedicine is a service innovation [28] and not a technological innovation. The technology most commonly used for telemedicine services is relatively simple. Hence, the TMSMM measures the maturity of the telemedicine service and as such considers the appropriateness, maintainability, availability and interoperability of the device and software.

According to the layered telemedicine implementation model [27] during the prototype phase, the focus is on the technological feasibility. Technological feasibility includes aspects such as the availability, reliability, and maintainability (RAM) of the used technology. Until this is achieved, the maturity of the telemedicine service, in terms of devices and software, is pitched at level 1 (ad hoc).

For a managed telemedicine service (level 2) the telemedicine device and/or software must be regularly available and maintained and user support must be available within the context in which it is to be used. This is typical in the pilot phase. In South Africa [21] and throughout the world [27] it seems that the initial enthusiasm of the 1990s has given way to.more reflective views of the place of telemedicine in healthcare delivery. This is mostly due to the fact that the majority of pilot projects have failed to be sustained. Yunkap Kwankam, eHealth coordinator of the World Health Organisation, ironically described this situation as "suffering from pilotitis" [29].

A telemedicine device or software application is only considered to be standard (level 3) if it is standardised, interoperable and integrated with other systems in the healthcare system. Keeping track of standard software upgrades entails technology maintenance (level 3).

A maturity level of 4 is reached if systems are in place to monitor the reliability, availability and maintainability of the technology, whilst a maturity level of 5 indicates that hardware and software are continuously upgraded, where appropriated.

### 4.3. Electronic health records (*Material*-domain)

The telemedicine service converts raw data into useful information, similar to any manufacturing process, in which raw material is converted into a useful product. Hence, "material" is included as a domain in the final TMSMM, referring to electronic health records (micro-level) and local EHR systems (meso-level) and national EHR systems (macro-level). The maturity capability statements of individual EHRs (micro-level) appear in Figure 8.

A maturity level of 3 is awarded to the "capture data", "perform diagnosis" and "react" processes if the EHRs are compiled according to a standard data format. If no intentional record keeping protocol is in place, the maturity of these three processes is gauged at 1. A maturity

| electronic health records | | | Capture, Diagnose/ Analyse, React processes | Data Transmission processes |
|---|---|---|---|---|
| | | | EHR data/ images/ video ect. | EHR-type data/ images/ video |
| Level 0 | no | no EHR | No record keeping whatsoever | No electronic transmission of data |
| Level 1 | ad hoc | uncertain quality | is of varying and most often unacceptable quality. | is sometimes unrightfully intercepted as part of transmission process. |
| | | | is of varying but most often acceptable quality. | sometime get list during transmission, but it is not unrightfully intercepted. |
| Level 2 | managed | consitent quality | are created repeatably with consistently acceptable quality. | is secured in terms of user control. |
| | | | are created repeatably. Consistent and acceptable (fit-for-purpose) quality of EHR record. | is secured in terms of encription and decription. |
| Level 3 | standard | quality standards | 's quality standards are clearly defined within context of this service. | is secured according to standards within context of the service. |
| | | | 's quality standards are clearly defined within a larger context. | is interoperating syntactically with other EHRs within context of this service. |
| Level 4 | measured | quality control | 's quality are measured as part of the standard process. | can be tracked throughout the telemedicine service. |
| | | | 's quality measures are effectively reported. | and identities of persons who viewed and edited it, can be tracked. |
| Level 5 | optimising | quality improvement | : Causes for unacceptable quality are continuously identified. | : Causes for delays and incorrectly transmitted EHRs are identified. |
| | | | : Causes for unacceptable are continuously and effectively addressed. | : Causes for delays and incorrectly transmitted EHRs are continuously addressed. |

**Figure 8.** Maturity capability statements for the micro-level processes of the "Material" domain

level of 2 indicates a consistent and repeatable record keeping process, but without considering standard data formats.

It is important that personal data about patients are transmitted securely and the privacy of data be ensured. This includes the raw data which is used for diagnosis, as well as the prognosis and information which is sent back to the person who needs to react. If this is accomplished according to encryption and decryption standards of the governing institution, the "transmit data" and "transmit feedback" processes are placed on maturity level 3. A maturity level of 1 indicates that data security protocols are not considered, whatsoever. A maturity level of 2 is awarded if security protocols are considered, but not necessarily managed by the governing institution.

Level 4 pertains to the tracking of electronic health records, whilst level 5 indicates deliberate attempts to increase the quality of electronic health records.

### 4.4. Work protocols (*Methods*-domain)

Refer to Figure 9 for the maturity capability statements for the micro-level processes of the "methods" domain, namely work protocols.

| work procedures | | | Capture, Diagnose/ Analyse, React processes | Data Transmission processes |
|---|---|---|---|---|
| | | | work procedure | network service |
| Level 0 | no innovation | no innovation | is exactly the same as without ICT. | does not exist. |
| Level 1 | ad hoc | ad hoc | is executed on and a trial and error basis. | is sometimes available. Not a specific service provider. |
| | | | differs from person to person and case to case. | is mostly available. Not a specific service provider. |
| Level 2 | managed | consistent execution | is executed consitently. | is delivered by a specific (set of) service provider(s) with varying service levels. |
| | | | is executed consitently and this process is documented. | is delivered by a specific (set of) service provider(s) with consistent service levels. |
| Level 3 | standard | work standards | is defined as a work standard for this service. | level agreements (SLAs) are defined. |
| | | | is acceptable within context of relevant ethical guidelines and legal frameworks. | level agreements (SLAs) are contractually agreed upon. |
| Level 4 | measured | performance control | 's effectiveness is continously monitored. | -levels are measured. |
| | | | 's efficiency is continuously monitored. | -levels are continuously monitored. |
| Level 5 | optimising | continuous improvement | : causes for ineffectiveness are continuously addressed. | -levels are continuously maintained. |
| | | | : continuous improvement in terms of process efficiency. | levels are continuously improved. |

**Figure 9.** Maturity capability statements for the micro-level processes of the "Methods" domain.

Any healthcare service needs to be executed according to a certain set of well defined protocols in order to ensure consistency, integrity and ethical conduct. In most cases these protocols was defined, before ICT made telemedicine possible. In many cases the telemedicine service deviates significantly from the original way of doing and a new protocol for the telemedicine service does not exists. In this case, a maturity level of 1 is allocated. A maturity level of 2 indicates that the telemedicine process is executed consistently and repeatably, but the protocol is not formally defined. Once it is formally defined the maturity is guaged at 3. Performance control metrics enables the consistent measurement of the effectiveness of the protocol (maturity level 4). A maturity level of 5 is reached as soon as the causes of performance deviations are continuously identified and rectified.

### 4.5. Costs (*Money*-domain)

The *money*-domain (considers maturity in terms of operational cost (micro-level), business model (meso-level) and health economics (macro-level). Figure 10 shows the maturity capability statements for the micro-level processes of the "money" domain.

| costs | | | Capture, Diagnose/ Analyse, React processes | Data Transmission processes |
|---|---|---|---|---|
| | | | operational and maintenance costs | cost of transmission service |
| Level 0 | no | no | : The service is still only in conceptual phase. | : The service is still only in conceptual phase. |
| Level 1 | ad hoc | R and D / entrepeneur | are not considered by developers/ entrepeneur. | are not considered by developers/ entrepeneur. |
| | | | are considered and covered by seed funds whilst service is in development phase. | are considered and covered by seed funds whilst service is in development phase. |
| Level 2 | managed | consitent, but temporary | will be covered on short term by seed funds. | will be covered on short term by seed funds. |
| | | | will be covered on long term by seed funds. | will be covered on long term by seed funds. |
| Level 3 | standard | consitent and permanent | are included partially as a standard budget item. | are included partially as a standard budget item. |
| | | | are included fully as a standard budget item. | are included fully as a standard budget item. |
| Level 4 | measured | accountability | are a reporting item of the accounting system. | are a reporting item of the accounting system. |
| | | | s reports are routinely scrutinized to ensure optimal use of funds. | s reports are routinely scrutinized to ensure optimal use of funds. |
| Level 5 | optimising | cost optimisation | : Non-value adding activities are continuously identified. | : Continuous efforts by service provider to bring down costs. |
| | | | : Non-value adding activities are continuously eliminated. | : Continuous efforts by service provider to bring down costs filtered through to service context. |

**Figure 10.** Maturity capability statements for the micro-level processes of the "Money" domain.

Maturity level 1 and 2 applies when the operational costs are provided by external entities, either for purposes of research and development (level 1) or for philantropic reasons by external donors. These funding modes are not sustainable. For financial sustainability, is it compulsory the operational expenses are covered as part of the standard budgeting process of the governing organization (maturity level 3). Maturity level 4 concerns accountability. It must be possible to measure and report on the costs related to this process. On maturity level 5 the cost effectiveness of the process are continuously improved.

## 5. Maturity capability statements for the meso and macro level processes of each domain

The scope of this chapter does not allow for detail maturity capability statements for meso- and macro-level processes. In this section follows a brief discussion on each of these processes.

### 5.1. User communities (*Man*-domain)

Telemedicine services inevitably cut across epistemic communities, for example medical practitioners, engineers, patients or public health actors [29]. The users of each step of the telemedicine process are members of one of these communities. The health worker / patient community and the society as a whole are added as respectively as meso-level and macro-level telemedicine systems, within the context of the user domain, since the maturity of the telemedicine service is dependent on the extent to which this service is accepted within these communities [27].

Maturity level 3 indicates that this activity is accepted as standard practice by the entire community. For example, if healthcare professionals are exposed to this telemedicine service as part of their training and if these practices are accepted by their professional societies or a it socially acceptable to use technology to communicate healthcare information.

*Evidence-based practice* is an interdisciplinary approach, which started in medicine as *evidence-based medicine* and spread across other fields over the past two decades [30]. Evidence based medicine aims for the ideal that healthcare professionals should make "conscientious, explicit, and judicious use of current best evidence in everyday practice." As such, healthcare workers and other professionals are familiar with this concept.

Evidence-based practice dictates that all practical decisions made should (1) be based on research studies and (2) that these research studies are selected and interpreted to some specific and quantitative norm. A maturity level of 4 applies if such research studies are successfully being executed with context of the respective user community.

According to the World Health Organization task shifting entails the reallocation of certain tasks from more-specialised to less-specialised health care workers across the board. For example, tasks are shifted from the physician to the non-professional health care worker [31, 32]. A maturity level of 5 indicates that the telemedicine service deliberately causes task shifts for an entire professional community.

### 5.2. Information and Communication Technology (ICT) infrastructure (*Machine*-domain)

ICT infrastructure refers to all of the hardware, software, networks, facilities etc. that are required to develop, test, deliver, monitor, control or support applications and IT services. [33].

The maturity of the ICT infrastructure depends on its availability, reliability and maintainability (maturity level 3) as well as the measurement thereof (maturity level 4). Continuous improvement (maturity level 5) within this context relates to technology upgrades and scalability.

### 5.3. EHR systems (*Material*-domain)

The maturity scale described below applies equally to meso-level, local EHR systems and the macro-level, national EHR systems.

Syntactic interoperability involves a common data format and common protocol to structure any data so that the manner of processing the information will be interpretable. When the different systems involved in a telemedicine service are capable of communicating and exchaning data, they are syntactically interoperable [35] and a maturity level of 2 is indicated.

„Beyond the ability of two or more computer systems to exchange information, semantic interoperability is the ability to automatically interpret the exchanged information meaningfully and accurately in order to produce useful results as defined by the end users of both systems" [35]. A maturity level of 3 is awarded if semantic interoperability is achieved. If no intentional record keeping protocol is in place, the maturity of these three processes is gauged at 1.

Business intelligence (BI) is a broad category of applications and technologies for gathering, storing, analyzing, and providing access to data to help enterprise users make better business decisions. A maturity level of 4 indicates that such applications and technologies existsBusiness analytics (BA) is often used as synonymn for BI. However, for purposes of the chapter, it is recognized that for BA statistical methods are used to develop an understanding of business performance and to provide a feedback loop towards continuous business improvement.

### 5.4. Change management (*Methods*-domain)

The need for deliberate and effective change management is echoed throughout studies on the implementation of telemedicine services [1-4, 23, 26, 37]. Change management is the process of changing processes. Within context of the TMSMM, change management is positioned as meso-level process of the Methods-domain (Figure 9).

The majority of telemedicine services do not sustain after pilot phase [22, 27, 26] even though the concept was technologically proved during prototype and pilot phase. In those cases, the change management process was ineffective (maturity level 1).

A champion is a user from the community who takes the role of innovator and advocate. Many authors [1, 25, 26] mention the involvement of a so-called champion as a critical success factor to the successful implementation of telemedicine services. Maturity level 2 applies when such a champion is either self-appointed or appointed by the institution.

A maturity level of 3 indicates sustainable institutional commitment to accomplish change. This commitment is firstly demonstrated by the formal and permanent appoint of a change agent (champion) and secondly if the change management process also manifests in other business processes, for example, during the budget process or facilities design process.

The effectiveness of the change management process is measured in terms of performance indicators (maturity level 4). Maturity level 5 implies that processes are in place to ensure continuous improvement in terms of these performance indicators.

### 5.5. Financial sustainability (*Money*-domain)

The maturity of the micro-level telemedicine service – as far as the *money*-domain is concerned – is measured in terms of the costs to operate and maintain this service. On macro-level the financial sustainability of the *money*-domain is considered, firstly, with respect to the specific telemedicine service and, secondly, on a higher level, with respect to the macro-economic healthcare system.

This subdomain of the TMSMM is the concern of health economics, which is a branch of economics concerned with the functioning of macro-economic healthcare systems as well as health affecting behaviours and interventions – such as the use of technology [36]. Health economists throughout the world still graple with challenges to find financial justification for telemedicine services [37, 38]. No clear-cut financial model has yet been developed. It is also not the intension of the TMSMM to provide answers concerning *how* the financial sustainability and return on investment can be measured and managed, but merely *if* it is being managed and measured.

A maturity level of 1 is typical to projects in the research and development or pilot phases, where the focus is on technical feasibility [27]. At level 2 some form of financial management system is in place. However, the service relies on donor or R&D funding. A maturity level of 3 indicates that the telemedicine service will sustain financially, without external funding.

With the context of health economics, many approaches can be found with respect to the measurement of the return on investment(ROI). The TMSMM does not dictate the method of ROI-measurement. Rather, a maturity level of 4 indicates that such measure is decided upon and these measures are indeed realized.

Macro-level continuous improvement and optimization within context of the *money* domain requires not only financial sustainability, but also reinvestment – in which case a maturity level of 5 is allocated.

## 6. Conclusion

In this chapter a telemedicine service maturity model (TMSMM) is presented. This TMSMM is developed in response to the need for a framework according to which the maturity of existing and proposed telemedicine projects can be measured with the purpose of supporting decision making towards sustained telemedicine services.

The TMSMM was developed by following an iterative process involving telemedicine practitioners from five different South African provincial departments of health (DoH). With each iteration a cross-functional group was involved in workshop format. Self-assessment maturity models, like the TMSMM proved to be particularly effective with cross-functional and interdisciplinary groups.

This descriptive maturity model can be used as basis for the development of a prescriptive and eventually comparative maturity model for which the following design principles applies [39]: Firstly, decision calculus is included the assist in the evaluation of different alternatives. Secondly, an adoption methodology is included which features a procedure model, advice on how to concretize and adapt improvement measures.

## Acknowledgements

The work presented in this article is based on research for purposes of the PhD thesis of Liezl van Dyk, for which financial support was provided by the National Research Foundation (NRF) of South Africa. The authors also wishes to acknowledge Jill Fortuin (Medical Research Council of South Africa) for her role in the initial workshops that lead to the development of the TMSMM as well as Kim Viljoen and André Hartmann (Stellenbosch University), who contributed to the definition of the capability statements through the execution of their respective MEng projects.

## Author details

Liezl van Dyk and Cornelius S.L. Schutte

Department of Industrial Engineering, Stellenbosch University, South Africa

## References

[1] Yellowlees, P. Successfully developing a telemedicine system. Journal of Telemedicine Telecare, Bd. 11, Nr. 7, pp. 331-336, 2005.

[2] Edwards, J. Hype Cycle for Telemedicine (G00214814). Gartner Industry Research, 28 July 2011. [Online]. Available: http://my.gartner.com/resources/214800/214814/hype_cycle_for_telemedicine__214814.pdf?li=1. [Retrieved on 8 March 2012].

[3] Khoja, S., Scott, R., Casebeer, A., Mohsin, M., Ishaq, A. and Gilani, S. E-health readiness assessment tools for healthcare institutions in developing countries. Telemedicine e-Health, Bd. 13, Nr. 4, pp. 425-432, 2007.

[4] Van Gemert-Pijnen, J.E., Nijl, N., Van Limburg, M., Ossebaard, H.C., Kelders, S.M., Eysenbach, G., and Seydel, E.R. A Holistic Framework to Improve the Uptake Impact

of eHealth Technologies. Journal of Medical Internet Research, Bd. 13, Nr. 4, p. Publised online, 2011.

[5] Crosby, P.B. Quality is still free : making quality certain in uncertain times, ISBN: 0070145326 : McGraw-Hill, 1996.

[6] De Bruin, T., Freeze, R., Kaulkarni, U., and Rosemann, M. Andersting the Main Phases of Developing a Maturity Assessment Model. in Australasian Chapter of the Association for Information Systems, Sydney, 2005.

[7] Wikipedia. Capability Maturity Model. Wikipedia, 26 June 2012. [Online]. Available: en.wikipedia.org/wiki/Capability_Maturity_Model. [Retrieved on 26 June 2012].

[8] Essman, H. Toward innovation capability maturity. Stellenbosch University, PhD Thesis, 2009.

[9] Fraser, P., Moultrie, J., and Gregory, J. The use of maturity models/grids as a tool in assessing product development capability. Engineering Management Conference, Bd. 1, Nr. Cambridge University, UK, pp. 244-249, 2002.

[10] Maier, A.M., Moultrie, J., and Clarkson, J.P. Assessing Organizational Capabilities: Reviewein Guiding the Development of Maturity Grids. IEEE Transactions on Engineering Management, Bd. 59, Nr. 1, pp. 138-159, 2012.

[11] Mettler, T., Rohner, P., and Winter, R. Towards a Classification of Maturity Models in Information Systems".

[12] Jennett, P., Gagnon, M., and Brandstadt, H. Readiness models for rural telehealth. Journal of Postgraduate Medicine, Bd. 51, Nr. 4, pp. 279-283, 2010.

[13] Legare, E., Vincent, C., Lehoux, P., Person, D., Kairy, D. and Gagnon, M et al. Telehealth readiness assessment tools. J Telemed Telecare 2010;16(3):107.. Journal of Telemedicine Telecare, Bd. 16, Nr. 3, pp. 107-115, 2010.

[14] Sharma, B. Electronic Healthcare Maturity model (eHMMM). June 2008. [Online]. Available: http://www.quintegrasolutions.com/eHMM%20White%20Paper.pdf. [Retrieved on 10 April 2012].

[15] Holl, M., Piai, S., Dunbrack, L.A. Healthcare IT Maturity Model: Western European Hospitals - the Leading Countries. IDC Health Insights, Framingham, MA, Tech. Rep No. H1210231.

[16] Van de Wetering, R. and Batenburg, R. A PACS maturity model: A systematic meta-analytic review on maturation evolvability of PACS in the hospital enterprise. International Journal of Medical Informatics, Bd. 78, pp. 127-140, 2009.

[17] Solli-Sæther, H., and Göttschalk, P. The Modeling Process for Stage Models. Journal of Organizational Computing Electronic Commerce, Bd. 20, Nr. 2010, pp. 279-293, 2010.

[18] Von Wangenheim, C.G., Hauch, J.C., Zoucas, A., Salviano, C.A., McCafferty, F. and Shull, F. Creating Software Process Capability/Maturity Models. IEEE Computer Society, Bd. Voice of Evidence, Nr. July/August 2010, pp. 92-94, 2010.

[19] Mettler, T. Maturity Assessment Models: A Design Science Research Approach. Internation Journal of Society Systems Science, Bd. 3, Nr. 1-2, pp. 81-98, 2011.

[20] Van der Zee, D. Developing participative simulation models—framing decomposition principles forjoint andersting. Journal of Simulation, Bd. 1, pp. 187-202, 2009.

[21] Van Dyk, L., Fortuin, J.B. and Schutte, C.S.L. A Systems Engineering Approach to Telemedicine System Implementation. in International Conference on Industrial Engineering, Systems Engineering Engineering Management for Sustainable Global Development, Spier, 2011.

[22] Van Dyk, L., Schutte, C.S.L. and Fortuin, J.B. A Maturity Model for Telemedicine Implementation. in The Fourth International Conference on eHealth, Telemedicine Social Medicine, Valencia, Spain, 2012.

[23] Van Dyk, L. and Schutte, C.S.L. Development of a Maturity Model for Telemedicine. Southern African Journal for Telemedicine, Bd. 23, Nr. 2, pp. 61-72, 2012.

[24] Van Zyl, A.J. and Van Dyk, L. An information system to support telemedicine projects in South Africa, Bd. MScEng Thesis, Stellenbosch: Stellenbosch University, 2012, pp. 1-151.

[25] Araki, Y., Scott. R.E. and Lear, S. Challenges of telehealth research in clinical setting. Journal of Telemedicine Telecare, pp. 425-426, 2007.

[26] Mars, M. Telemedicine in South Africa. in Telehealth in the Developing World , Online, OECD, 2009, pp. 222-231.

[27] Broens, T.H.F., Vollenbroek-Hutten, M.M.R., Hermens, H.J., Van Halteren, A.T., Nieuwenhuis, L.J.M. et al. Determinants of successful telemedicine implementations. Journal of Telemedicine Telecare, Bd. 6, Nr. 303, p. 13, 2007.

[28] Kuusisto, J., Den Hertog, P., Berghäll, S., Hjelt, M., Ahvenharju, S. and Van der Aa, W. Service Typologies tools for effective innovatation policy development. European policies intruments to support service innovation (EPISIS), Pro Inno Europe, 27 May 2011.

[29] Schrapel, N. Connecting Africa - African Connections: Africa's engagement with ICTs their role for development - the case of telemedicine in South Africa. in ICT Development - Research Voices from Africa, Makerere University, Uga, International Federation for Information Processing (IFIP), Technical Commission 9 - Relationship between Computers Society, 22-23 March 2010, pp. 1-11.

[30] Wikipedia. Evidence-based practice. Wikipedia, 27 June 2012. [Online]. Available: http://en.wikipedia.org/wiki/Evidence-based_practice. [Retrieved on 27 June 2012].

[31] Hermann, K., Van Damme, W., Pariyo, G.W., Schouten, E., Assefa, Y., Cirera, A. and Massavon, W. Community health workers for ART in sub-saharan Africa: learning from experience = capitalizing on new opportunities. Human Resources for Health, Bd. 7, Nr. 31, pp. 1-11, 9 April 2009.

[32] Fulton, B.D., Scheffler, R.M., Sparkes, S.P., Auh, E.Y., Vujicic, M. and Soucat. Health workforce skill mix task shifting in low income countries: a review of recent evidence. Human Resources for Health, Bd. 9, Nr. 1, pp. 1-11, 2011.

[33] Information Technology Infrastructure Library. Information Technology Infrastructure Library glossary abbreviations. 2011. [Online]. Available: http://www.itil-officialsite.com/. [Retrieved on 28 June 2012].

[34] Business dictionary. Legacy. [Online]. Available: http://www.businessdictionary.com/definition/legacy-system.html#ixzz23Qi1etZq.

[35] Wikipedia. Interoperability. Wikipedia, 12 August 2012. [Online]. Available: www.wikipedia.org/interoperability. [Retrieved on 2012 August 2012].

[36] Wikipedia. Health Economics. Wikipedia, 2 August 2012. [Online]. Available: www.wikipedia.org/health_economics. [Retrieved on 2012 August 2012].

[37] Bashshur, R., Shannon, G. Hasan, S.H. Telemedicine evaluation. Telemedicine Journal & e-Health, Bd. 11, Nr. 3, pp. 296-316, 2005.

[38] World Health Organization. Health Economics Research Group. [Online].

[39] Reuglinger, J. Pöppelbuss and Becker, J. Maturity models in business process management. Business Process Management Journal, Bd. 18, Nr. 2, pp. 328-346, 2012.

# 8

# PITES: Telemedicine and e-Health Innovation Platform

José Luis Monteagudo, Mario Pascual,
Adolfo Muñoz, Pilar G. Sagredo,
Ricardo Sánchez de Madariaga and
Carlos H. Salvador

## 1. Introduction

A considerable amount of R&D&I has been carried out in recent years in the area of telemedicine and e-Health directed at supporting innovative health care models for people with chronic health conditions such as hypertension, cardiac insufficiency, chronic pulmonary obstruction, asthma, diabetes, cancer, dementia and other ailments [1]. The objective is to implement more appropriate and effective health care models in order to maintain health under everyday conditions, avoiding serious complications and without the need to resort to emergency services and hospital admittances. One priority is to avoid or delay for as long as possible the situation of dependence on the health care system for pluripathological conditions.

The development of telehealth applications is guided by its potential to confront the challenges brought about by the aging of the population and financial restrictions together with the need to satisfy the population for better services and access to them.

In this context, a convergence can be observed between the transformation movement of health care systems, the development of new information and communication technologies (Internet, Web 2.0, 3G and 4G mobile communications, touch-screen terminals, etc.) which have a high support potential for new ideas in the field of health care implying the active support of the patients and facilitating collaboration environments between all of the actors involved.

It must be borne in mind that telehealth systems and services are in the definition and positioning phase in traditional health care systems and coexist with other systems such as Telecare, Personal Health Systems (PHS), mobile Health (mHealth) and Personal Health Applications (PHAs) with which often overlap [2,3].

It is important to consider that innovation in telehealth does not only rest in technological advances. The system of innovation in this domain is very complex and interdependent. A fusion of technology with health care knowledge and the organization of health care systems is necessary together with measures to empower the users and a redefinition of the contact of the professionals with the patients.

In this chapter, an experience is described in the conception, design, implementation and evaluation of a Platform of Innovation in Telehealth Systems (PITES) oriented at improving the health care of chronic, fragile and dependent patients.

The PITES platform is a stable and public innovation infrastructure. It is made up of a technological platform, services and tools, with its use directed at research groups, public or private entities and organizations, with the objective of offering support for the obtaining of evidence on new models for health care provision based on ICT (Telehealth) in scenarios related to chronic illness and dependency.

PITES is directed at broaching two main objectives: a) facilitating and accelerating the development of telehealth applications by making available technological infrastructures which in another way would not be tackled or would have to be designed and constructed from scratch by each project, and b) promote interoperability through the adoption of open standards for the communication of medical data and information (semantic interoperability).

PITES stems from experience and lessons learned over 15 years in the design, implementation and use of telehealth applications in different environments and contexts of real application, supported by a large number of pilot projects and trials. PITES currently serves as an infrastructure for diverse projects in different locations in Spain. PITES also forms part of the Accion B3 of the European Innovation Partnership for Active and Healthy Ageing [4].

The PITES platform supports research or innovation projects, not health care activities nor commercial services. The platform permits different telehealth projects to be implemented in a flexible and transparent manner using different local approximations and contexts of use for both professionals and patients. PITES incorporates the philosophy of separating the applications of the infrastructures that support them.

As an R&D&I platform it has been conceived to be flexible, functionally transparent, secure and with the capacity to evolve and coexist with other platforms (for research or clinical use) by means of technical and semantic operability mechanisms based on standards. Technologically, it is aligned with the current convergence framework for the provision of digital services on IP networks using Web technologies and SOA.

PITES follows an open innovation model promoted from the knowledge of the professional health users for the application of secure, accessible and interoperable telehealth environments using open standards. The PITES digital ecosystem gives each Project the freedom to design and implement its protocols.

The structure of the chapter is as follows: The two goals of the PITES innovation activities are described in section 2. The obtaining of evidence (section 2.1) and the interoperability of the clinical information (section 2.2). As regards the obtaining of evidence, we begin by presenting the current context of the evaluation in e-services (section 2.1.1) and methodological basis which has shown to be more suitable for the obtaining of evidence (section 2.1.2). The challenges that persist are highlighted, brought about by the intrinsic complexity of the environments in which the evaluations have to be carried out. The need for implementation in the organizations stands out as the factor that most compromises the viability and validity of the process (section 2.1.3). The methodology designed and proposed in PITES is then described in order to tackle the complexity of the search for evidence on the e-services process (section 2.1.4). As regards interoperability, the fundamental aspects of interoperability in clinical information (section 2.2.1) and the interoperability framework of the platform (section 2.2.2)

The PITES platform is presented in section 3. Firstly, a conceptual model of the organizational and functional framework is described as a proposal for the reduction in users, resources and its interactions to which the interventions must be adapted to be able to be evaluated with the support of the platform (section 3.1). After that, the architecture of the PITES platform is presented as an open system of distributed services and its advantages in collaborative research and innovation in this field (section 3.2). Finally, some of the services that currently support the platform and which already act as permanent components supporting the projects are described (section 3.3).

In section 4, as a result of the platform, a description of some of the already finished projects is included together with very brief descriptions of some of the current projects that our unit is working on plus a list of current projects of other research groups.

## 2. Context of innovation within the PITES scenario

### 2.1. Evaluation of services based on telemedicine

#### *2.1.1. Current context of the evaluation of e-services*

One of the permanent challenges facing e-health, and therefore telemedicine and its effects is the obtaining of scientific, generalized and reliable evidence (transferable between different contexts) on it. There are numerous reasons for evaluation: promotional, pragmatic, ethical, medical-legal, even academic. The objective is to promote and legitimize practices of excellence, evaluate the policies, regulations and national legislations on e-health and value its impact in terms of efficiency and technical and clinical effectiveness, impact on the organization, health staff, costs, patient satisfaction and personal ethical health aspects, confidentiality and safety.

The recommendation for evaluation has been endorsed from multiple authorities and international organizations such as the World Health Organization in its "eHealth Program for Health-Care Delivery" (eHCD) [5] and the "Global Observatory for eHealth" [6], which established that services based on e-health will be essential when they demonstrate that they are based on evidence, requiring well-defined agreed specifications and criteria for it, and validated by means of controlled experimental trials or by consensus widely accepted by experts. Also within the ambit of the European Union, by means of eEurope initiatives [7] or i2010 [8], the need to strengthen the aspects of demonstration and evaluation in projects has been made clear to allow the complete analysis of the results to be undertaken and make available the evidence of quality for the drawing up and dissemination of directives on good practices.

Traditionally, the evaluation of e-health services has brought to light significant difficulties giving rise to uncertainties and thus resistance to its implementation by consultants and managers. The belief that the implementation of formal evaluation processes constitutes an obstacle for developers and the commercial and economic context is currently being dismissed. It has come to light through demonstration that the systems are effective, cost-effective safe, robust, accessible, and usable, as well as a source of benefits and knowledge, an aspect which is known in the technological sector as "evidence-based business" [9]. Nevertheless, it is evident that the organizations and health systems determine a priori numerous factors that, in evaluation interventions, condition the work frameworks and their implementation, and therefore the potential final results. In this sense, there still remain significant methodological challenges and practical implementations mainly related to two aspects: 1) the interdisciplinary nature of the field of e-health, and 2) the intrinsic complexity of the context in which the evaluations have to be carried out.

As regards the first aspect, it is an obvious fact that e-health constitutes a heterogeneous and interdisciplinary field of science with which two areas of research converge fundamentally (in turn, trans-disciplinary): the computer aspects of health (technological ambit) and research into health services (socio-health ambit). Traditionally, all of them use different languages, cultures, reasons and operating conditions which have generated divergent working templates [10]. These silos of parallel competencies are a cause of additional difficulties in the development of e-health. In the past decades efforts have been directed at achieving a mutual recognition between the respective disciplines and a search for synergies and single paradigms [11].

The second aspect refers to the intrinsic complexity of the context in which the evaluations have to be carried out. During the past two decades, the results achieved related to the dissemination of the innovation, knowledge and experience in the ambit of health have not all been as satisfactory as was hoped. The cause would have to be sought in some of the work strategies more orientated towards the resolution of complicated problems rather than a complex problem [12]. Starting from this idea, different authors have carried out an approximation of the organizations and health practice from the perspective of complexity theory, contemplating them as adaptive complex systems [13, 14, 15, 16, 17]. Parallelisms related to questions such as changing behaviors, interrelated, yet not totally predicable, whose evolution and behavior patterns respond to the relationships between their components on the basis of non-explicit rules, the appearance of emerging behaviors, "attractor patterns", effects of self-organization, the influence of "shadow systems", etc. have come to light. By means of the aforementioned work, it has become possible to explain different aspects of behavior dynamics in relation to clinical care, education, leadership and management in health environments, which have opened up new ways and action strategies related to evaluation, as well as improving the quality and adoption of innovations.

### 2.1.2. *Complex interventions and hybrid evaluation methodologies*

In the health environment, an intervention is a deliberate action through which it is hoped to bring about an effect or change in any aspect of health which is the object of the aforementioned action. The intervention may be directed at individuals, collectives or at a population level; and the purpose may be a pathology, a behavior, etc. The concept of a "complex intervention" [17] arises from the evolution of the interventions that are extended or influenced by or immersed in organizational aspects, processes, and technological adoption. From the perspective of complexity theory, a "complex intervention" is an intervention in which components that act independently and interdependently become involved, and are characterized by the difficulty in determining which participating agents are active elements in the intervention and how some are related to others and with the rest of the agents, and this represents a challenge as regards the definition, development, documentation, reproduction and evaluation of the intervention.

It is evident that any intervention based on e-health services constitutes in itself a "complex intervention" [18]. Research into interventions has been a natural field of development of research into health services and its objective has been to gain knowledge into the impact of these interventions at a population level. Traditionally within the ambit of health, the clinical-epidemiology evaluation methodology most widely recognized and accepted as the "gold standard" in order to obtain evidence of the maximum quality is the Randomized Controlled Trial (RCT) [19]. By means of an RCT the validity and effectiveness of an intervention is determined quantitatively as are the possibilities of the transfer or generalization of the results obtained.

Historically, RCTs have been used in the evaluation of interventions in the context of acute illnesses, consequently, in short-term interventions and acute care hospital environments. It is a well-described fact that when this evaluation methodology is adopted in other context that imply periods of mid- to long-term intervention, such as, for example in the case of chronic illnesses, or complex environments such as e-health interventions (complex interventions), intrinsic practical limitations emerge [20]. These limitations have to be taken into account not only in the design of the studies and the evaluation of the results, but also the planning of the intervention itself [21], which has to adopt centered services design on the user [10], which also take into consideration the organization in which the new services are going to be implemented together with social aspects [22] and even the implementation process itself [23].

As a response to these challenges, and inspired in some cases in the industrial processes [24], the evaluation strategies that are shown to be potentially more efficient in the evaluation of e-health services are those which combine longitudinal synergy [25], itinerary [26], progressiveness [27], dissemination of the innovation [28], and a simultaneous consideration of the organizational aspects and human behavior from the perspective of complexity and complex adaptive systems [29]. Following these directives, "hybrid" evaluation models have been proposed that, setting out from an eclectic point of view, combine the characteristics of the traditional evaluation models (such as RCT) and the different perspectives of each of the "stakeholders" related to the process [10, 30-33].

The "hybrid models" have the capacity to tackle the evaluation as a successive process, in stages, to obtain the evidence in different ambits, by distinguishing at each phase which collectives have to be undoubtedly satisfied with the new resource, and for which ones is achieving the optimum result optional [25]. This division of the evaluation into consecutive stages or phases (see Figure 1) is a response to the complexity that is dealt with as a generation process and successive accumulation of knowledge of the interventions making each phase correspond to a different ambit of evidence. In general three generic phases are established: the first one related to the evaluation of the concept and the prototype of the service, the second one related to the evaluation of the results relative to the impact of the service in innovation in processes and health results in controlled environments, and a third pragmatic evaluation phase related to the long-term impact in production environments.

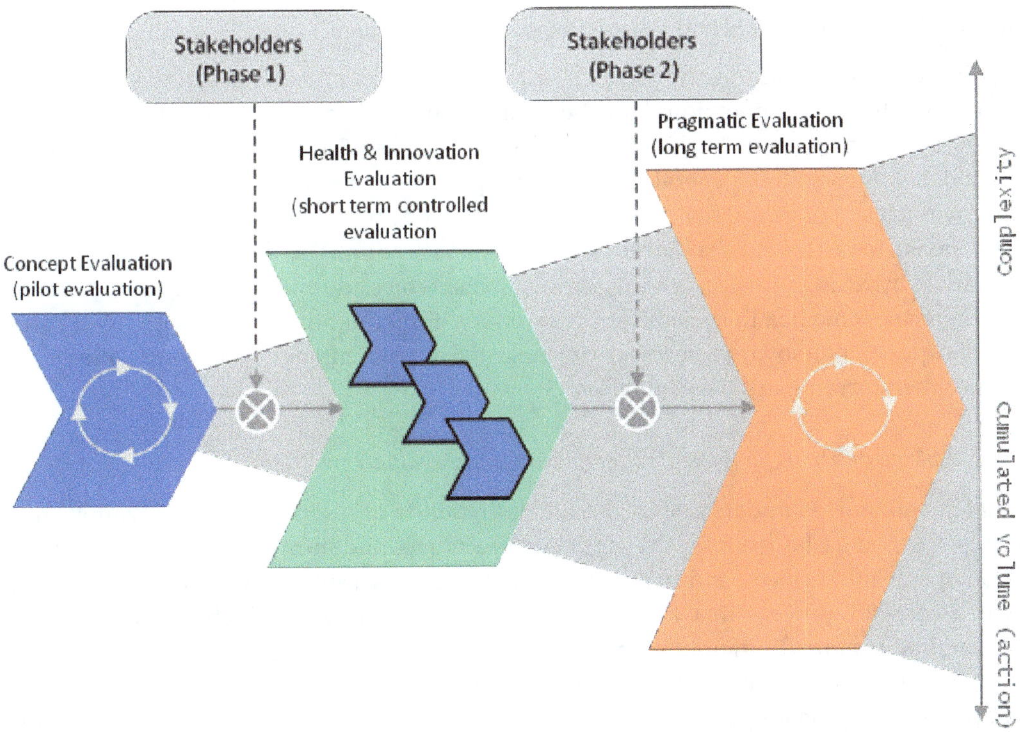


**Figure 1.** Generic structure of the hybrid models.

The progress of the evaluation is materialized by generating useful information, appropriate for each phase, and in this way reducing the profile of uncertainty or ambiguity in successive phases. It is, in short, a question of a gradual increase in knowledge on the intervention by predicting valuable information in advance which allows the risk to be reduced in successive phases. In this context, the risk is related to the resources invested in the evaluation: economic, infrastructures, human, etc. These progressive evaluation models establish decision-making elements between successive stages ("stakeholders") who, on the one hand, are recipients of the evaluation results of the previous phase. On the other hand, between its functions, it may be that which decides whether the evaluation progresses or not to the following phase, or if it is necessary to activate an iterative cycle with the objective of modifying some aspects of the service and restart or resume the evaluation at a determined stage or point.

In these methodologies an interdisciplinary vision of the process is combined assuming the diversity and complexity of the environment by means of aspects such as: 1) dealing with the evaluation process in successive phases by contemplating an ambit of differentiated evidence at each stage, 2) consider at each stage that the "stakeholders" are more suitable for deciding the continuation, closure or repetition (health and non-health professionals, patients, carers/caretakers, evaluation agencies, health authorities, the research group) and 3) make it possible to gain progressive knowledge on the intervention which at the same time acts as a risk control mechanism which establishes a road map for the actors and agents involved, offering a clear idea of where the project is and what is required at each stage.

The proposal for "hybrid methodologies" assumes a significant advance in the evaluation of "complex e-health interventions" in the health context, conciliating holistic focuses with widely-accepted traditional validation procedures such as RCT. However, to date, the hybrid methodologies constitute general and not very specific proposals. In spite of setting out clear objectives in each of its phases, they are clearly non-specific in some relevant aspects lending it a generic character and therefore a non-direct application. The difficulties are aggravated even more by taking into account that the context in which the evaluations have to be carried out, there are some health systems unprepared for it, highlighting in the majority of cases, a lack of support and recourses necessariy to make the implementation of the interventions more visible when carrying out the evaluation.

### *2.1.3. Implementation as an element of complexity in the evaluation*

"Implementation" is understood as the full assimilation of a service by organizations for its routine use and sustained from the permanent recourses and infrastructures. The implementation of e-health services, and in a wide sense the ICTs as a support to health attention, is in itself a complex process that has to be managed [34, 35], and which implies numerous determining factors in different ambits: organizational, technological, work and work flows and the individuals themselves. The implementation of e-services assumes the insertion of technology, reengineering of assistance processes, redistribution of resources, modification or addition of new roles, articulation of processes and collaboration models between different assistance levels, etc. Currently, the implementation of e-health services is still too slow and it is a fact that the said process is unsuccessful on a large number of occasions [36]: the lack of suitable infrastructures, the impossibility of finding financing, complications with the scalability and uncertainty of efficiency and sustainability.

In this sense the strategy of disseminating innovation and the management of change is relevant in organizations such as the "Breakthrough Series Learning Model" [28, 37], "Continuous Quality Improvement Model" [38], "Performance Improvement Model" [39], "Deming Model" [26], among others. Equally the combination and putting into practice of "top-down" and "bottom-up" strategies with solid institutional support (political and organizational), leadership and participation of health and non-health professionals, the specification of clear programs for change and the maintenance of permanent "feedback" from all of the stakeholders.

There is the opinion in which it is necessary to deal with implementation strategies that accompany design and development, in such a way that the new e-services are compatible with the infrastructures, purposes and local demands, and that the organization and the main "stakeholders" are involved in the local context and extended by adopting wide-ranging focuses so that the solutions are not extremely localized [35].

It seems evident then that implementation is probably the process that contributes the greatest complexity to the insertion of new e-services into the organizations, and therefore has a significant impact on the strategies for the search for evidence and evaluation on the said e-services. Nevertheless, the implementation forms part of the longitudinal evaluation process and therefore cannot be left out; the evaluation process cannot conclude until the e-service has been totally implemented into the organization and has had a mutual integration with the work flows, since there are extremes that cannot be determined without an adaptation being reached at a local context.

However, assuming the need to carry out an early implementation of the e-service into the health organization in order to be evaluated, it would have implications that might compromise the internal and external validity of the said evaluations, and even the feasibility itself of carrying it out. Among others, the most relevant implications are:

- To deal "suddenly" with the complexity of the implementation process
- Carry out local adaptations of the intervention, which could compromise the capacity for the generalization of the results obtained and therefore its transfer capacity
- Extend the envisaged period of time prior to the beginning of the evaluation, a fact that might compromise the committed administrative periods, especially in the context of research projects
- Make public the high risk of not achieving homogeneous deployments in interventions which, in order to achieve a sufficient volume of users, require multicentre scenarios

Therefore, it is relevant to develop proposals on how to make the need for the implementation and evaluation of an e-service in an organization compatible. In other words, within the framework of the "hybrid methodologies", search for evidence on an e-service at the same time by controlling the complexity that the implementation process introduces [40].

In this sense the following questions are posed: Is it possible to delay or at least contain within some essential minimums the implementation of the intervention in the health organization until the final stages of the evaluation? What type of resources or infrastructures is it necessary to authorize to make the deployment of these conditions viable? And under these conditions:

What type of evidence on the intervention can be reached? Finally, what are the advantages of achieving a certain level of evidence on the intervention during the early stages of the evaluation?

The adoption of a strategy of "minimum implementation" during the initial phases of the evaluation offers the following advantages:

- It makes an initial distancing of the conditions of the local outline possible, facilitating the work of identifying the functional components of the intervention and in this way obtain greater general or transferable transparency evidence.
- Increase the possibility of success in multicentre interventions since a greater homogeneity in the interventions can be achieved without compromising either its internal or external validity.
- It reduces institutional resistance due to the lesser commitment to initial resources.
- It implies the professionals (health and non-health) before getting to full implementations, thus facilitating the "top-down", "bottom-up" and "peer-to-peer" dynamic during the process
- It increases the confidence of the promoters and "stakeholders" to continue the evaluation of the intervention on making it possible to obtain early evidence. If the evidence obtained is negative, it permits: 1) to have the possibility and margin of maneuver to carry out rethinks of the intervention that will still be viable; 2) if it were inevitable, interrupt the progress of the evaluation of the intervention having been committed to up to the moment of minimum resources.

Finally, the following considerations have to be taken into account:

- The putting into practice of a strategy of "minimum implementation" in the initial phases of the evaluation requires the resources and infrastructures required to make the deployment of the intervention viable to be contributed to the organization externally for the aforementioned period of time. Under ideal conditions, it would only need the participation of the health and non-health professionals and as an organizational resource, facilitating externally all of the support necessary for the deployment of the experimental studies as part of the methodological support
- A "minimum implementation" during the initial phases does not shorten the total evaluation period since the process does not conclude until a complete adaptation of the intervention at the local context is achieved. However, it does make the progressive obtaining of evidence on the intervention possible by maintaining of the resources committed in the initial phases since they are those that contribute the greatest uncertainty and risk and therefore those that have to be the most protected from the effects of additional complexity that contribute a more wide-ranging implementation process.

The PITES platform responds to the aspects below:

- It proposes an evaluation strategy in interventions based on e-health based on the hybrid models that make the obtaining of evidence possible in the early stages implying some minimal institutional resources ("minimum implementation") in such a way that knowledge may be obtained, and at the same time, contain the complexity of the implementation process (section 2.1.4)
- It contributes a technological platform that, based on a generic conceptual model, makes possible the deployment of interventions become evaluated under conditions of "minimum implementation" during the initial phases, externally facilitating the resources and infrastructures necessary to the organizations, in such a way that for the health professionals, patients or other participating users, the intervention is perceived as an assistance service integrated into the health context (section 3)

### *2.1.4. Evaluation methodology of e-services in PITES*

Within the framework of the PITES platform the specification of an evaluation methodology has been carried out aligned with the hybrid methodologies for the search for evidence into the new assistance services based on telemedicine directed at chronic illness.

The PITES evaluation methodology is made up of four consecutive pages (Figure 2): pilot phase, exploratory trial phase, clinical trial phase, and the implementation phase. Responding to the classic sequence in hybrid models, an initial stage related to the evaluation of the concept and the configuration of the intervention prototype (pilot phase), followed by an intermediate step related to the evaluation of the results relative to the impact of the intervention in the innovation in health processes and results (exploratory trial and clinical trial phases), and a third pragmatic evaluation stage related to the long-term impact of the intervention in production environments (implementation phase).

By means of the support of infrastructures and resources that the PITES platform contributes, it is possible to carry out phases 1 to 3 (pilot, exploratory trial and clinical trial) under conditions of "minimum implementation".

The description of the phases is as follows:

**Pilot phase**

The objective of this phase is the evaluation of the technological prototype that is going to support the intervention as regards the quality and functioning of the prototype, usability, and satisfaction of the users of the prototype. Internally the process involves two consecutive tasks. Firstly, the design and development of the technological prototype under optimal laboratory conditions. This first task has the character of a concept trial, exploratory and iterative until the optimum prototype is configured. For this, it is necessary to carry out a study on the state of the art, available technologies, medical devices, communications, etc. In second place, the carrying out of a feasibility study under controlled practical conditions outside the laboratory. Few participants are required to carry out this initial field trial (It would be valid for the proposal of the basic model to not exceed 20 patients nor more than 5 health professionals), as is the availability of equipment under optimum

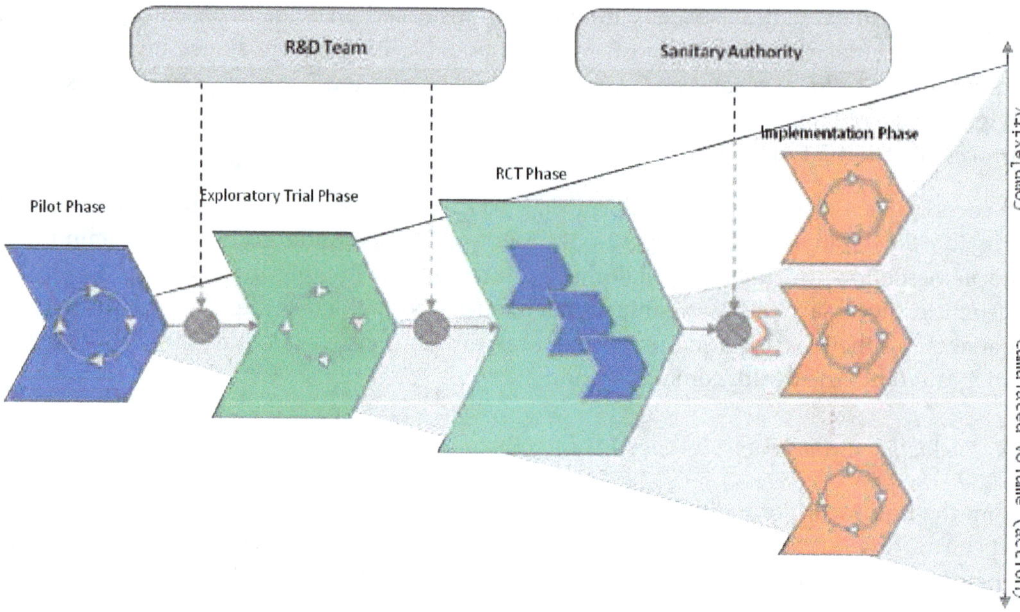


**Figure 2.** The PITES evaluation methodology.

working conditions, together with well-trained and motivated users. It is not a question of carrying out a comparison study since the focus continues to be on the technological system and its optimization; therefore throughout the development of this phase, proposals for improving the prototype are gathered and then sent to the laboratory. The technological prototype is developed externally to the health organization with the participation of health professionals among which include those belonging to the research group and the resources and infrastructures required are facilitated externally to the health organization by the PITES platform.

To pass from phase 1 to phase 2 a positive evaluation of the results of phase 1 is necessary in relation to: the test of the concept, the technical viability, the acceptability of the health professionals, and the satisfaction of the users of the system. The decision is brought about within the ambit of the research group itself and is made effective by the promoting or financing entity.

**Exploratory trial phase**

Once the technological prototype has been optimized, it is time to begin the evaluation of the intervention in the health aspect of clinical efficiency. For this and, in agreement with the requirement to maintain a controlled complexity by means of a "minimum implementation" in the health organization, it is necessary to establish the provision model by means of carrying out the intervention emphasizing the resources and infrastructures required that are going to be facilitated externally to the health organization by the PITES platform. To carry out this task the proposed procedure is the carrying out of one or more exploratory trials whose objective is to experiment with the intervention, varying the deferent components and alternatives, to observe the effect of the intervention in its entirety and its consistency in different contexts, viability, participant acceptability, etc. As a result, evidence has to be obtained on the most suitable parameterization of the clinical trial (the following phase), to specify the intervention and the optimum studies.

Aspects such as identifying the key processes and results of the intervention, identifying the mechanisms through which the intervention would lead to an improvement in the results, the identification of the application difficulties or implementation of the intervention, the establishment of the collectives or groups on those that influence the intervention by optimizing its probability of response, the determination of the components and the intensity of the intervention in accordance with the available possibilities and resources, or the evaluation of the learning curve of the skills of the users are basic aspects to be determined in order to be able to guarantee the performance in the suitable intervention in the clinical trial phase. It is also not necessary to perform an analysis and modeling of the intervention that is required to be evaluated. If it is going to be compared with a practical standard, or an improved practice (for example, the same intervention with and without the support of telemedicine), it will also be necessary to model the comparison intervention which might be the same or even more complex. As well as the modeling process, if it is possible, it may be very interesting to carry out a simulation of the intervention by means of experimenting functional aspects of the scenario, the modeling of components, the statistical and mathematical model, etc.

As regards the methodology of the exploratory trial phase, the same degree of quality of evidence is not demanded as in a controlled randomized clinical trial; while it is inacceptable methodologically to modify an intervention during the course of the controlled randomized clinical trial, a study in this phase may be developed precisely to carry out trials on the variations in the intervention and clarify which are the most appropriate with views to the clinical trial. The criterion is to carry out one or more studies with a more adaptable development especially as regards the rigidity of the protocols and the inclusion of patients. The carrying out of quasi-experimental studies with sample sizes that do not exceed 100 patients and 10 health professionals may be suitable in this phase.

The availability of "Living Labs" as a community experimentation context may result in an appropriate option as it would carry out formal studies in social environments with a controlled complexity. If this is not possible, it would be advisable to carry out an analysis on the context in which the intervention is going to be evaluated since the degrees of complexity which show the different health problems are diverse and dependent on the context. It is recommended to consider aspects related to: the illness itself (risk factors, co-morbidity, prevalence, etc.), the patient (lifestyle, adherence to the treatment, symptoms, etc.), and the social context (social support, socio-economic level, cultural level, etc.).

The support of the exploratory trial and the corresponding interventions (resources, logistics, and infrastructures), is carried out externally of the health organizations involved and counting exclusively on the participation of health professionals belonging to the said organizations and contributing the resources and infrastructures required by the PITES platform.

To pass from phase 2 to phase 3 a positive evaluation of the results of the experimental studies carried out in phase 2 is needed which guarantees the viability of carrying out the controlled randomized clinical trial in order to evaluate the intervention in terms of efficiency. The decision is made within the ambit of the research group itself and put into effect by the promoting or financing entity.

**Clinical trial phase**

This phase is key to the evaluation of the efficiency of the complex interventions and consists of carrying out a controlled randomized trial with all of the rigor and power required, assuming the standard design aspects that require these types of trial: inclusion and exclusion criteria, sample size, criteria and duration of the intervention, randomization and informed consent of the participants, etc. From the knowledge accumulated in phase 2, definitive decisions must be taken on the nature of the intervention in order to standardize the intervention going to be evaluated and minimize the biases that limit not only the internal but also the external validity.

During this phase, unlike the previous ones, it is absolutely prohibited to make modifications in the protocol of the intervention. The minimum sample size determines the statistical power of the clinical trial and there must be the possibility of carrying out a replication of the intervention in multiple centers (multicentre trial), maintain its uniformity of implementation to guarantee the internal and external validity of the study and the generalization of the results. The participation of multiple centers contributes an additional value as it makes possible the study in different contexts of established patterns and emerging self-organization behaviors shown by the health professionals that are of doubtable use in phase 4.

The support of the clinical trial and the corresponding interventions (resources, logistics, and infrastructures), are carried out externally to the health organizations involved and counting exclusively on the participation of health professionals belonging to the said organizations and contributing the resources and infrastructures required by the PITES platform. It is essential that the resources and infrastructures external to the health organization do not represent a direct object of evaluation in the clinical trial, and act exclusively as a support to the operational deployment of the intervention.

To pass from phase 3 to phase 4 a positive evaluation of the efficiency of the intervention in the results of the trial, together with a decision from the health authority to adopt, is necessary (for example, an autonomous health service) with the support or endorsement of a Health Technology Evaluation Agency. Therefore, the ambit of the decision is outside the scope of the research group, although its continuity and participation in phase 4 may still be relevant.

**Implementation phase**

Once the evidence on the efficiency of the health of the intervention is demanded, it is necessary to adapt it to the local contexts in order to deal with two objectives: the full implementation of the intervention in the health organization in its technologic and health ambits, in such a way that it constitutes a health procedure more as regards the provision of all of the resources and infrastructures required at the margin of the external supports, and from that, the carrying out of financial cost studies and long-term studies to determine the efficiency of the intervention.

For this, it is necessary to count on a significant and essential institutional support that promotes and manages the change and the dissemination of the innovation to the health organizations participating in this phase, and preferably from legal and financial instruments that regulate the introduction of new technologies in the National Health System as a factor essential for the progression of the intervention as a routine health procedure.

The total effect of knowledge that would contribute to carrying out the local implementation in different socio-health contexts from the participation of several organizations, would contribute to the convergence of the intervention towards the standardized health procedure. Taking the methods and other knowledge accumulated during the development of phases 2 and 3 as reference, it is necessary to carry out an analysis on the operative feasibility of the service that adapts the intervention in specific health contexts, together with a deployment project and all of them particularized for the conditions of each participating organization. In this process it would constitute a valuable contribution of the health professionals who would act as active agents of the health process in the previous phases due to their knowledge on the intervention and the health context, and as the promoters of complementary strategies for the dissemination of the innovation.

## 2.2. Interoperability

### *2.2.1. Interoperability of the clinical information*

The interoperability of the clinical information is one of the requirements of the health continuity [41]. The current paradigms of the health put the patient at the centre of a process around which are located the organizations and professionals who provide them with their services independently of their geographical or temporary location. For this strategy to be effective it needs the information to flow between the different nodes in such a way that it is automatically interpretable by them. Thus the professionals will have all of the information that they require to carry out their work, avoiding problems of duplicating the test for the patient to increase his/her safety, statistical studies can be carried out more easily on having the normalized information available and are able to plan the action to be carried out automatically.

Also for a platform like the one presented here, or for any other medical telecare service, this question is essential, as one of the problems that usually comes up is that of its isolation as regards other information systems, since on being systems created specifically for carrying out the support work of the service, the possibility of communicating with others is not normally taken into account and the information generated in these services usually stays in their own storage systems, without reaching the patient's records unless a manual introduction of the required data is written [42]. The interoperability of these platforms, therefore, is a fundamental requirement if it is required to integrate into the trends of the health continuity.

With these premises the PITES platform has been provided with an interoperability framework to facilitate the sharing of the information between the different nodes that are connected to the platform, as is its interconnection with other information systems such as the clinical records of the health organizations and for the use of the information for secondary uses.

But, what is interoperability? the ISO (specifically the Information Technology Vocabulary – Fundamental Terms, or ISO/IEC 2382-01) defines the interoperability as the "capacity to communicate, implement applications or transfer data between sever functional units without the user needing to know the particular characteristics of the said units". The definition is fairly clear, but perhaps insufficient. The first thing that has to be specified is that there are several types of interoperability: the classic technical, syntactical and semantic; the organizational has recently been merged, and there are authors that go further and even speak of political interoperability, whose existence depends rather on where the limit of the definition of the organization is placed. Let us see what each of these "interoperabilities" are.

Technical Interoperability: this is the basis on which the connection between systems is supported. Technical interoperability defines the interfaces, both physical and logical, which allow the aforementioned functional definition to be able to exchange information. It is currently well advanced, since, it is not exclusive to the health scenario and its development has been necessary for many other fields. Regulations such as 802.3, 802.11, TCP/IP, HTTP, the Zigbee Bluetooth specification, the low levels of the ISO 11073, SOAP family, etc. are those that are used to achieve technical interoperability.

Syntactical Interoperability: Syntactical interoperability deals with the formats of the exchanged files or of the types of data used, making them able to make translations between formats depending on those used for each system involving the communication. The systems that only provide this type of interoperability act as mere messengers without intervening in the content of the information communicated without being able to react depending on it. This type of interoperability also has a high level of development, although in the health field some evolution is still necessary. Within the range of regulations on which they are based so as to achieve syntactical interoperability can be found XML, the specifications for types of data such as TS 14796 from CEN or the ISO 21090, the specifications of messages of versions 2.x of HL7 or the reference models of HL7 V3 or UNE-EN ISO 13606, although the latter are also the basis of the semantic interoperability, as can be seen below.

Semantic Interoperability: according to the definition of the 251 Technical Committee of CEN, it is the state that exists between the two entities-applications when, with respect to a specific task, an application can accept data from the other and carry out this task satisfactorily without the need for the intervention of an external operator. That is, two systems will be semantically interoperable if the information circulates between them without the original meaning being altered and each of them understanding by itself what the other sends and is consequently able to act. It is that which it would permit, for example, that the dispersed information of a patient, generated in many different sources, in different places, systems and moments, may be shared. It also needs to be at the disposal of the professionals where they need it or can be used easily in secondary uses such as research or statistics. Contrary to what is frequently believed, the use of terminologies to encode the information is not sufficient to achieve semantic interoperability since clinical information consists of much more than just words. At the times of expressing the clinical information the vocabulary is necessary, as well as being able to express the context in which the information has been generated (who, when, with which objective, about whom, the level of viability, etc.) as well as being able to formalize that which must be gathered for each concept handled so that it makes sense (it must contain a summary of the records, a discharge report, the Barthel index, etc.). For the first necessity, the terminologies (SNOMED-CT, CIE-10, LOINC, etc.) can be used to express the context; (UNE-EN ISO 13606:1, RIM, CDA, etc.) reference models are used and there are mechanisms as archetypes to formalize and share the concepts (for example those defined in UNE-EN ISO 13606:2) or the detailed clinical models (DCM).

Organizational Interoperability: summarizing considerably, it may be said that the organizational interoperability is supported by business rules. In order for two organizations to be able to cooperate they must share a common context in their procedures and work flows. It will be difficult to interoperate, for example, if the definitions of the process, health plan or health order are different or incompatibles. The definitions of some of these concepts are currently imposed by the information systems that are used in the different organizations and that the providers have included in their developments without previously formalizing them. Other concepts are established by the health policies developed by the different administrations on which the organizations depend (that is the concept that some political interoperability authors use). There is still much more to be done in this field, although in the environment of standardization there are works such as the EN 12967 HISA (Health Informatics - Service Architecture) regulation which, in its first part, deals with the business point of view, and mainly the UNE-EN ISO 13940 regulation (system of concepts to give support to the continuity of the health).

### *2.2.2. Definition of the Interoperability Framework of the Platform*

The design of the interoperability layer of the PITES platform is dealt with by taking its objective into account (open platform to support e-health services) such as the special characteristics of the scenario in which its activity is developed, as well as the peculiarities in Spain, where the existence of autonomous regional governments (known as Comunidades Autónomas), with different languages and the health responsibilities transferred, conditions to a large extent the approach to be implemented:

- PITES is an open platform to give support to a large variety of research groups belonging to different organizations.
- The organizations participating in PITES belong to different Comunidades Autónomas with the health powers transferred and with different languages.
- The information systems of the different nodes may be manufactured differently and be based on different models.
- The list of organizations participating in PITES is not closed, but it is envisaged that in future calls new nodes will be incorporated, a question that also forms part of the philosophy of the platform. That is, the solution that is adopted for the interoperability must be capable of incorporating new elements probably based on systems and models different from those that currently exist.

In such a scenario it would be very difficult to establish a rigid framework for the exchange of information to be set, for example, a series of predefined messages to which any user of the platform, present or future should attend, especially in the health field in which the complexity of the information dealt with is a determinant factor at the time of finding satisfactory communications solutions, as is also the speed of changing the domain knowledge.

In this sphere, current trends point to the use of strategies that permit the information to be separated (which is known from a certain entity and is not going to vary over time) from the knowledge (that which is valid for all of the entities of the domain but which is subject to variations as the research advances or new techniques are developed). These double-model strategies (information or reference model and knowledge model or archetypes) [43] allow, on the one hand, the variations systems in the knowledge to be protected and, on the other hand, separate the actions of the experts in the technical field (they develop the systems based on the reference model) of the domain experts (the health professionals that define the concepts to be used by means of archetypes). This is the strategy that, for example, the UNE-EN ISO 13606 regulation implements.

Under these premises, the main requirement that the standardization framework must achieve is to provide interoperability to the information systems involved, independently of the moment in which the scenario is used, and with the best possible impact both in the configuration of its teams and in the way of working or organizing the information. In order to achieve it, the use of a series of international regulations has been opted for: ISO 21090 for the types of data, UNE-EN ISO 13606 for the transfer of the clinical information and the EN 13940 regulation as a series of concepts to give support to the health continuity.

#### 2.2.2.1. *Interoperability framework: syntactical interoperability*

Syntactical interoperability strengthens the use of XML to encode the messages. This is done in accordance with the reference model of the UNE-EN ISO 13606 regulation using the type of information defined in ISO 21090. Given that the UNE-EN ISO 13606 regulation remains agnostic as regards the technology (and does not define what has to be used to carry out the final encoding), some common XML Schemas are used for the reference model created by Dr. Dipak Kalra's group (leader of the EHRCom task force that developed the regulation), which is being converted into the de facto regulation, as they are currently being used in a multitude of both national and international projects.

As regards the types of data specified by the ISO 21090 regulation [44], the XML Schema which proposes the regulation in its informative part is used. In this case, a reduction has been made in the types available to facilitate the implementation, always maintaining the compatibility with the regulation, as well as the possibility of easily adding the new types that are necessary.

#### 2.2.2.2. *Interoperability framework: semantic interoperability*

Semantic interoperability is supported on two pillars: the use of terminologies together with the double reference model and archetypes of the UNE-EN ISO 13606 regulation [45, 46].

#### 2.2.2.2.1. *Use of terminologies*

The first basis for the semantic interoperability of the clinical information is the encoding of the terms used in the domain. For this it has become necessary to use the standardized terminologies. The proposed PITES interoperability framework, the use of SNOMED CT and its link with the archetypes defined as one of the means of supporting the semantic interoperability [47]. This is implemented by means of the creation of the corresponding subsets of terms. Equally, in those cases in which the use of SNOMED CT does not cover the terminological necessities, and given that the 13606 regulation does not impose any specific terminology, the terminologies suitable for each domain are used.

#### 2.2.2.2.2. *Reference models and archetypes*

The reference model is in charge of representing the general characteristics of the components of the ECR, how they are organized, and the context information necessary to satisfy the requirements both ethical and legal of the register. The model defines the series of classes that make up the constituent blocks of the register, that is, gather its stable characteristics.

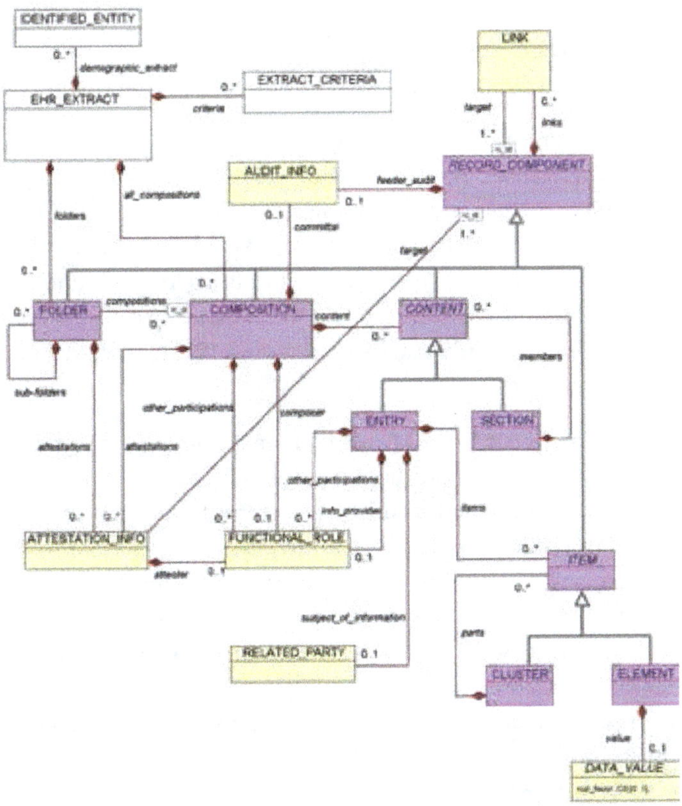


**Figure 3.** Simplified diagram of the UNE-EN ISO 13606 model reference (obtained from (2))

The reference model of the 13606 regulation organizes information in the following way (see Figure 3): the summary, which forms part of a message is the container of the information referring to a patient (the whole file or part of it) that is going to be transmitted. This information includes the demographic data (the identification of the people and entities are separated from the clinic in order to satisfy legal requirements), the access policies and the clinical information, which is organized thus: the summary contains a series of compositions (information on the subject gathered during the meeting, a report, etc.) which are adapted to be able to reconstruct the history of the data. The compositions store simple statements on observations, evaluations or instructions (entry), which may be grouped together in sections to represent the internal organization of the documents as their headings are made. Finally, the entries contain elements, in each of which a specific datum is stored. The elements may be grouped together in clusters to represent more complex structures of data, such as temporary series or tables. The regulation provides a way of additional organization high level which permits the compositions to be grouped together in folders, to be able to reproduce the organizational criteria of each centre (per episode, per service, per meeting, etc.). The clinical information is accompanied by another type of context information to complement its meaning or comply with the legal requirements. Thus any component can contain information on who completed it (audit_info), it can be signed (attestation_info) or be linked to other components (link), to express cause-effect relationships, problem-solución, etc. It also gathers information on the environment in which an activity is developed (clinical_session), who participated in it (functional_role) or if the information refers to the patient or another entity (related_party).

In order to achieve interoperability, a model such as this one has to be complemented in the knowledge domain with a formal model to transmit and share structures of predefined classes, agreed to by a community, corresponding to fragments of the registry created under specific clinical situations: the archetypes. An archetype is the definition of a hierarchical combination of components or the reference model, to which it restricts (given their names, types of possible data, default values, cardinality, etc.), to model clinical concepts of the knowledge domain. These structures, although sufficiently stable, can be modified or substituted by other through the evolution of clinical practice.

The knowledge model (archetype model) implements the separation of information and knowledge and the strategy of the generation of systems to be changed. According to this new strategy, the technological professionals build the systems based only on the reference model. This provides protection against changes in the knowledge. If the domain concepts do not form part of the design of the systems, it will not be necessary to update these if those change. In the same way, the same system may be used by different organizations although they use different documents (that is, concepts of a different domain). On the other hand, the health professionals model the concepts of the domain using tools based on the knowledge model that will have generated the technologies for but without the need to have a profound knowledge of the technological artifacts on which they are based, being only concerned about correctly defining the concepts that they use. It is worth summarizing that these models (archetypes) can be created at any time, since the systems use them in real time to generate requests for data in accordance with them, they verify the validity of the requests received, interpret them automatically from the semantic point of view, build applications for entering data, etc.

By using this double model, it is not necessary to have a prior total agreement between the organizations participating in the communication, since they have the mechanism of the archetypes as a formalized way of sharing the concepts that are being used and that the receptor is capable of correctly interpreting, the information received automatically. In Figure 4 it can be seen how the communication process would be:

**a.** When system A is going to send information to system D, it will turn to a repository of archetypes in order to obtain the model corresponding to the concepts that are wished to be sent.

**b.** Using the corresponding archetype, system A will generate a message in real time.

**c.** The message is sent to system D, which...

**d.** will check according to which archetype has generated the information and will request it from the corresponding repository (or the organization that sent the information)

**e.** System D obtains the requested archetype...

**f.** and with it, it correctly interprets the information received to incorporate it automatically into its own storage system.

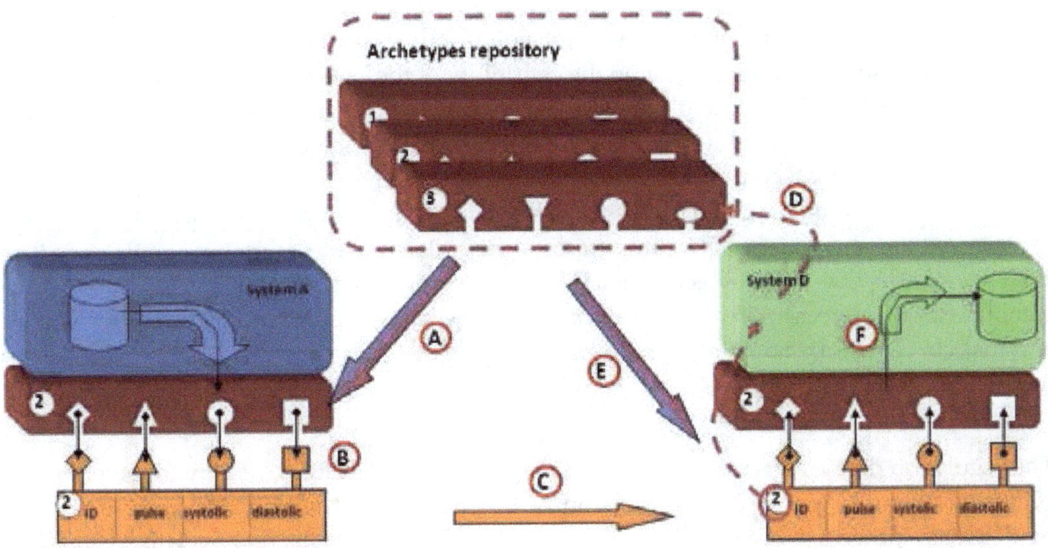


**Figure 4.** Communications model with archetypes

The archetypes have to be completed with the terminologies. This process consists essentially of the association of an element of the archetype defined by the ADL language (Archetype Description Language) [48] to a SNOMED CT concept or to an expression following the grammatical regulations specified in the terminological standard.

Therefore, in accordance with the defined interoperability framework, the health professionals of the different nodes participating in the PITES platform generate the models (archetypes) of the concepts that handle in their domain and, from this moment on, the rest of the nodes are able to correctly interpret the messages that are transmitted. This process may be carried out at any time to adapt the concepts to the changes in the knowledge that come about.

#### 2.2.2.3. *Interoperability framework: organizational interoperability*

The interoperability of the health information is not only based on syntactical and semantic interoperability. In its COM(2008)3282 recommendation the European Commission recommends that the member states act on different planes, the organizational between themselves, to achieve trans-border interoperability of the health information in Europe [49]. Equally, in the final report of the Semantic Health project that proposes a road map to achieve the semantic interoperability in Europe. Organizational interoperability is cited as of the factors necessary to achieve it (1).

The scenario proposed by the PITES project, in which the participating nodes belong to different autonomous communities, with their powers transferred and, therefore, with the capacity to take their own decisions as regard health policy and how to implement the communications in their territory and using different languages, it becomes very similar to the general European scenario, therefore the organizational interoperability also becomes of great importance. This is why it is proposed to use the UN-EN ISO 13940 regulation [50]. The said regulation defines the types of concept and the descriptive associations, as regards the health processes with special consideration on the continuity of the care centered on the patient, and the shared care. Its objective is to carry out a description and formalization of the continuity of the care in the context of information systems, implying the definition of concepts and descriptive terms that contribute to establishing a common conceptual framework that overcomes national, cultural and professional barriers. That is why a set of concepts is designed to represent the phenomena of the attention process, related to the subject of attention. In this case, the focus is not on the subject in itself but on its condition or state. It applies a modeling technique of the processes in order to identify the objectives of the process, the sub-processes and the activities, also taking into account aspects on the resources, responsibilities and means for patient participation in his or her own care. In those points in which social health is necessary, there activities also appear as well as its work flow.

The regulation defines an attention organization as "an organization directly involved in the provision of care". Within an organization of this type, the provision of health services is modeled as a process of organization of the attention (Figure 5). This process will contain one or more attention processes. Similarly, it will also contain an administration process and probably a research process (aimed at improving medical knowledge) and a training process (with the object of improving the capacities of the health professionals by applying medical knowledge). The health care process constitutes the heart of the health care organizations and, at the same time, it is made up of a clinical process and a resources management process, which is in charge of the logistic of the activity. Finally, the clinical process contains a clinical management process, a documentation and communication process and management of the quality of attention process. The documentation process is essential in the entire clinical act. It is that which allows the activity to be registered and able to communicate its results to other activities, giving support to the health care continuity.

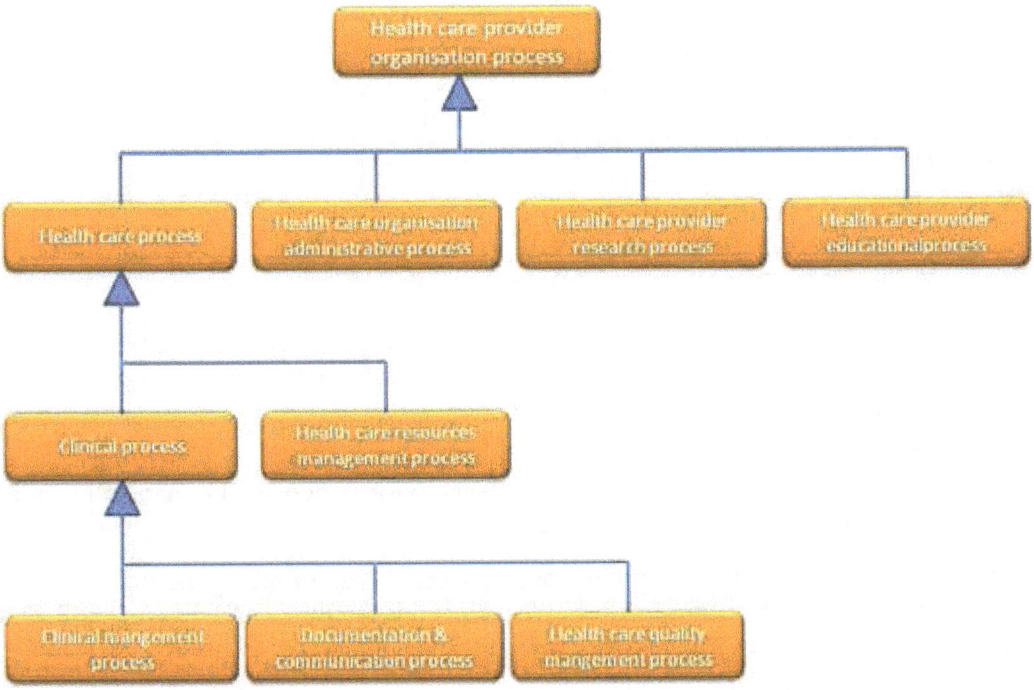


**Figure 5.** Components of the organization of the attention process in accordance with EN 13940

### 2.2.3. *Summary: the PITES interoperability framework*

In summary, in the following Table 1 the interoperability model defined for the PITES project can be specifically seen

| INTEROPERABILITY | ACTIONS | REGULATIONS |
|---|---|---|
| Syntactical | •Encoding messages in XML<br>•Use of a series of types of data proposed by ISO 21090<br>•Messages in accordance with the 13606 XML Schema as defined by Dipak Kalra's group and that proposed by the computing part of ISO | •XML<br>•XML Schema UNE-EN ISO13606.1<br>•XML Schema ISO 21090 |
| Semantic | •Generation of subsets of terms from SNOMED - CT<br>•Use of other specific terminologies according to need<br>•Definition of the local concepts by means of archetypes in accordance with UNE-EN ISO 13606.<br>•Linking of the terminologies and the subsets defined with the archetypes | •UNE-EN ISO 13606.1: Reference model<br>•UNE-EN ISO 13606.2: Archetype model<br>•SNOMED-CT<br>* Other terminologies |
| Organizational | •Definition of a common conceptual framework based on UNE-EN ISO 13940<br>•Definition of an inter-organizational processes based on UNE-EN ISO 13940<br>•Definition of inter-organizational work flows based on UNE-EN ISO 13940 | •UNE-EN 13940: System of<br>•UNE-EN 13940: Processes and work flows |

**Table 1.** Specification of the PITES interoperability framework

## 3. Description of the platform

Within the ambit of new services based on telemedicine, the generic overall scenario constitutes a heterogeneous and diverse ecosystem (Figure 6):

- Patients and citizens in different environments, With different health conditions and health care necessities, different degrees of dependence, age and family context, different skills and technological availability, different living and social habits, etc.
- Health and non-health professionals and with different professional profiles, different skills, attitudes, and technological availability in their environments.
- The world of medical devices, mainly for personal and domestic use, with an enormous diversity, a more and more extensive catalogue becoming even more essential so as to be able to put new health care models into practice, mainly for those whose self-treatment is the main therapeutic option
- Technological platforms of different types: health platforms, non-platforms, private monitoring platforms, research platforms, etc. These platforms make a ubiquitous access possible and provide personalized services in a complex environment in a solvent manner.
- Some communications networks with a high level of capillarity which makes the Internet possible and with support by means of high-capacity, fixed wireless and digital networks

in an environment of convergence and the provision of services on an IP protocol. In this environment, the platforms act as elements of interrelation or an interface between them. The users already have more and more availability to network access technology and are familiarized with it.

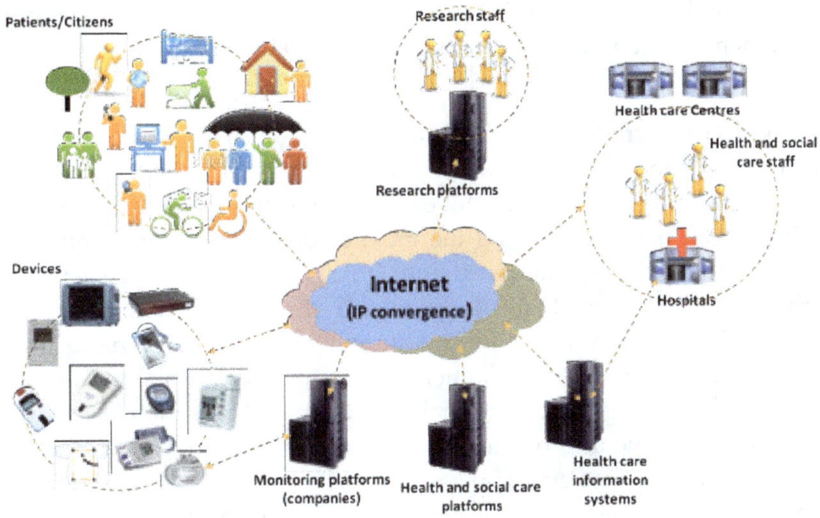


**Figure 6.** Technological environment of the PITES platform

In this complex environment, the PITES platform is constituted as a stable public infrastructure technology, aimed at research groups with innovation nodes located in Health Centers, with the objective of making support possible to collaborative research and for the obtaining of evidence on new models for the health care provision based on ICT in scenarios related to chronic illness and dependency.

The design of the platform is sensitive to the complexity of the socio-health system and the difficulties and limitations that the implementation process of e-services has on the organizations. Within the framework of experimental studies, the platform provides support to the first three phases of the aforementioned evaluation methodology of e-services, that is, authorize the resources and infrastructures necessary to deploy interventions with minimum implementation necessities in the socio-health organizations.

The PITES platform is designed to support research projects; not health care activity in "clinical routine". As a research platform it responds to several requirements different from those platforms orientated to "clinical routine". These peculiarities manifest themselves, on the one hand, in a conceptual model of entities that constitute a proposal for a reduction in users, resources and their interactions in the design process of the e-services and, on the other hand, an architecture based on available technologies and those which are nowadays mature such as Web technologies, SOA (Service Oriented Architecture) and the "Cloud Computing" model.

### 3.1. Conceptual entities model

In the context of complex interventions it is fundamental to detect and make clear as soon as possible which agents participate actively in the intervention and its action and interaction mechanisms [29]. Once the said active agents are detected it facilitates the definition, design, development, implementation, and evaluation process of the intervention itself. In this sense, the Chronic Care Model (CCM) [51] [52] from the aspects that propose on the organization, interaction and identification of actors, contributes a good orientation to carry out this initial task.

The CCM has been considered a general reference model on a global level that represents an organizational focus of the health care and tries to act as a guide for the activities aimed at improving the quality and the management of the chronic health care. It is the most studied model and that which has accumulated the most evidence, in more countries and health systems, illnesses and patient collectives, and which have derived the large part of the organizational models and models for the provision of chronic health care that have been proposed. The CCM establishes that in any chronic patient care scenario three contexts participate or interact: society (with its numerous resources and public and private policies), the health system, and the health professionals and the patients as direct actors of the health care. It is established that the improvements in the results of the chronic health care come to light by means of productive interactions between some informed and active patients and some prepared health teams together with a proactive attitude, which are promoted by the coordination of additional resources at a social and health level. In this sense, the CCM specifies six categories of resources: the policies and social resources, the organization of the health care, help to self-management, the systems of provision of health care and help in the decision and the clinical information systems. Thus, it implicitly establishes a classification of entities from which it is possible to identify the agents participating in the interventions aimed at an improvement in the chronic health care. The patients and health professionals are always active agents of direct participation in any intervention, and the rest of the resources are agents or optionally active subsystems (they do not need to be present in all of the interventions) that play a support or promoter role.

Taking the focus of the CCM as reference in the design process of the e-services, the PITES platform establishes a conceptual entities model that constitutes a user abstraction proposal, resources and their interactions. The model (Figure 7) is made up of six entities: patient entity, health care professional entity, external resource entity, health care information system entity, intervention management entity and technological platform entity. Each of the conceptual entities of the model represents a view or perspective of the health care provision model that is wished to evaluate by means of the intervention.

The patient entity encompasses the patient and all of the resources assigned to him or her for the intervention. The patient entity is usually made up of:

- A patient protocol usually consists of periodically carrying out biometric measurements (arterial pressure, weight, pulse, ECG, spirometry, lipid profile, activity, etc.), and replies to questionnaires on symptoms or actions.

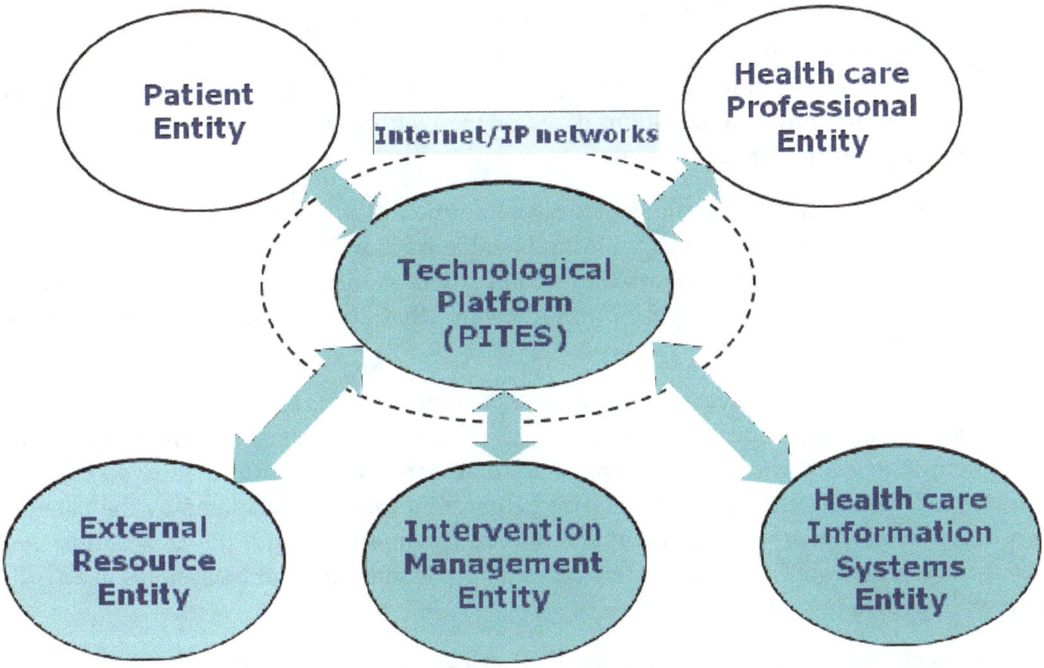


**Figure 7.** PITES conceptual entities

- Some biomedical monitoring equipment for personal use (sphygmomanometer, pulse oximeter, scales, thermometer, etc.) or environmental monitoring, to carry out the measurements required by the patient protocol
- Communications equipment to carry out the periodical sending of protocol information. The equipment must be suitable to interact with the interfaces authorized by the platform.

The health care professional entity represents the perspective of the health professionals and is made up of the series of tools and resources required to carry out the health care protocol established by the intervention. In general, it is applications adapted to the specific patient protocols by means of which the monitoring is carried out including help tools and functionalities that make an indirect communication possible with the patient (advice, warnings, etc.). These applications are usually accessible by means of the Internet with the appropriate access controls. The reply messages to the patients are sent by means of personalized services such as SMS, e-mail, interactive voice systems, etc.

The external resource entity represents any support resource additional to the intervention on the health or community environment. That is health centers, pharmacies, consultations, geriatric residencies, other platforms, etc. The function of this entity is usually to represent any infrastructure that acts as a resource shared between patients, because it supposes some type of logistic advantage (economical, location, etc.). They can act as external resources, for example:

- Residential homes, in which there is the possibility of attending the patients collectively by means of shared equipment, for example, patients with oral anticoagulation therapy who share the INR monitor and the communications equipment. The interfaces with this type of external resource may be applications based on the Web, designed so that a person responsible manages the patient collectives.

- Platforms for external monitoring that receive information of specific patient collectives, for example, a collective of patients with implantable cardioverter-defibrillator (ICD) monitored from a platform that authorizes the company providing the ICD. In these cases, the interface would be based on specific "middleware" that makes it possible to interoperate with the said external platform.

The health care information system entity essentially represents the Electronic Clinical Records of the Patient and the perspective from the health information systems. The function that this entity contributes is that of making it possible to exchange clinical information on the said systems and the ECR essentially summarized clinical information generated by the patients and health professionals during the interventions. The interfaces with the ECR entities are based on "middleware" specific to interoperate with the said information systems in accordance with regulations.

The intervention management entity supports a series of roles and resources that are required to carry out the intervention and that are not available or cannot be carried out suitable either by the health system or the community. The services provided by this entity are of two kinds:

- Support to the deployment of the intervention: it provides resources to make it possible to train the health professionals, patients, families; resources for the maintenance and management of the equipment used; tools for the monitoring of the compliance with patient protocols, etc.

- Support methodology of the experimental evaluation study: it provides resources for the support methodology of the clinical trials and experimental studies. For example, drawing up and management of the documentation (Case Report Forms), applications for the Electronic Data Capture, services for the centralized randomization, recompilation and analysis of results, among others.

The Technological Platform Entity represents the ICT nucleus that supports the functional interfaces, the coordination of activities and finally the telematic infrastructure that require the interventions to be implemented during its evaluation. The services provided by the platform are provided mainly by means of the Internet, digital cellular networks or basic telephone network; the architecture of the platform is described in the following section.

When it is desired to evaluate the health care provision model with the support of the platform, the steps to be followed are as follows: define the intervention that leads to the practice of the health care model and the experimental evaluation study (type of study, variables, measurement instruments, dimension of the study as regards the sample and duration of the intervention, etc.) and define and design the new e-service which will give support to the intervention. To carry out this second stage, the actors involved must be determined (direct and indirect); this datum will establish the entities of the conceptual model that participate. Below, from the perspective of each of the participating entities, we have to establish:

- the specifications of the interfaces, applications and services based on the roles that each participant contributes in the health care process,
- the interactions with the patient as subject of the health care and their environment,
- the temporary aspects of the provision of health care,
- the organization and management of the health care, the aspects of support to the decision and monitoring of the activity, and
- the aspects related to responsibilities, flows and management of the information.

Finally, the provision model establishes an organizational and functional framework to which the intervention and experimental evaluation study must be adapted, to be able to carry out a joint deployment which may be supported by the PITES technological platform, and therefore develop it in the context that establishes that of the evaluation methodology.

### 3.2. Architecture

As has already been said, the PITES platform is a platform for research, not a support to health care activity in "clinical routine". As a research platform, its design responds to some requirements that are additional to those adopted by the platforms oriented to "clinical routine" and which condition architecture decisions.

The platforms oriented to "clinical routine" must provide greater attention to aspects such as scalability maintainability and availability. The research platforms, also:

- Must be conceived from their basis in order to change, evolve and interoperate;
- Must contemplate intrinsically evaluation mechanisms in the widest sense, and
- Must be capable of coexisting with the "clinical routine" platforms to make the mutual interaction possible together with the progressive implementation of e-services.

Under these conditions, the requisites demanded by the PITES platform and which constitute the references for the design of its architecture, are as follows:

- Functionality independent of the technological infrastructure of the environment in which the e-services are going to be deployed: the platform must guarantee some homogeneous functional deployment conditions during the evaluation of the interventions, especially on those that imply geographical dispersion so as to be more sensitive to this aspect
- Scalability: the platform must be capable of supporting from small pilot projects and concept trials, up to multi-centered interventions that involve hundreds of users (patients, professionals, etc.).
- Dynamism and flexibility: the platform must have the capacity for rapid adaptation and evolution, the incorporation of new functionalities and the reuse of components, incorporation of technological opportunities, etc.

- Operative transparency in the access and location of the resources: the platform must deploy the services in such a way that they are perceived by the users as incorporated or integrated in the socio-health care. This requirement is of greater relevance during the evaluation phases on clinical effectiveness. In the said phases, the platform must not constitute an element that commits the validity of the studies
- Interoperability: capacity to interoperate with heterogeneous components, distributions, inherited, other platforms/devices. The interoperability is contemplated in a wide sense (syntactic and semantic level) and tied to the conformity with regulations.
- Robustness, safety, maintainability and high availability: just as in a clinical routine use, the platform must maintain operating production conditions in experimental studies whose interventions can be extended for months, even years, as well as having the capacity to support multiple interventions simultaneously
- Conformity with international regulations and developments based on "open-source" software: both as recommendations of the European interoperability framework and of the WHO for e-health [53]. Conformity with regulations is an essential element to have generalizable and interoperable solutions, as well as a promoter factor of the success in the implementations and a reduction in costs. Questions related to the regulation in the exchange of data (ECR), and the interoperability between platforms/devices must be attended to.

These requirements are currently completely reachable by means of available and mature technologies such as:

- The Web technologies as a series of services associated with the Internet for the provision of e-services to users and interoperability support;
- SOA as an architecture paradigm to implement open systems and distributed services
- The "Cloud Computing" model, as a paradigm for the provision of services and technologies through the Internet, which in collaborative research environments such as PITES, allows the platform to be able to act as a "hub" for the dynamic provision of services
- A basic Internet network infrastructure based on the current convergence of the ubiquitous provision of services on IP networks.

With the support of these technologies and from the requirements, the platform has been designed as an open system of distributed services on communications based on the IP protocol. Any e-service supported by the PITES platform adopts an architecture oriented to services (SOA) and design paradigms established on the web 2.0: weak connection between services, interfaces based on "web-services", "hybrid" web applications (mashups), etc. As additional priority directives, the developments on the PITES platform must be based on "open-source" and obtaining conformity with international regulations.

The architecture of the platform is distributed on two levels (see Figure 8):

- the "front-end" of the platform, that encompasses the interaction mechanisms of the platform with the users of the system, that is, the interfaces of the entities (people or other platforms/services), and
- the "back-end", which constitutes the heart of the platform in which the structure has been defined, integration, and interdependence of the internal components of the platform and those of the "front-end" components, that is, the support of the logic of the e-services that support the interventions

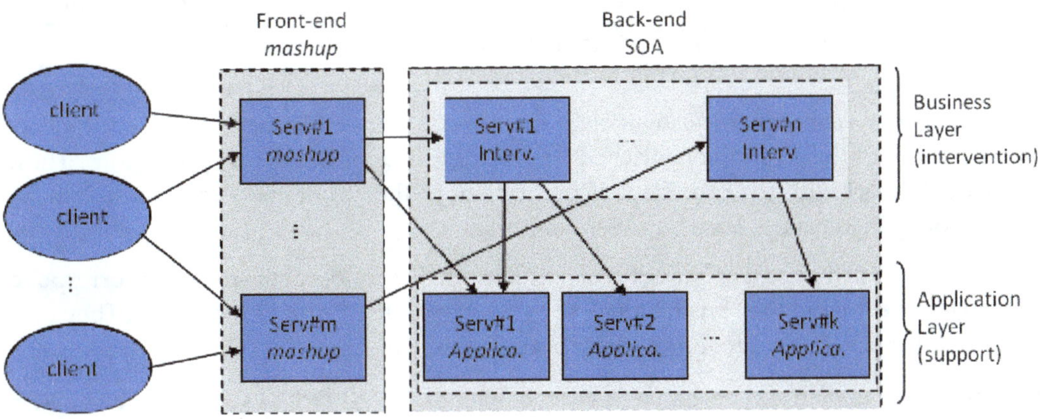


**Figure 8.** Architecture of the PITES technological platform

The "front-end" interfaces are based on applications, services and protocols based on Internet and digital cellular networks and commutated telephone networks. The platform, has a base services to support these types of intervention by means of content, server, Web SMS gateways, IVR system(Interactive Voice Response), TTS services (Text-to-speech), services ASR (Automatic Voice Recognition), streaming server managers, etc.

The design of the platform in "back-end" adopts an architecture oriented to services in two layers:

- "Business layer", in which the functionalities/services specific to the support of the interventions, the business logic of the applications and services directly linked to each intervention and which implement the requirements proper to them are deployed
- "Application layer", where the additional services with functionalities of a special and specialized character and oriented to its use by the services of the "business layer" and of the "front-end" are located. The objective of this layer is to constitute an extendable, diverse and detached series of functionalities that give support to the e-services supported by the platform in the research projects. The provision of these services is transparent and with open interfaces based on "web-services" (SOAP and REST on HTTP/HTTPS protocols). These support services can be made public (beyond the PITES community) by moving the access interface to the "front-end" layer.

From the point of view of the users to whom they are aimed, the support services and applications for the platform are of two types: those directed to the users-person, that is, patients, health professionals, health carers/caretakers or families and support staff for the experimental studies, and those directed to the users-machine, that is, to other platforms, services or monitoring devices.

The architecture adopted for the user-person applications follow a "mashup" model based on three components:

- client application, in the "front-end" of the platform, based on different technologies: WWW, WAP, J2ME, SMS, VoiceXML, accessible from commercial devices such as PC, conventional or mobile telephones, "smartphones" (Android), IP telephones, etc. These applications are located in the "front-end" of the platform
- The "mashup" component also in the "front-end", whose function is the addition of information for the creation of enriched content destined for the client applications. These services interact with the providers of the content in the "front-end" and "back-end" by means of open interfaces based on Web services.
- The providers of the content, made up of the "back-end" services of the platform correspond to the intervention in the "business layer" or services of the "application layer". They may also be other services content providers located in the "front-end".

The services of the platform designed to interact with the user-machines are those directed at monitoring devices and external services platforms (health or non-health). They have a classic "middleware" architecture so as to eliminate heterogeneous points with the external entities, brought about by the manufacturer's or third-party software, networks or different community protocols. The "middleware" is implemented by means of "gateway" type services specific to each case. These "gateway" type services can be assimilated as new "application layer" services in the "back-end", so that in this way they are available to new services in the "business layer" or "front-end" applications and therefore for any e-service that requires it.

The following example is proposed to illustrate the functioning of this architecture, consisting of the architecture required for a remote activity monitoring e-service of ICDs (Figure 9). Imagine that we want to evaluate the clinical effectiveness of a remote ICD monitoring service by means of an experimental study. The objective would be to measure the possible improvement in the health results of a group of patients to whom this type of monitoring is carried out (intervention), as opposed to another group in which a conventional monitoring is based on hospital visits. We suppose that there is a remote monitoring platform deployed by the manufacturer of the ICD that gathers the information generated by these devices and stores it in its information system (ICD Monitoring Platform). The health professional needs to periodically analyze the activity generated by the ICDs in the patients of the intervention group and combine it with other clinical information through other means. As well as this, the health professional needs to be able to send messages to these patients to give them advice, warnings, etc. As the study is framed within a clinical trial, the health professional needs to be able to carry out a random assignment of the patients in an flexible and safe manner before being included in the study as well as guaranteeing an anonymity of the identification of the patients every time it is necessary to get access to their demographic information by searching the information system of the hospital. Finally the health professional has to periodically send a summary of the clinical activity generated in the study to the ECR of the patients so that it does not become isolated in the platform that supports the intervention.

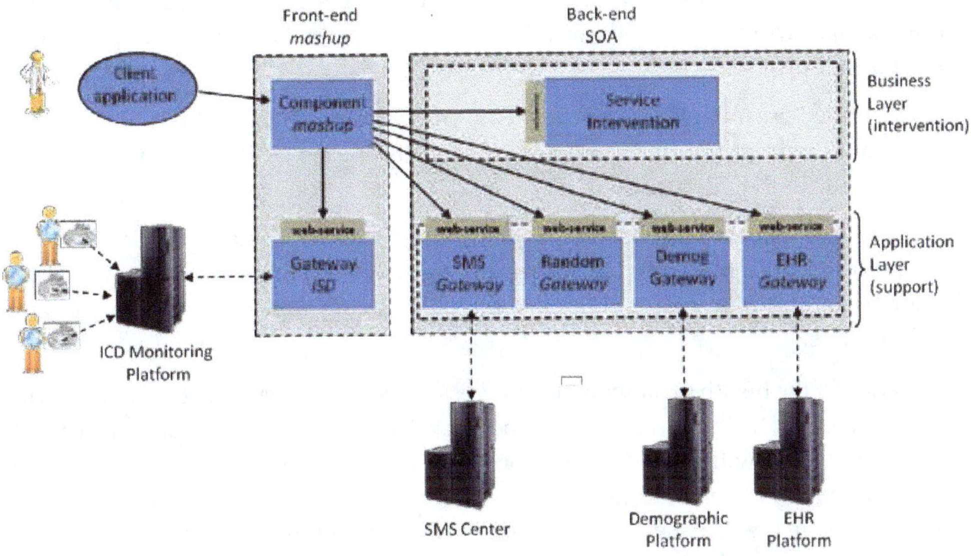


**Figure 9.** Example of the ICD e-service monitoring architecture

Within the framework of the architecture of the PITES platform, for the health professional, a client application would be implemented based on the Web to which it would be accessed securely (access control and HTTPS protocol). This application (client application) would be managed by a "mashup", component in the "front-end" of the platform that provides it access to the different sources of distributed data:

- a gateway service at the "front-end" based on "middleware" (Gateway ICD) which has the capacity to access an external monitoring ICD platform in such a way that from the client application client, the health professional can obtain information on the ICD activity of the patients of the intervention group
- a gateway service in the "application layer" of the "back-end" (SMS Gateway) which permits the sending of SMS messages. This gateway service consists of a "middleware" which manages the transactions with the SMS Center of the mobile telephone provider
- a gateway service in the "application layer" of the "back-end" (Demog Gateway) which permits access to the demographic information of the patients located in the information system of its organization. On the one hand, the "middleware" accesses the said system by means of a proprietary protocol and, on the other hand, as regards the platform, it authorizes

an interface based on the ISO EN 13606 regulation that standardizes access to this information.

- a gateway service in the "application layer" of the "back-end" (EHR Gateway) which permits the sending of summaries of the clinical activity generated by the users during the intervention to the ECR of the organization. Once the clinical information is validated by the health professional, the gateway receives an extract in accordance with the a ISO-EN 13606 regulation by means of an interface based on Web services which contains the said information and which the "middleware" sends to the hospital information system through the established protocol.
- a service in the "business layer" of the "back-end" (Service Intervention) that established the operating logic of the intervention managed by means of data bases and processes aspects specific to the intervention
- a gateway service in the "application layer" of the "back-end" (Random Gateway) which permits access through an interface based on Web services to a centralized randomizing service making the robust distribution of the patients in the two established assignment groups possible.

The application of the health professional has access to a specific service in the "business layer" (service intervention), to a specific service in the "front-end" (ICD gateway) and to four services oriented to general use within the "application layer" of the "back-end" by means of his or her "mashup" component. While the client application together with the "mashup" component′, the service located in the "business layer" and the gateway ICD, are specific to the intervention, the gateway services of the "application layer" are also resources accessible for any other intervention that supports the platform. As an additional element, it is evident that to carry out the implementation of the study, the minimum is to commit resources to be contributed to the structure of the health organization.

The SOA architecture of the PITES platform makes it possible for the services that are initially specified for an intervention to be able to be promoted to services of general use because of its interest, use, and functionality. The weak connection between the services through the Web services interfaces allows functionalities to be added or taken away with relative ease. Following the "cloud computing" paradigm, these services can be used and evolved for future experiments in the PITES community, even making them accessible to the global community. This possibility gives the platform a significant advantage in the promotion of collaborative research in this field as well as being able to put the progressive implementation strategies into practice so that the platform can act as a temporary support to platforms in "clinical routine".

#### *3.2.1. Component hardware*

The PITES platform has an autonomous functioning (without the need for operators) on a 24x7 regime. The platform is accessible through Internet by means of a redundant link and has the capacity to establish point-to-point VPN with other networks. In order to achieve this demanding working regime, there is a robust telematic infrastructure available in many of its components (communications, storage).

The platform consists at the physical level of a segmented Internet-accessible network including: 9 physical and virtual servers (Xen) on IBM xSeries equipment over Linux OS (Suse Linux Enterprise); SAN/NAS (IBM N3600) redundant storage networks; backup library systems (TSM and IBM System Storage TS3200 Tape Library).

As basic support for e-services the platform provides a number of different general services: WWW service (Apache), DBMS (MySQL, PostgreSQL), applications managers (Tomcat), content managers (Drupal, LifeRay), "e-learning" server (Moodle), VoiceXML/IVR (VXI*/ Asterisk) service, TTS/ASR (Verbio) engines.

The platform includes security elements at different levels: control access (physical and telematic) policies, (storage and communications) redundancy and monitoring tools (Nagios/ Cacti).

### 3.3. Services

The specific services currently provided by the platform include:

Messenger service: telematic service accessible through the Internet which implements the possibility of sending short SMS messages, usually from the health professionals sent to the patients for notifications, warnings, advice, etc. The service interacts with the SMS Centers of the telephone operators via GSMs available on the platform.

Two conditions are demanded from the SMS service:

- that the SMS messages are delivered to the addressee and if not, get notification that it has not (together with the causes) and
- that the SMS messages are delivered after a certain period of time so that the validity of its content is not indefinite.

Obviously the SMS service offered by the GSM is highly reliable although none of the two conditions demanded can be guaranteed 100%. However, the SMS service has mechanisms available that make it possible to know the current state of the SMS messages together with the occasional incidents that could take place in transit to the destination terminal. The SMS Centers offer the possibility of sending reports to the sender on the progress of the SMS (DLR, Delivery Reports). By means of the DLR request by message, the SMS service of the central station is capable of knowing whether a message is still in transit, has been delivered to the addressee (with time and date of receipt), or not or has been eliminated (together with its cause).

Equally, the SMS service is capable of establishing the period of validity ("validity period") of each message, exceeding which, if it has not been delivered to the addressee, it instructs the SMS Center in order to eliminate the said message from its lists (accompanied by the corresponding DLR report). The period of validity chosen depends on different factors and can vary from just a few hours to several days; its choice for example, in the case of communications to patients, depends on the medical protocol followed in the specific scenario. However, it is not a critical aspect in other types of task, and the default expiry period is not extended.

Another limitation of SMS messages is the nominal limitation in the total number of characters that can be included in each message, and which is fixed at 160. This length is very limiting in the majority of notifications from the doctor to the patient. It is also impractical for the doctor to send consecutive messages to the patient referring to the same matter (one of them might not arrive or arrive in the wrong order, etc.). However, there is the technical possibility of generating messages that are longer than usual ( "long SMS" calls) and which are segmented at the origin and later reassembled by the patient's mobile telephone in a way transparent to the user, and therefore permitting the sending of arbitrarily long messages. This functionality is supported by the SMS service of the platform.

Functionally, access to the SMS messages server is carried out by means of the HTTP/SOAP1.1/1.2. "web-services" interface. In each request to send, the following is indicated: addressee of the message, text of the message, need for confirmation of delivery, period of validity and preferred time period for sending the message (or immediate delivery). Once the request is accepted a univocal identifier is generated with the service applicant and the sending procedure commences with an adjustment of the parameters of the message (establishment of the output queue, internal register, etc). The SMS service is in charge of sending the message through one of the available GSM modems. From the moment of sending the message to the corresponding SMS Center, the progress of the SMS is monitored through to the reception of the corresponding DLR. Before the arrival of each DLR message, the SMS messages server analyzes its content and notifies the state to the corresponding service that requested its sending in such a way that the state of the messages can be known at all times.

By means of a widely available mobile service, this service authorizes, by means of an open interface, a way of indirect communication between health professionals and patients with a high level of security (delivery security and range of validity), and personalization (flexibility in the size of the message and the establishment of the preferred period of time for delivery).

Randomizing service: telematic service accessible through the Internet that implements support to the randomizing process of clinical trials in a centralized way. The service deploys the following functionalities:

- Simultaneous support to randomizing in multiple studies
- Complete management of the randomizing process by the promoter of the clinical trial
- Randomizing support in different modalities: simple, by block, stratified, centralized and blind
- Assignation lists of up to 6 groups with the capacity for self-replication
- Control of transactions to guarantee the integrity for the applicants of the assignation
- Generation statistics of the randomizing progress upon request

The service establishes three levels of privilege (overall administrator, project administrator, project user):

- The "overall administrator" user (level 1), has the capacity to create new projects and administer the functioning of the overall service; each project corresponds to a clinical trial.

The process of creating a new project has the aim of authorizing the permission, structures and data necessary for its configuration in the service. Once the new project is created, the figure of the administrator "project administrator" already associated to a specific study is established.

- The "project administrator" (level 2), has the capacity to create the structure of the process of randomizing the clinical trial: total sample, number of assigned groups (identified successively by: A, B, C, D, E, F), variable block sizes (multiples of the number of assignation groups), and the stratification tree (if required). The "project administrator" has the capacity to open/interrupt/close the randomizing process, and request progress statistics on the randomizing (overall, by time intervals, by stratum, etc.)
- The "project user" (level 3), whose function is basically to request the assignments to groups in a specific study.

The service does not establish limits on the studies in relation to the total number of stratification levels. A random assignment list is generated for each stratification branch with as many assignment groups as have been established to guarantee the assignment balance in groups of varying sized blocks. Each randomizing request that the service carries out is associated to a transaction identifier which the service may propose or generated dynamically, in such a way that it is possible to control each assignment individually in relation not only to the activity register but also the recovery in real time of errors in the process. The randomizing service includes internal functionalities for the register of auditing in each clinical trial. In relation to the generation of the project and the assignment tables, the randomizing seed is stored which makes it possible to guarantee the integrity of the assignment lists and their reproduction. It also generates a series of daily files on the degree of activity and functioning of the server, created and updated dynamically by date/time/project/user access/action carried out.

The service is accessible through an interface based on Web services by means of the SOAP (1.1/1.2) protocol and transport on the HTTPS service. This randomizing service has the advantage of basing its functionality on an open interface for the integral management of the process. This approximation makes it possible to promote the clinical trial, design and develop client applications in the measurement of their requirements and resources, incorporating the randomizing process transparently as another element/service in the management of its clinical trial.

Clinical information service: telematic service which stores and retrieves clinical information compliant with the ISO EN 13606 standard. In is based upon a web services structure with two groups of functionalities: the input of information and its querying/retrieval. The input of information is performed through an interface compliant with part 5 of the standard which accepts extracts codified in XML. The service processes the received information before storing it in order to obtain features which permit to classify it and enable its ulterior querying and retrieval. To do so for one side complete extracts are stored (preserving the integrity of the information) and for the other a relational database is built where the obtained features are kept in order. The querying/retrieval of information presents three options:

- Querying of the information through a graphical interface: the user, after identification, has access to a browser which permits him or her to navigate through the information, but only to that part on which it has permissions depending on his/her role (access control compliant with part 4 of the 13606 standard). This functionality makes use of the archetype server service in order to obtain those used in the generation of the information and be able to present the data in a complete manner and in the language or using the terminologies desired by the user (if they are defined and mapped in the archetype).
- Retrieval of a patient's information: web service which permits to request a given patient's information using an interface compliant with part 5 of the standard. Through this service the user can request (utilizing other application, service or system) the whole information stored in a person's record or a part of it, obtaining an extract with the requested compositions and complaining the corresponding access restrictions.
- Information queries: the service also offers the possibility to pose specific queries oriented to the statistical processing of the total population in the repository and yielding numerical results about prevalence of diseases or concurrence of problems.

Archetype repository service: telematic service which stores and retrieves archetypes compliant with the model established in the standard: archetypes are transferred in text files codified in the ADL language and using an interface compatible with part 5 of the 13606 standard. The system stores archetypes according the reference model normalized in part 2, which enables to perform searches using any identification data or any state of the archetype and also through the meaning of the nodes (specified as restrictions to the RECORD_COMPONENT class of the reference model of the extracts) defined in it. The retrieval/querying of archetypes permits two possibilities:

- Retrieval of archetypes: following the specifications of the interface defined in part 5 of the standard this automatic service enables to retrieve archetypes through its identifier, concept, terminology, language or those that are specializations or have been specialized by another archetype. This service is oriented to its use by other services, applications or even other external systems.
- Archetype querying: the server offers a web graphical browser for users to navigate through the archetypes repository; to query them through concept or type; see their specializations and download them to be used in their own projects.

Following the philosophy of the double model in the standard, this service permits the archetype querying in an open fashion.

Demographic information service: this service stores and provides demographic information of the entities involved in the clinical information systems. It is based upon the demographic information model included in the reference model of part 1 in the standard; this permits to deal with persons (patients and health professionals) and also with organizations or devices and programs in use. This service keeps track of all the identifiers assigned to each entity, including official entities but also those assigned internally by organizations, for instance in specific projects. This working method allows to separate demographic information from the rest of data facilitating to make information anonym. For security reasons this service is not accessible from the outside of the platform so that its possible clients may only be its running applications or other supplied services.

Anonymisation service: this service enables to make anonym clinical information to be used in secondary uses such as research or statistics. This service accepts and returns extracts compliant with the standard reference model, codified in XML. Received extracts are analyzed to suppress the identification of the patient including demographic information codified in class IDENTIFIED_ENTITY of the reference model, even though the year of birthday (not including day and month) and the sex of the patient may be preserved for statistical purposes. To do so, a new randomized identifier is assigned and substituted in the extract. This service makes use of the demographic service in order to maintain a record of the identifiers in use so that if further information about the same patient arrives its identifier can be assigned and the health information repository remains coherent. For this reason it is possible to install this service and the demographic service in the client side so that the information about the person does not leave the organization where it was generated and the clinical information is presented anonym to the outside world.

## 4. Results of the platform

Projects supported by the PITES platform since 2004 are described below. The list is not exhaustive. Those that have been considered as of greater interest have been included. From 2009 the platform has been open to other Spanish research groups.

### 4.1. Finalized projects

- Impact of Patient–General Practitioner Short-Messages-Based Interaction on the Control of Hypertension in a Follow-up Service for Low-to-Medium Risk Hypertensive Patients: A Randomized Controlled Trial. (FIS 01/0915. SEP 1201/02. AIRMED II Program). [54]

– Main objective. To evaluate a telemedicine system for Primary Attention; improve the control and monitoring of arterial hypertension. Secondary objectives: Measure its effect on perceived health and anxiety.

– Type of study. Multicenter randomized controlled trial. 285 patients were enrolled by 38 GPs from 21 health centers in four different health areas in Madrid, Spain. October 2004-June 2006. Intervention period, 6 months.

– Description intervention. The coordination office set up appointments with the patients of both the TmG and the CG for training in self-blood pressure monitoring (SBPM) and the use of the digital sphygmomanometer (both groups) and the telephone (only TmG). During the six-month follow-up period, the TmG patients sent their mean self-measured SBP (sSBP) and DBP (sDBP), based on three measurements made at 3-min intervals under fasting conditions in the morning and at night, four times a week (Monday and Thursday, morning and night), and their pulse rate and weight once a week. During each WAP session, they had the option of responding to a simple questionnaire. At some later moment, with no obligation imposed by the protocol in terms of frequency of access to the CS, the GPs accessed the data sent by their patients via the Web. According to his or her own criteria, the GP could send an SMS regarding any related issue to the patient's phone. The CG patients followed the same SBPM protocol, with the exception that the results were recorded on paper in a data collection notebook; they sent no data to the CS, and thus, had no interaction with their GPs. They continued to make their scheduled visits to their GPs at their corresponding center, as they had done prior to the study.

– Study variables. The main outcome measure, referred to by us as the degree of hypertension control, was the percentage of patients who were not optimally controlled at the time of the final visit. Optimal control was defined as a mean of three arterial pressure determinations carried out by a professional during the final visit, resulting in pSBP ≤ 140 mmHg and pDBP ≤90 mmHg. The secondary outcome measures were: 1) the changes in pSBP and pDBP between the initial and final visits measured in the office of the GP; 2) the changes in the mean self-measured sSBP, sDBP, and HR throughout the intervention period; 3) the changes in the dimensions of the brief profiles of the SF-36 Health Survey physical component summary (PCS) and mental component summary (MCS) and in the state anxiety (SA) and trait anxiety (TA), according to the State–Trait Anxiety Inventory (STAI); and 4) the number of consultations and hospital admissions in the two groups.

– Results. A) Degree of hypertension control. The number of patients exhibiting poor control at the final visit, was the case in 31.7% of the patients in the TmG and in 35.7% of those in the CG, (difference: 4.0%, 95% CI: −7.0% to 14.9%) there being no significant difference (p = 0.47). B) Change in hypertension during follow-up. In the comparison of the measurements carried out by the GPs at the initial and final visits, the TmG presented a decrease in pSBP of 15.5 mmHg and a decrease in pDBP of 9.6 mmHg, while in the CG, the pSBP decreased by 11.9 mmHg and the pDBP by 4.4 mmHg, decreases that did not differ significantly (pSBP: p=0.13; pDBP: p=0.40). The mean values for self-measured sSBP, sDBP, and HR (TmG: 131.6, 78.7, 70.1; CG: 132.4, 78.0, 69.7) throughout the six-month period, calculated according to the area under the curve, were not significantly different between the two groups (sSBP: p = 0.52; sDBP: p = 0.50; and HR: p = 0.79).

– Comments. There are no significant differences between the two groups in terms of the degree of hypertension control, measured as the number of poorly controlled patients at the final visit, given that the intention to treat analysis adds those that dropped out prior to the initial visit (TmG: n = 11; CG: n = 1) and those occurring during follow-up (TmG: n = 4; CG: n = 10) to the number of poorly controlled patients who underwent follow-up (TmG: n = 30; CG: n = 40). However self-blood pressure monitoring brings about improvements in hypertension control, given that the percentage of controlled patients in the final visit is greater in TmG. The reduction obtained in pSBP and pDBP in the TmG are consistent with the values reported by other authors, independent of the intervention selected.

- Evaluation of a Telemedicine-Based Service for the Follow-Up and Monitoring of Patients Treated With Oral Anticoagulant Therapy. (FIS 02/1156. SEP 1201/02. AIRMED II Program). [55]

– Main objective: To find out the acceptability and satisfaction of the patients who have a supervised system of self-controlled INR measurement, with home follow up by means of telemedicine based on mobile telephony within the ambit of Primary Attention. Secondary objectives: To determine the degree of control suitable for oral anticoagulant treatment achieved by patients, users of the system. To describe the eventual factors which condition a bad control. Clinically relevant possible accidents (hemorrhage and thrombosis) suffered by the patients in the study.

– Type of study. Quasi-experimental study, with two differentiated groups. 108 patients included in a Health Center in Pozuelo, Madrid, Spain. December 2004 -March 2006. Intervention period, 12 months

– Description intervention. The patients in the TmG were trained in the use of the coagulometer and the cellular phone by staff from the coordination office. At the beginning and end of the study, the patients in both the groups completed the quality of life questionnaire specific to anticoagulated patients designed by Sawicki; the SF-12 quality of life questionnaire for application in the general population; and the STAI to assess anxiety. The patients in the TmG measured their own INR every 3 weeks if they met the criteria for good control; otherwise, their GP proposed the date for the next determination and modification of the TWD. After each self-measurement, the patients sent their INR values and responded yes or no via a safe WAP session, to questions concerning another six clinical parameters, such as omission or duplication of doses, ingestion of new drugs, alcohol intake, changes in diet, fever, and intercurrent diseases, in order to define the causes of poor control.

– Study variables. Data on safety and the degree of control: a) Number of determinations made by each patient and their correlation with adequate INR control; b) number of determinations falling in and out of the target INR range, with the possible reasons for poor control; c) time during which each patient was in or out of the target INR range, measured using standard methods--linear interpolation and in or out of range; and d) the incidence of adverse events associated with OAT (death, hemorrhagic complications, and thrombosis) in the two groups. Data concerning the acceptability of the change: a) The degree of compliance with the protocol in the TmG, measured both in the patients and the GPs and b) changes in the results of the three questionnaires provided at the beginning and end of the study.

– Results. (A) Degree of INR control. There were no significant differences between the two groups in terms of INR control. In all, 57.6% of the determinations in the TmG and 60.1% of those made in the CG were within this range. The patients in the TmG were in the target range (linear interpolation method) 65.4% of the time over a mean participation in the project of 329.4 days. In the CG, the patients were within the range 68.0% of the time over a mean duration of participation of 310.1 days. For the same variable measured by means of the in or out of range method, the rates were 66.6% in the TmG and 68.9% in the CG, over the same mean participation time. The number of INR determinations within the target range, the number of days spent within the range according to the two conventional methods, and the distance, defined as the deviation of the INR determination from the center of the range for each patient, were also assessed. (B) Deaths, Complications, and Hospital Admissions. There were three deaths in each group; there were no major complications in the TmG and only one in the CG. There were six minor complications, four in the TmG and two in the CG, and three cases of thromboembolism, one in the TmG and two in the CG. In the TmG, there was one hospital admission associated with OAT versus two due to other causes; in the CG, the incidence was three versus one, respectively. (C) Acceptability of the Change. With the exception of two patients, who received no help from the family and rejected the proposal for fear of being incapable of using the coagulometer and the cellular phone, all the patients were capable of self-testing and remained active in the project throughout the entire intervention period. The training sessions, held in groups of five patients, were approximately 2 h long, and were followed by a preregistered period of 1–2 weeks. In five cases, the INR measurement and WAP sessions were always carried out by a relative; in three cases, the patients did not even attend the training sessions, given their instability.

The patients in the TmG determined their INR on or around the date that had been indicated by the GP; 45.5% of the determinations were carried out on the designated day and 74.8% were carried out within 3 days, either before or after, of that date, indicating a high rate of adherence to the protocol, despite the freedom granted to the patients.

The degree of compliance on the part of the GPs, measured as the time elapsed before they responded to a message from a patient, was very high; 48.5% of the total weekly dosage was sent on the same day and 43.8% within 3 days of the reception of the message.

– Comments. The e-service exhibits highly positive features in terms of acceptability of the procedure, satisfaction, and quality of life, and reduces the number of visits to the healthcare center.

- Evaluation of a Telemedicine Service for the Secondary Prevention of Coronary Artery Disease. (TSI2005-02682. FIS PI05-1882. Programa MOBIS). [56]

– Main objective. To analyze the efficacy of a new telemonitoring system for the following up of patients with coronary heart disease (CHD), connecting patients, provided with self-measurement devices, and care managers through mobile phone messages over the Web, and integrating the monitoring of several cardiovascular risk factors (CRF), as a toll for secondary prevention.

– Type of study. A single-blind, randomized controlled, clinical trial. 203 acute coronary syndrome (ACS) survivors, was conducted at a hospital in Madrid, Spain. December 2007 - January 2010. Intervention period: 12 months.

– Description intervention. TmG patients were temporarily provided with an automatic sphygmomanometer, a glucose and lipid meter and a cellular phone, and support staff if needed, were taught to measure their blood pressure (BP), heart rate and weight (weekly), and glucose and lipids (monthly), and to send the results through their mobile phones following a structured questionnaire (WAP session). A cardiologist accessed the biological and clinical data via a secure Web application and, through this application, sent individualized short message service text messages with recommendations to the patients. At exit, subjects in the TmG completed an additional questionnaire to evaluate satisfaction with the program.

– Study variables. Outcome measures were resting BP, body mass index (BMI), smoking status, LDL-c, and glycated hemoglobin A1c (HbA1c), all measured at the initial and final visits for comparison. Their smoking status was determined by self-report and confirmed by a 1-step cotinine immunoassay in urine. The primary outcome was cardiovascular risk improvement (CRI), defined as the proportion of patients who achieve the goal of treatment in at least 1 CRF without exacerbation of any of the others. Treatment goals were as follows: (1) smoking cessation, (2) LDL-c less than 100 mg/dL, (3) BP lower than 140/90 mmHg, and (4) HbA1c less than 7%. Exacerbation of a CRF was defined as a 10% or more increase in BP, LDL-c, or HbA1c, with respect to initial levels. Secondary outcomes were: the proportion of patients achieving the treatment goal in each of the outcome measurements, quantitative changes in LDL-c, BP, BMI, and HbA1c (in diabetic patients), and changes in quality of life and level of anxiety.

– Results. Four patients were lost in the followup (1.9%) and 5 died (2.5%), all in the CG. Seventeen patients left the study (8.4%), 12 in the TmG (11.8%) and 5 in the CG (4.9%) (RR = 2.38; 95% CI = 0.87-6.50; P =.08). Reasons for leaving the program in the TmG were stress associated with the use of the telemonitoring equipment in 3 patients, personal reasons in 7, and inability to handle the equipment in 2 patients; in the CG, all 5 attributed it to personal reasons.

Analysis on the basis of intention to treat showed that patients in the TmG were more likely (RR = 1.4; 95% CI = 1.1-1.7) to experience improvement in their CRF profile than patients in the CG (P =.010) at the end of 12 months. More TmG patients achieved the treatment goal in BP (62.1% vs 42.9%, P =.012; RR =1.4, 95% CI = 1.1-1.9) and in HbA1c among diabetic patients (86.4% vs 54.2%, P =.018; RR = 1.6; 95% CI = 1.1-2.4); there were no between-group differences for smoking cessation (80.7% vs 81.0%, P =.964; RR = 1.0; 95% CI = 0.9-1.1) or LDL-c (76.2% vs 76.6%, P =.948; RR = 1.0; 95% CI = 0.9-1.2).

Quantitative changes in continuous variables with comparison of the difference between the groups: Patients in the TmG showed significant changes in all variables with the exception of diastolic BP (DBP) (systolic BP [SBP], P =.0460; DBP, P =.237; LDL-c, P =.027; HbA1c, P =.001; BMI in overweight patients P =.003). In the CG, significant reductions were obtained in LDL-c and DBP (SBP, P =.780; DBP, P =.001; LDL-c, P =.098; HbA1c, P =.239; BMI, P =.299). Body mass index diminished in the TmG and increased slightly in the CG. Triglyceride levels also decreased significantly in the TmG (P =.0001), but not in the CG (P =.435). No differences between-groups were found in physical activity (75% TmG vs 73% CG, P =.756) or medication adherence (99% in both groups, P =.980) both self-reported by patients. Nutritional habits were not explored. There were no significant differences between the scores obtained in SF-36 and State-Trait Anxiety Inventory tests at the initial visit in the 2 groups and changes were not significant between groups. At 12 months, the SF-36 "physical health" scale showed a 2.8-point increase in the TmG (P =.011) and a 1.5-point increase in the CG (P =.16). The change was smaller in the "mental health" scale, with a 0.5-point increase in the TMG (P =.64) and a 0.5-point decrease (P =.73) in the CG.

(B) Protocol acceptability: Adherence to protocol was measured by the percentage of WAP sessions held (89.2% ± 16.0). Almost all patients (98%) completed more than 50% of WAP sessions and more than 83% completed more than 75% of them. Only 0.5 messages per patient were missed, due to the mobile phone being turned off. Family support of the TmG patients was analyzed at 4 different levels: never (58% of patients), first week only (10%), 1 month (7%), and always (25%).

– Comments. A telemonitoring program, via mobile phone messages, appears to be useful for improving the risk profile in ACS survivors and can be an effective tool for secondary prevention, especially for overweight patients.

Other already carried out and finished projects are described briefly below

- Control and monitoring of self-care plans in asthma by means of a telemedicine platform. (FIS 02/1391. SEP 1201/02. AIRMED II Program). [57].

– Main objective. To evaluate the efficacy of a monitoring and self-care program for asthmatic patients based on telemedicine services. Secondary objectives: To evaluate the efficacy of the program as regards the adhesion to the self-care plans and to the adhesion to the monitoring of the FEM and FEV1. To evaluate the efficacy of the program as regards the clinical evolution of the asthma and quality of life of the patients with asthma.

– Type of study. Quasi-experimental project with two differentiated groups: study and control. 37 patients of the Pneumology Unit of the Hospital Universitario Puerta de Hierro, Madrid, Spain. October 2004 –May 2007. Intervention period, 12 months.

– Description intervention. All of the patients have their FEM and FEV1 monitored daily (morning and evening) (volume expired in the first second), by means of a portable spirometer, their symptoms and the medication taken. Those of the CG entered their data manually on ad-hoc designed forms and acted in accordance with the guidelines given during the consultation. The patients of the TmG followed the same medical protocol, although unlike the control group, they had the permanent support of the telemedicine platform which sent the protocol information by means of a mobile telephone (spirometry through CSD-GSM transmission, and symptoms and actions by means of a WAP session on GPRS-GSM). The patients of the TmG immediately and automatically received an SMS message as a reply which included information on their current state and the recommended medication guidelines in accordance with their personalized plan. The doctor also has permanent access to the information sent and evolution of each TmG patient so that he or she could individually supervise the development of the self-care plans.

– Results. There we no significant differences as regards the monitoring of the FEV1 at home and in the consultations of the study group. Compliance with the self-care plans was 70% in more than half of the patients. Adherence to the self-treatment plans was greater in the study group (95.28%) than in the control (93.09%).

– Comments. The tool that was designed to help in the decision-making process was highly evaluated by both the patients and professionals.

- AmIVital. Digital personal environment for health and wellbeing. (CENIT2007-1010). [58].

Within the (2008-2011) framework of a great technological project in which companies such as Siemens, Telefónica, Ericsson and Telvent have participated, together with 4 SMEs and 8 Universities and Public research Centers, our group has carried out the following studies:

– Study of the prevalence and co-morbidity of heart failure in the family practice. [59].

– Type of study. A cross-sectional, observational descriptive study set in a health area of the Community of Madrid, Spain. The study was carried out in a population of 198 670 individuals over 14 years of age, attended to by 129 specialists in family medicine. The patient was considered to have HF when this diagnosis (ICPC code K77) appeared in his or her electronic medical record. The prevalence of HF was quantified and its association with another 25 chronic diseases was analyzed.

– Results. The prevalence of HF was 6.9%, 7.9% among women and 5.9% among men. Patients with HF had a high rate of chronic co-morbidity, with an average of 5.2 + 2.1 chronic diseases. Only 3% of the patients present with isolated HF and >60% have four or more additional chronic problems. Hypertension, cardiac arrhythmias, hyperlipidaemia, obesity and diabetes mellitus are the chronic diseases most frequently detected in HF patients.

– Comments. Patients with HF frequently visit the offices of family physicians, presenting with a high rate of cardiac and non-cardiac co-morbidity that proves to be a challenge on the clinical level and in terms of the organization of health care services.

– Study of disability measured by WHO-DAS II. [60].

– Type of study. Samples of consecutive patients diagnosed with COPD (102), CHF (99), and stroke (99) were taken from 1,053 primary care users in the southern area of the autonomous region of Madrid. The patients were informed of the study and were assessed in their homes by trained field workers using the World Health Organization Disability Assessment Schedule II (WHO-DAS II).

– Results. None of the groups had extreme disability on their overall WHO-DAS II scores. The prevalence of severe disability differed among the groups and was highest for stroke and CHF (33.33% and 29.29%, respectively) and lowest for COPD (14.71%). The three groups shared two similar traits, namely, a higher prevalence of disability among women than men, and a specific pattern by domain, with the highest prevalence of severe/extreme limitations being found in household life activities and mobility. Severe restrictions in Social Participation were more frequent in patients with stroke and CHF. The group with moderate disability according to the overall WHODAS II score (n=94) showed a high prevalence of severe limitations in mobility, life activities and self-care.

– Comments. Disability among non-institutionalized persons with COPD, CHF and stroke is frequent and shows gender- and domain-related patterns similar to those described in a population-based study performed using the WHO-DAS II in elderly persons in Spain. ICF-validated disability categories could be useful in epidemiological surveys, individual assessments and primary care data monitoring systems.

– Co-morbidity Patterns in Patients with Chronic Diseases in General Practice. [61].

– Type of study. A cross-sectional study was conducted in a health-area setting of the Madrid Autonomous Region, covering a population of 198,670 individuals aged over 14 years old. Multiple correspondences were analyzed to identify the clustering patterns of the conditions targeted.

– Results. Forty-two percent (95% confidence interval [CI]: 41.8–42.2) of the registered population had at least one chronic condition. In all, 24.5% (95% CI: 24.3–24.6) of the population presented with multi-morbidity. In the correspondence analysis, 98.3% of the total information was accounted for by three dimensions. The following four, age- and sex-related co-morbidity patterns were identified: pattern B, showing a high co-morbidity rate; pattern C, showing a low co-morbidity rate; and two patterns, A and D, showing intermediate co-morbidity rates.

– Comments. Four co-morbidity patterns could be identified which grouped diseases as follows: one showing diseases with a high co-morbidity burden; one showing diseases with a low co-morbidity burden; and two showing diseases with an intermediate co-morbidity burden.

### 4.2. Current projects

#### *4.2.1. Our own projects*

Current projects as envisaged projects of our group are described briefly below.

- Monitoring of the elderly in assisted spaces for independent living. [FIS PI08-0435]

– Main objective. : To study how the monitoring of domestic activities may help to achieve a better overall geriatric evaluation and better attention to the elderly in their homes.

– Type of study. Pilot study with 30 patients at a geriatric unit at the Hospital Universitario Ramón y Cajal, Madrid, Spain. Commencement: February 2010.

– Intervention description. Two information methods were used: one subjective, by means of an integrated evaluation scale: Barthel, Lawton-Brody, Mini-Nutritional, Mini-Mental State Exam, Geriatric Depression Scale, Morisky-Green and Short Physical Performance Battery). Another objective: by means of an environmental monitoring. The following was installed in the homes of each patient: 5 presence detectors, 2 magnetic door opening sensors (refrigerator and front door), 2 pressure sensors (bed and armchair), 1 sensor in their pill box, 1 for the use of the telephone, for a week-10 days to obtain basic values for the behavior pattern.

– Study variables. 15 items were analyzed related to: Therapeutic Control, In-house Mobility, Outdoor Mobility, Personal Hygiene, Cleanliness: Urination/Bowel movements, Dressing, Domestic activities, Emotional, Memory, Orientation, Meals, Personal, Telephone use.

– Comments. Finalization 1st phase envisaged December 2012.

– Monitoring of an advanced Spanish EPOC cohort (CEPA). [FIS PS09-01787].

– Main objective. Describe the clinical course of the EPOC in terms of clinical data, functional and radiological. Secondary objectives: Describe the incident mortality and causes of death.

Describe the phenotypic features and group them together in their respective dimensions or factors. Describe the assorted and incident morbidity. Describe the health care load on the health system (use of medication and frequency of doctor and hospitals consultations). Explore the viability of the application of the weekly questionnaires.

– Type of study. Observational study, longitudinal and concurrent of two groups of patients with advanced EPOC. 214 patients were enrolled by 32 pneumologists and followed by 32 nurses from 32 hospitals from all of the regions, Spain. Commenced November 2011. Intervention period: 18 months.

– Intervention description. In both groups: Programmed weekly visits to pneumonological services of the corresponding hospital. The TmG patients will answer a weekly questionnaire from home of 12 questions related to their state of health. They can choose the internet, mobile telephone or interactive voice by means of a fixed or mobile telephone (IVR) to fill in and send their weekly questionnaire.

– Study variables. In the weekly visits of both groups: personal and demographic data, health model, diagnostics, risk factors, symptoms, signs, current treatment, use of resources, quality of life (CAT), anxiety/depression (HAD), as well as tests to determine biochemical and blood count, pulmonary function, blood-gas analysis, BODE, blood, TAC, echocardiogram. In the weekly questionnaire: a) degree of breathlessness, b) fever, c) expectoration, d) nocturnal symptoms, e) treatment, f) level of activity, g) tobacco, and h) use of health resources.

– Comments. Finalization envisaged in October 2013.

- REHABILITA. Disruptive technologies for future rehabilitation. [CENIT2009-1043]. [62]

Support the interoperability in the development of the project by means of the use of medical report services and archetypes of the PITES platform. The medical report services and archetypes are used as a support for the sending and consulting of information from the monitoring devices of the patients during the development of the REHABILITA services platform.

Semantically interoperable interconnection of the servers of the REHABILITA platform with the information systems of the health centers involved. The PITES platform is being used as an information and archetypes buffer for the reading of the information of the systems of the health organizations (acquisition of data for the preparation of therapeutic explanations) and for the storage of the results of the rehabilitation sessions in the electronic clinical records storage systems.

Development in the PITES platform of an observatory of disruptive technologies in rehabilitation as a collaboration Web space of the researchers of the project; by means of its analysis and study; then applying it in the aspects of use for innovation activities in the said domain.

– Comments. Finalization envisaged April 2013.

- PITES-ISA. Innovation platform in new telemedicine and e-health services: Definition, design and development of tools for interoperability, patient safety and help in decision making. [FIS PI12-00508.]

– Main objective. Updating of the PITES platform through the creation of an environment for the development of technological support of new devices for biomedical, contextual and environmental monitoring, and new applications and services based on Internet and Internet devices. The inclusion of new archetypes and knowledge management server and a new medical report and information management server. Development of: a) new client applications for access to both servers, b) safety policy in accordance with ISO EN 13606, and c) applications for advanced visualization.

– Comments. Commencement envisaged January 2013.

*4.2.2. Projects of other groups*

In 2009 the possibility opened up for the PITES platform to be used by other research groups within the Spanish National Health Service. Without describing them for reasons of confidentiality, current projects and envisaged projects are cited below.

- Current projects, which are envisaged to finish throughout 2013.
- Monitoring and control based on telemedicine patients with (TAO-E) oral anticoagulation treatment. [FIS PI09-90094]. Bioengineering and Telemedicine Unit. Hospital Universitario Puerta de Hierro. Majadahonda. Madrid.
- Methods and tools for the design and implementation of telemedicine and e-health services for the attention of chronic patients. [FIS PI09-90518]. Hospital Universitario Virgen del Rocío. Sevilla. Andalucía.
- Integral attention to aged chronic-dependent people. Evaluation of the interlinked provision of health and social services - (AYUDA). [FIS PI09-90549]. Barbastro Health Sector. Huesca. Aragón.
- Hospitalization at home and rare illnesses in Navarra. Evaluation of the home health care and identification of added-value e-health services. [FIS PI09-90317]. Medical-Technological Complex of Navarra. Pamplona. Navarra.
- Innovative health care services integrated for chronic patients. [FIS PI09-90634]. Hospital Clinic. Barcelona. Cataluña.
- Effectiveness of a telemedicine program in the monitoring and control de patients con metabolic syndrome within the ambit of primary attention. [FIS PI09/90285]. Management of Primary Attention. Albacete. Castilla la Mancha.
- Approved projects, envisaged to begin throughout 2013.
- T-CUIDAENCASA: Innovation platform at home telemedicine services. [FIS PI12/00673]. Barbastro Health Sector. Huesca. Aragón
- Regional scalability of the integrated attention services and aid in the clinical decision. [FIS PI12-01241]. Hospital Clínic de Barcelona. Cataluña.

- Implementation of tools to aid in the decision, interoperability and safety for an e-service for the early detection of exacerbations in EPOC patients "frequent-user phenotype ". [FIS PI12/01305]. Hospital Universitario Puerta de Hierro. Majadahonda. Madrid.
- Development de a system of at home attention for rheumatologic patients. [FIS PI2-01415]. Hospitalario Universitario Complex A Coruña. Galicia.
- PREVICA MULTICANAL. Contribution of telemedicine to the health care continuity of the complex chronic patient. [FIS PI12-01433]. Hospital Universitario Marqués de Valdecilla. Santander. Cantabria.
- Definition, design and development of tools and services based on standards for the support of the clinical decision and personalized medicine. [FIS PI12-01571]. Hospital Universitario Virgen del Rocío. Sevilla. Andalucía.

## 5. Conclusion

This chapter shows how an infrastructure composed of an open systems technological platform and an interdisciplinary team of technologist researchers and health and social sciences specialists aimed at research groups and public and private organizations and entities as described in the Description section can support simultaneous telemedicine-based services deployment in order to obtain evidence through the execution of experimental studies in chronicity and associated disabilities-related healthcare provision scenarios such as those presented in the Results section.

## Author details

José Luis Monteagudo*, Mario Pascual, Adolfo Muñoz, Pilar G. Sagredo,
Ricardo Sánchez de Madariaga and Carlos H. Salvador

*Address all correspondence to: jlm@isciii.es

Telemedicine and e-Health Research Unit, Instituto de Salud Carlos III, Madrid, Spain

## References

[1] Salvador CH., editor. Innovación TIC para las personas mayores. Situación, Requerimientos y Soluciones en la Atención Integral de la Cronicidad y la Dependencia. Fundación Vodafone; 2011.

[2] Smith JM. The doctor will see you ALWAYS. IEEE Spectrum 2011;48(10) 56-62.

[3] Haverhals LM, Lee CA, Siek KA, Darr CA, Linnebur SA, Ruscin JM, Ross SE Older Adults with Multi-Morbidity: Medication Management Processes and Design Implications for Personal Health Applications J Med Internet Res 2011;13(2):e44

[4] Communication from the Commission to the European Parliament and the Council. Taking forward the Strategic Implementation Plan of the European Innovation Partnership on Active and Healthy Ageing. COM/2012/083 final. 2012.

[5] World Health Organization WHO: Essential Health Technologies. (2003). Strategy 2004-2007: e-Health for Health-care Delivery. http://www.who.int/entity/eht/en/eHealth_HCD.pdf (accessed 5 December 2007).

[6] Report of the WHO Global Observatory for e-Health Building Foundations for e-Health: Progress of Member States. 2006.

[7] European Union EU: Initiative e-Europe 2005. http://eur-lex.europa.eu/LexUriServ/LexUriServ.do?uri= COM:2002:0263:FIN:ES:PDF (accessed 6 December 2007).

[8] European Union EU: Initiative i2010. http://ec.europa.eu/information_society/eeurope/i2010/index_ en.htm (accessed 6 December 2007).

[9] Innovation Report UK Department of Trade and Industry. Competing the Global Economy: The Innovation Challenge. London, UK: HMSO. 2003.

[10] Pagliari C. Design and Evaluation in e-Health: Challenges and Implications for an Interdisciplinary Field. J Med Internet Res 2007;9(2): e15.

[11] Weingart P. Interdisciplinarity: the paradoxical discourse. Practising interdisciplinarity. Toronto, ON: University of Toronto Press; 2000. p25-42.

[12] Glouberman S, Zimmerman B.J. Complicated and complex systems: What would successful reform of Medicare look like? Discussion paper #8 Commission on the Future of Health Care in Canada. 2002.

[13] Plsek PE, Greenhalgh T. The challenge of complexity in health care. British Medical Journal 2001 323:625-8.

[14] Millar WL, McDaniel RR, Crabtree B.F. Practice Jazz: Understanding Variation in Family Practices Using Complexity Science. Journal of Family Practice 2001;50(10).

[15] Sweeney K, Griffiths F. Complexity and Healthcare: An Introduction. London: Radcliff, 2002.

[16] Litaker D, Tomolo A, Liberatore V, Stange KC, Aron D. Using complexity theory to build interventions that improve health care delivery in primary care. J Gen Intern Med 2006;21 30-34.

[17] Medical Research Council. A framework for development and evaluation of RTCs for complex interventions to improve health. 2000.

[18] Holbrook A, Thabane L, Shcherbatykh I, O'Reilly D. E-Health Interventions as Complex Interventions: Improving the Quality of Methods of Assessment. AMIA 2006 Symposium Proceedings. 2006.

[19] Sacket DL. The competing objetives of randomized trials. N Eng J Med 1980;303(18) 1059-1060.

[20] Pincus T. Limitations of randomized Clinical Trials in Chronic Diseases: Explanations and Recommendations. Adv Mind Body Med 2002;18(2):14-21.

[21] Berg M, Aarts J, Van der Lei J. ICT in Health care: sociotechnical approaches (editorial), Methods Inf. Med. 2003;42 297-301.

[22] Kaplan B, Flatley PB, Dowling AF, Friedman CP, Peel V. Toward an Informatics Research Agenda: Key people and Organizational Issues. JAMIA 2001;8(3) 235-241.

[23] Karsh BT. Beyond usability: designing effective technology implementation systems to promote patient safety. Qual. Saf. Health Care 2004;13 338-394.

[24] Cooper RG. Stage-Gate Systems: A New Tool for Managing New Products. IEEE Engineering Management Review 1991;19 5-12.

[25] Friedman CP, Wyatt JC. Evaluation methods in biomedical informatics (Health informatics). New York: Springer-Verlag; 2006.

[26] The Deming Cicle. Plan – Do – Check – Act (PDCA). http://en.wikipedia.org/wiki/PDCA (accessed 11 October 2007).

[27] Martínez A, Rodríguez RJ, Infante A, Campillo C, Gattini C. Bases metodológicas para evaluar la viabilidad y el impacto de proyectos de telemedicina. Washington, D.C. Organización Panamericana de la Salud. 2001.

[28] Institute for Healthcare Improvement. http://www.ihi.org/ (accessed 11 October 2007).

[29] Campbell M, Fitzpatrick R, Haines A, Kinmonth AL, Sandercock P, Spiegelhalter D, Tyrer P. Framework for design and evaluation of complex interventions to improve health. BMJ 2000;321 694-696.

[30] Holle R, Zahlmann G. Evaluation of telemedical services. IEEE Trans Inf Technol Biomed. 1999;3(2) 84-91.

[31] Monteagudo JL, Salvador CH, García-López F. Metodología de introducción de servicios de e-salud para el seguimiento y control de pacientes crónicos. Rev Esp Salud Pública 2004;78 571-581.

[32] Catwell L, Sheikh A. Evaluating e-Health Interventions: The need for Continuous Systemic Evaluation. PLoS Medicine 2009;6(8) e1000126.

[33] EWC van Gemert-Pijnen J, Nijland N, van Limburg M, Ossebaard HC, Kelders SM, Eysenbach G, Seydel ER. A Holistic Framework to Improve the Uptake and Impact of e-Health Technologies. J Med Internet Res 2011;13(4) e111.

[34] Eason K. Changing perspectives on the organizational consequences of information technology. Behav Inform Technol 2001;20 323–8.

[35] van Limburg M, EWC van Gemert-Pijnen J, Nijland N, Ossebaard HC, Hendrix RMG, Seydel ER. Why Business Modeling is Crucial in the Development of e-Health Technologies. J Med Internet Res 2011;13(4) e124.

[36] Littlejohns P, Wyatt JC, Garvican L. Evaluating computerised health information systems: hard lessons still to be learnt. BMJ 2007;326 860-863.

[37] The Breakthrough Series: IHI's Collaborative Model for Achieving Breakthrough Improvement. IHI Innovation Series white paper. Boston: Institute for Healthcare Improvement. 2003.

[38] Kritchevsky SB, Simmons BP. Continuous Quality Improvement Concepts and Applications for Physician Care. JAMA 1991;266(13) 1817-1823.

[39] How to Improve. Institute for Healthcare Improvement. http://www.ihi.org/IHI/Topics/Improvement/ ImprovementMethods/HowToImprove (accessed 11 October 2007).

[40] Pascual Carrasco M. Aportaciones a un modelo de Inserción de servicios asistenciales basados en telemedicina para su uso y validación en el seguimiento de pacientes crónicos. PhD thesis. Technical University of Madrid; 2008. http://oa.upm.es/1875/1/MARIO_PASCUAL_CARRASCO.pdf

[41] SemanticHEALTH Project. Semantic Interoperability for Better Health and Safer Healthcare. Research and Deployment Roadmap for Europe. European Commission. Information and Society Media. 2009.

[42] Muñoz A, Somolinos R, Pascual M, Fragua JA, González MÁ, Monteagudo JL, et al. Proof-of-Concept Design and Development of an EN13606-based Electronic Healthcare Record Service. Journal of the American Medical Informatics Assocciation. 2007;14(1) 118-129.

[43] Beale T. Archetypes: constraints-based domain models for future-proof information systems. 2002. http://www.openehr.org/publications/archetypes/archetypes_beale_oopsla_2002.pdf (accessed 17 July 2012).

[44] SO. ISO 21090:2011. Health Informatics: Harmonized data types for information interchange. 2011.

[45] Kalra D, Lloyd D. ISO 13606 Electronic Health Record Communication Part 1: Reference Model. 2008.

[46] Kalra D, Beale T, Lloyd D. ISO 13606 Electronic Health Record Communication Part 2: Archetype Interchange Specification. 2008.

[47] Maldonado JA, Moner D, Tomás D, Angulo C, Robles M, Fernández JT. Framework for clinical data standardization based on archetypes. In MEDINFO 2007; 2007; Brisbane. p. 454-458.

[48] Beale T, Heard S. The OpenEHR Archetype Model. Archetype Definition Language. ADL 1.5. 2011. http://www.openehr.org/wiki/pages/viewpage.action? pageld=196633 (accessed 17 July 2012).

[49] Commission E. On telemedicine for the benefit of patients, healthcare systems and society. 2008. http://eurlex.europa.eu/LexUriServ/LexUriServ.do?uri=COM:2008:0689:FIN:EN:PDF. (accessed 17 July 2012).

[50] SO. ISO/CD 13940: Health Informatics -- System of concepts to support continuity of care. 2012.

[51] Wagner EH, Austin BT, Von Korff M. Improving outcomes in chronic care. Manag Care Q 1996;4(2) 12-25.

[52] Wagner EH, Austin BT, Von Korff M. Organizing care for patients with chronic illness. Milbank Q 1996;74(4) 511-544.

[53] World Health Organization, Report of the WHO Global Observatory for e-Health. "Building Foundations for e-Health: Progress of Member States". 2006.

[54] Pascual M, Salvador CH, García-Sagredo P, Márquez J, González MA, Fragua JA, Carmona M, García LM, García F, Muñoz A, Monteagudo JL. Impact of patient-general practitioner short-messages-based interaction on the control of hypertension in a follow-up service for low-to-medium risk hypertensive patients: a randomized controlled trial. IEEE Transactions on Information Technology in Biomedicine 2008;12(6) 780-791.

[55] Salvador CH, Ruiz A, González MA, Carmona M, Pascual M, García-Sagredo P, Fragua JA, Caballero F, García F, Márquez J, Monteagudo JL. Evaluation of a telemedicine-based service for the follow-up and monitoring of patients treated with oral anticoagulant therapy. IEEE Transactions on Information Technology in Biomedicine 2008;12(6) 696-706.

[56] Blasco A, Carmona M, Fernández-Lozano I, Salvador CH, Pascual M, Sagredo PG, Somolinos R, Muñoz A, García-López F, Escudier JM, Mingo S, Toquero J, Moñivas V, González MA, Fragua JA, López-Rodríguez F, Monteagudo JL, Alonso-Pulpón L. Evaluation of a Telemedicine Service for the Secondary Prevention of Coronary Artery Disease. Journal of Cardiopulmonary Rehabilitation and Prevention 2012;32(1) 25-31.

[57] Otero L, López-Viña A, Sánchez-Agudo L, Carmona M, Fragua JA, García-Sagredo P, González MA, Muñoz A, Pascual M, Salvador CH. El futuro de los cuidados "asma y telemedicina". Revista de Patología Respiratoria 2005;8(1) 62-63.

[58] AmIVital. Entorno personal digital para la salud y el bienestar. https://amivital.ugr.es/ index.php (accessed 14 june 2012).

[59] Carmona M, García-Olmos LM, Alberquilla A, Muñoz A, García-Sagredo P, Somolinos R, Pascual-Carrasco M, Salvador CH, Monteagudo JL. Heart failure in the family practice: a study of the prevalence and co-morbidity. Family Practice 2011;28(2) 128-133.

[60] De Pedro-Cuesta J, Alberquilla A, Virués-Ortega J, Carmona M, Alcalde-Cabero E, Bosca G, López-Rodríguez F, García-Sagredo P, García-Olmos L, Salvador CH, Monteagudo JL. ICF disability measured by WHO-DAS II in three community diagnostic groups in Madrid, Spain. Gaceta Sanitaria 2011;25(S) 21–28.

[61] García-Olmos L, Salvador CH, Alberquilla A, Lora D, Carmona M, García-Sagredo P, Pascual M, Muñoz A, Monteagudo JL, García-López F. Comorbidity patterns in patients with chronic diseases in general practice. PLoS ONE 2012;7(2) e32141. doi: 10.1371/journal.pone.0032141.

[62] Tecnologías disruptivas para la rehabilitación del futuro http:// rehabilita.gmv.com/web/guest (accessed 15 june 2012).

# 9

# Update on the Most Rural American Telemedicine Program — The Present and Future

Edward T. Zawada Jr, Dana Buus, Don Kosiak,
Pat Herr and Michael Heisler

## 1. Introduction

### 1.1. Review of previous experience and accomplishments

As previously published (1) the Avera Health system launched its telemedicine program by offering consultation by video connectivity from the main tertiary hospital in the largest city of the multi-state North Central Region of the United States to some of its smallest partner clinics and hospitals. Between 1993 and 2004, medical providers and patients learned what it was like to practice medicine and receive care via a telemedicine connection. A major growth spurt in Avera's rural telemedicine program came in 2004 after the initiation of a virtual ICU service staffed by intensivist physicians and critical care nurses; Avera *e*ICU CARE[TM1]. Since 2004, Avera has initiated and rapidly expanded multiple other telemedicine programs to meet demand for additional services and coverage. These around-the-clock, always available services are unique as stand-alone programs, but combined provide one of the most robust telemedicine platforms on the planet.

In the previous report, the goals, expectations and consequences of the Avera *e*ICU CARE program were described. Avera *e*ICU CARE initially started with the system's tertiary hospital, Avera McKennan Hospital & University Health Center, serving as the hub location for the provision of twenty-four hour per day remote patient care and monitoring of seriously ill patients in three medium-sized rural hospitals. Over time it evolved to include several more hospitals of that size called "Rural Regional Hospitals." Additionally, remote Critical Access Hospitals (CAHs) began to request *e*ICU coverage. Intensivist-led medical supervision and

1 Avera eICU CARE is a registered trademark of VISICU, Inc.

monitoring further expanded to hospitals outside of the Avera Health system, including those with different medical record or electronic record platforms. Finally, Avera *e*ICU services expanded into multiple states.

Avera *e*CARE™ has several years of experience in providing a broad expanse of telemedicine services. Each service has enjoyed similar growth and success. Avera's programs have also experienced similar and unique challenges in implementation, growth, and cultural adaptation. The expansion of Avera's telemedicine program was born in the success of Avera eICU CARE, and lead to the development and expansion of programs such as *e*Emergency and *e*Pharmacy. Like the Avera eICU CARE™ program, these services provide rural facilities access to additional health care services and providers. *e*Emergency and *e*Pharmacy have expanded faster and are more widely distributed than Avera *e*ICU CARE™. This could be the result of several factors, but one could postulate that perhaps these services have been more useful to rural sites of care. Today, a variety of services are being researched, designed and piloted to provide care to an amazing assortment of patients, medical providers, clinics, hospitals, and other health care facilities to be described later. Many of these pilots have been launched and have been well received. The goal of this chapter is to describe the status of the comprehensive Avera *e*CARE™ system and to hypothesize the future of this very successful paradigm of care.

As time progresses and needs arise, unique applications of telemedicine supervision are developed. Many of these applications are in the pilot stages of development as part of Avera's comprehensive program. Avera's suite of telemedicine services are now largely sustained without any outside financial support. Avera's telemedicine start-up costs have been off-set, in part, by grants and other funding opportunities. Avera's growing breadth and scope of telemedicine service offerings lead to a decision to bring *e*CARE together as a "Virtual Hospital". With this goal in mind, and generous financial support, Avera has developed a co-located telemedicine center that brings together all of Avera's telemedicine services under one roof, offsite from any traditional hospital or clinic location. Side-by-side, the medical providers, nurses and support staff work toward multidisciplinary success in each patient encounter. This telemedicine center is unique in the practice of telemedicine and is called the Avera *e*Helm™.

## 2. Current programs and their results

Figure 1 displays the geographic breadth of the Avera *e*CARE™ program which is of one of the most comprehensive rural telemedicine programs in the world by geographic breadth, number of sites served, and number of unique telemedicine services operating from one location. It can be noted from the figure that the greatest concentration of activity is along the borders of five states of the North Central region of the United States: South Dakota, North Dakota, Minnesota, Iowa, and Nebraska. However, the greatest recent growth is westward including expansion into the states of Wyoming and Montana.

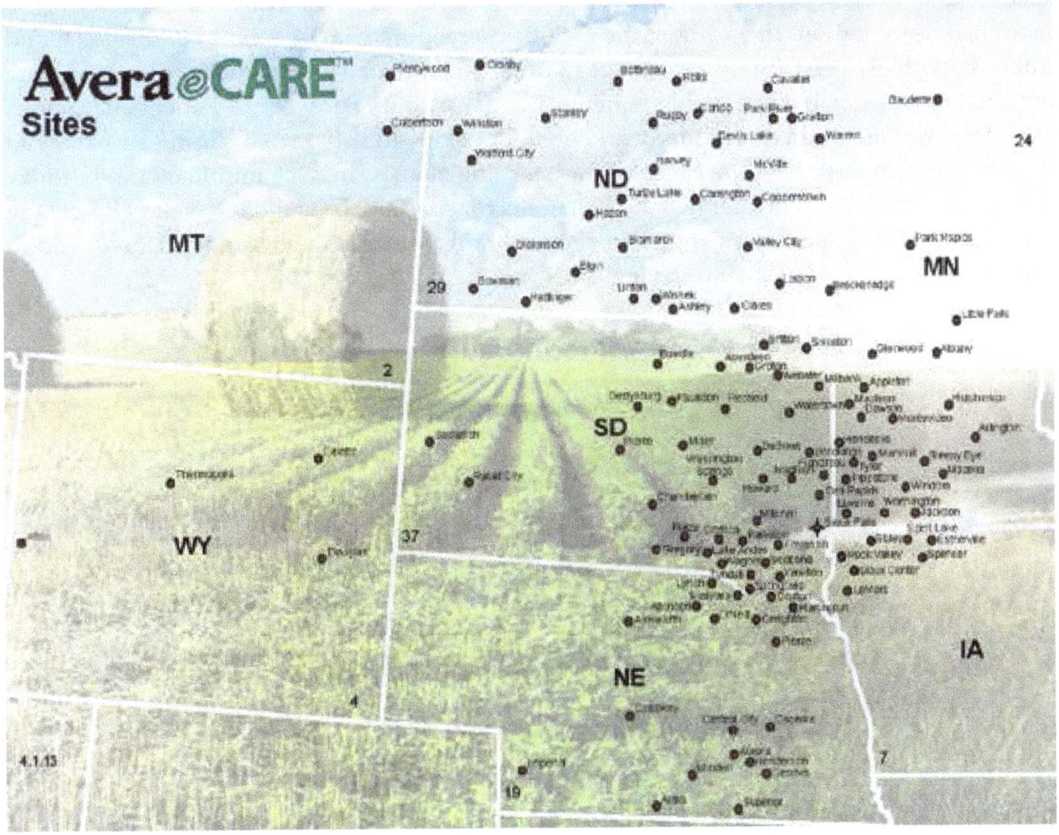


**Figure 1.** shows the seven states of the North Central United States which receive Avera eCARE™ services: Wyoming (WY), North Dakota (ND), South Dakota (SD), Nebraska (NE), Minnesota (MN), Montana (MT) and Iowa (IA).

Avera's telemedicine experience initially shows the seven states of the North Central United States which receive Avera *e*CARE™ services: Wyoming (WY), North Dakota (ND), South Dakota (SD), Nebraska (NE), Minnesota (MN), Montana (MT) and Iowa (IA).started by using video-conferencing equipment to facilitate medical consultations between primary care providers and patients in rural locations in South Dakota to specialists in a tertiary setting. It now is an active and robust program spanning seven states of the North Central region of the United States. Expansion of the type of programs and number of sites served has pushed Avera's total service area to include more than one hundred sixty-five hospitals and clinics within and outside of the Avera Health system.

The six primary *e*CARE services are shown in Figure 2: *e*Consult, *e*Pharmacy, *e*Emergency, *e*Long Term Care, and *e*Urgent Care in Correctional Facilities.

These telemedicine programs are shows the six telemedicine services offered by Avera *e*CARE™ to date.designed to benefit rural patients and medical providers by improving the speed of care delivery and helping ensure the highest quality of care is provided locally where the patient resides. For the remote medical provider, Avera *e*CARE services offset a lack of specialists in rural areas affected by fewer resources and limited medical professional assistance and consultation. In addition, the facilities served may lack access to educational and career growth opportunities. These medical providers often have large patient loads and are required to be available to provide patient care many hours per week[2],[3]. Patients in remote, rural locations are often more elderly and are more likely to suffer from chronic disease than their urban counterparts[4]. The cause of this startling statistic may be multifactorial but may include reasons such as greater distances to travel for specialty consultation, delays in seeking care due to higher rates of lacking primary health insurance or being underinsured, and in some cases inclement weather delaying access to care.

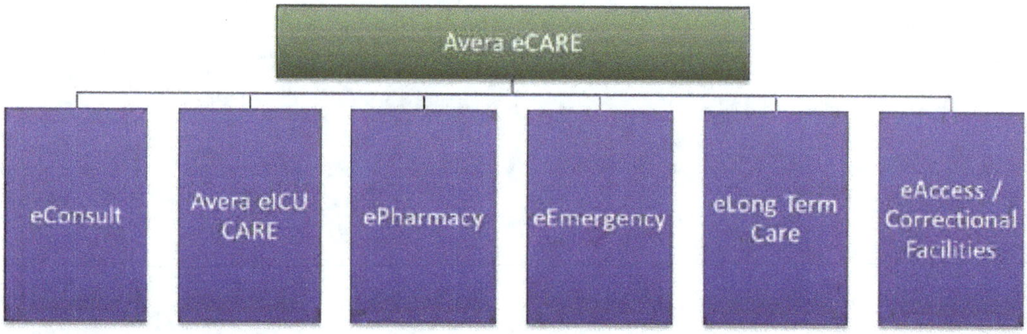


**Figure 2.** shows the six telemedicine services offered by Avera eCARE™ to date.

## 2.1. The Avera *e*CARE™ programs

*e*Consult allows patients to access scheduled specialty consults at their local facility through two-way video technology. These consults are supported by special telephonic stethoscopes, otoscopes, and examination cameras. Avera first began providing virtual visits in 1993. *e*Consult benefits patients by saving time away from school or work and by saving the expenses of roundtrip travel. Figure 3 illustrates the utilization of this service by specialty over the past twelve months. As can be seen, primary specialties such as pediatrics or mental health are regularly requested. Many rare subspecialties are also utilized monthly. Infectious disease expertise is the single most frequently scheduled telemedicine consult provided to rural medical providers and their patients.

The status of this program is summarized as of May 30, 2013. *e*Consult is live in 109 sites; 76 patient sites and 33 specialty sites. Over a twelve month period, 5,900 *e*Consults were conducted by 88 unique specialist providers. *e*Consult services have saved an estimated 28,500

2 Ormond, B., Wallin, S., Goldenson, S. (2000). Supporting the rural health care safety net. The Urban Institute, Occasional Paper 36.

3 2009. Rural practice, keeping physicians in. AAFP Position Paper. http://www.aafp.org/online.en/home/policy/policies/r/ruralpracticekeep.html

4 Joynt, K., Orav, J., and Jha (2013). Mortality rates for medicare beneficiaries admitted to critical access and non-critical access hospitals, 2002-2010.

patient travel hours and more than 1.8 million patient travel miles. Additionally, access to specialist care via *e*Consult has resulted in a cost savings of more than $425,970 for rural patients[5].

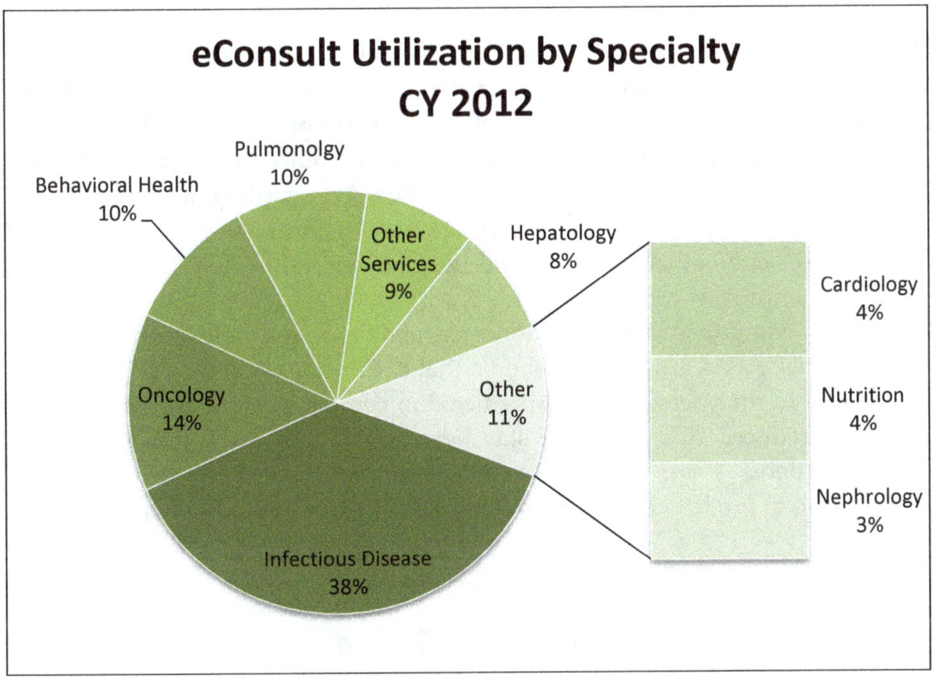


"Other Services" illustrates the utilization of telemedicine consultations by specialty over the past twelve months include those specialties that average <100 consults/year: Rehab, Internal Medicine, Gastroenterology, Occupational Medicine, Palliative Care, Women's Services, Dermatology, Pediatrics, Neonatology, Otolaryngology, Neurosurgery, Neurology, and Endocrinology

**Figure 3.** illustrates the utilization of telemedicine consultations by specialty over the past twelve months.

**Avera *e*ICU Care™ (*e*ICU)** began in 2004 and had accounted for the largest quantum of growth in the history of Avera's telemedicine services until just recently. As stated earlier, Avera *e*ICU CARE provides around-the-clock remote intensive care monitoring of seriously and critically ill patients in the thirty-three hospitals served. With the inception of this program, Avera was able to electronically quantitate the severity of illness for such patients by using an internationally known and validated severity adjustment methodology called the Acute Physiology and Chronic Health Evaluation (APACHE) scoring system. Patient data is automatically calculated from the data entered into the electronic medical record to generate APACHE predictions. The system also analyzes quality measures such as the frequency of ordering "best practice" national guidelines. Avera tracks outcomes such as severity-adjusted intensive care unit (ICU) length of stay, severity-adjusted ICU mortality, severity-adjusted hospital mortality,

5 eConsult Database (2013). Avera eCARE Services.

and severity adjusted hospital length of stay. Avera uses these analyses to design strategies to improve the care delivered to seriously and critically ill patients in the *e*ICU CARE system. Avera *e*ICU CARE has also provided education to medical providers across the region concerning this new high quality service by publishing results in the South Dakota Journal of Medicine (2).

From the initial forty beds, Avera *e*ICU CARE has expanded to include smaller hospitals within the Avera system, hospitals out of the Avera system, and even hospitals out of the state. Avera was one of the first in the nation to offer the *e*ICU service to patients in CAHs. Avera studied whether the Avera *e*ICU program had an impact on patient outcomes. Data revealed that after the program was implemented there was reduction in severity-adjusted ICU mortality, reduction in severity-adjusted ICU length of stay, reduction of severity adjusted hospital mortality, and reduction of severity-adjusted hospital length of stay (3). In addition, Avera *e*ICU CARE has improved compliance with best practice guidelines, and has achieved one hundred percent compliance with stress ulcer prophylaxis and DVT prophylaxis in *e*ICU-monitored patients. APACHE data has shown that ICU mortality among *e*ICU patients is an average of thirty to fifty percent below predicted in comparison to the APACHE database. Avera has also reduced ICU length of stay by an average of twenty-five percent. Using APACHE predictions, Avera has calculated the number of lives saved from the difference between observed to predicted mortality. Figure 4 shows those results from initial analysis to the current year.

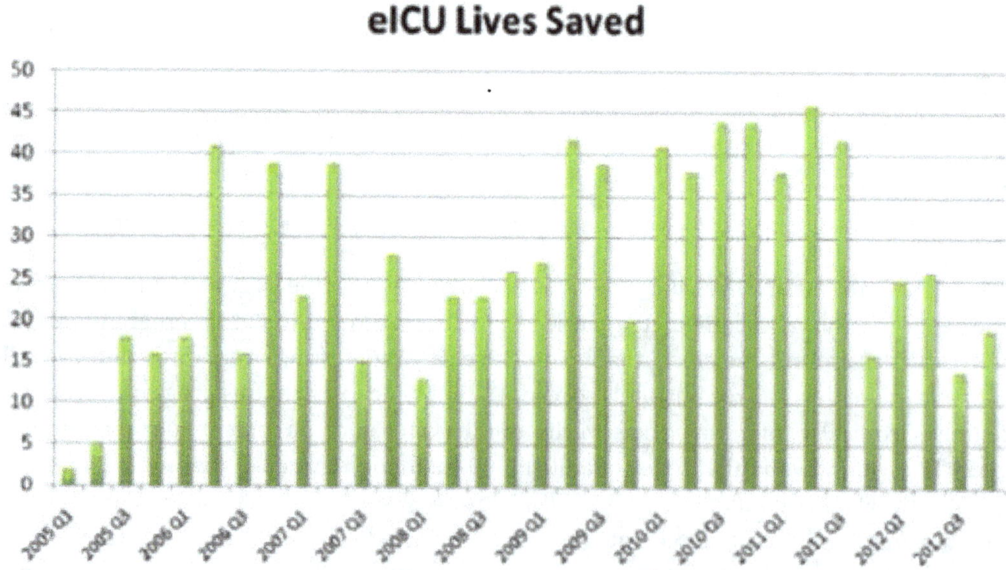


**Figure 4.** illustrates the number of lives saved quarterly from 2005 to the present.

The around-the illustrates the number of lives saved quarterly from 2005 to the present -clock, direct monitoring of critically ill and seriously ill patients by the intensivist-led team, supported by sophisticated technology that recognizes and alerts for negative trends in vital signs and abnormalities in laboratory tests is one of the primary reasons for such significant improvement in patient outcomes. The *e*ICU team of intensivists and critical care nurses is alerted to negative trends in patient status and can immediately be present in a patient's room by a two-way interactive televideo system to respond to emergencies. Additionally, Avera *e*ICU CARE supports consistent application of evidenced-based medicine through active rounding on patients, with a focus on ensuring such evidence-based measures are implemented and documented in the medical record.

Avera *e*ICU CARE currently provides coverage for one hundred thirty-two beds in thirty-three facilities across six states, spanning a geography from Wyoming to mid-Iowa and from North Dakota to Nebraska. The Avera *e*ICU CARE team monitors an average of sixty to sixty-five patients at any time, and averages twenty-two admissions per a twenty-four hour period. *e*ICU intensivist physicians write an average of 1,400 orders per month. This greatly exceeds the average number of interventions for other tele-intensivist programs (4), which attests to the welcome invitation by rural sites for continous coverage when primary providers cannot be available. There are no charges to patients for this service.

Although the number of ICU telemedicine programs in the United States has continued to grow rapidly, our program has been recognized for its coverage to the least densely populated geographic rural region (5) and to the largest number of critical access hospitals (those receiving federal pass-through payments for services but limited to 20 beds or less).

***e*Pharmacy was** developed shortly after the quantum expansion of the Avera *e*ICU CARE™ service. Many rural sites experienced long periods of time when a local pharmacist was not available, highlighting a need for this service. Avera's virtual pharmacy service provides remote medication order review and approval before a first dose of medication is administered. ePharmacy uses automated dispensing equipment and remote provider order entry which has led to a reduction in serious safety events related to duplication of medication therapies, allergies, and drug-to-drug interactions. Currently ePharmacy service is provided to forty-six sites. Since its inception in 2009, more than 83,300 patients have been served by ePharmacy. To date more than 1,054,000 orders have been reviewed, and more than 14,200 serious safety events avoided. Each month, the ePharmacy team of pharmacists reviews more than 44,000 orders and documents 800 interventions to promote medication safety and efficacy.

Figure 5 illustrates the breakdown of adverse events noted in a single month.

**eEmergency (eED)** illustrates the types of errors which have been detected by the ePharmacy service line in a single month.has had the greatest success with expansion and requests for service. As of June 1, 2013, seventy-six sites utilize eEmergency services. Figure 6 illustrates the pace of growth of this highly requested program to the rural communities of the North Central region of the United States. The *e*ED provides immediate, two-way video access to a board-certified emergency physician and a core of experienced emergency nurses. They assist in the management of a multitude of medical emergencies such as trauma, acute myocardial infarction and stroke, to name a few.

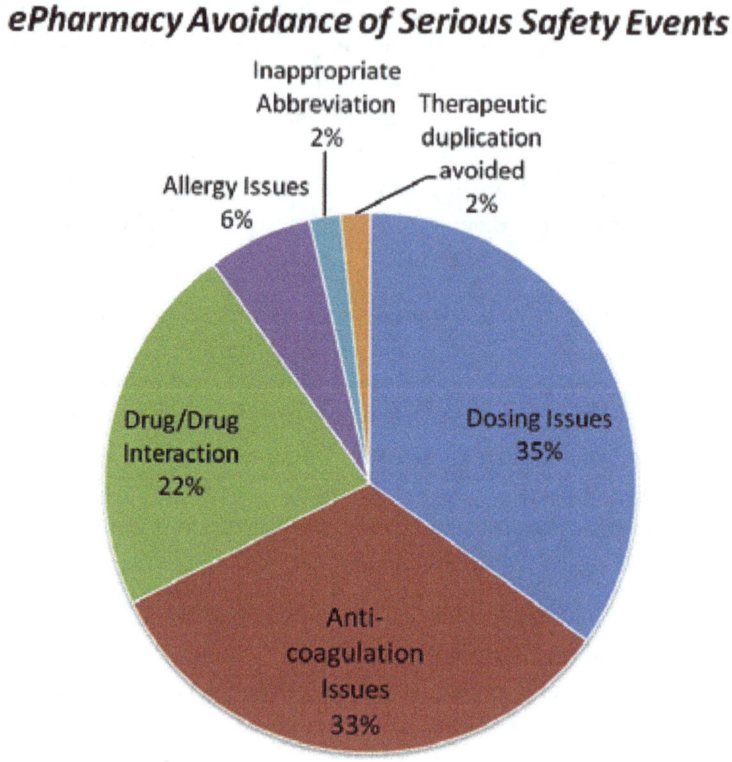


**Figure 5.** illustrates the types of errors which have been detected by the ePharmacy service line in a single month.

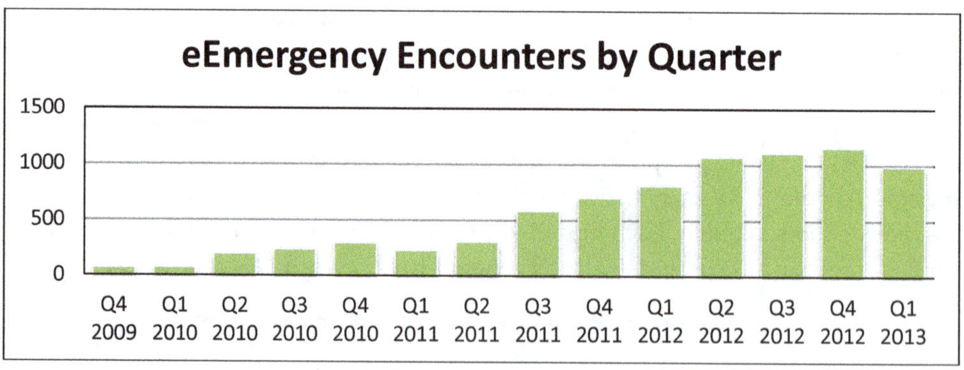


**Figure 6.** demonstrates the pace of growth of eEmergency services aided by the Helmsley grant to be described below.

*e*Emergency allows for the demonstrates the pace of growth of eEmergency services aided by the Helmsley grant to be described below.initiation of accurate diagnostic testing before local provider arrival, streamlines emergency transfer arrangements, and eliminates unnecessary transfers. Since inception in 2009 through May 30, 2013, more than 5,900 patients have been treated, over 10,800 transfers have been arranged, and over 980 transfers have been avoided, resulting in a savings of $7.85 million. Figure 7 breaks down the types of complaints routinely handled by the *e*ED.

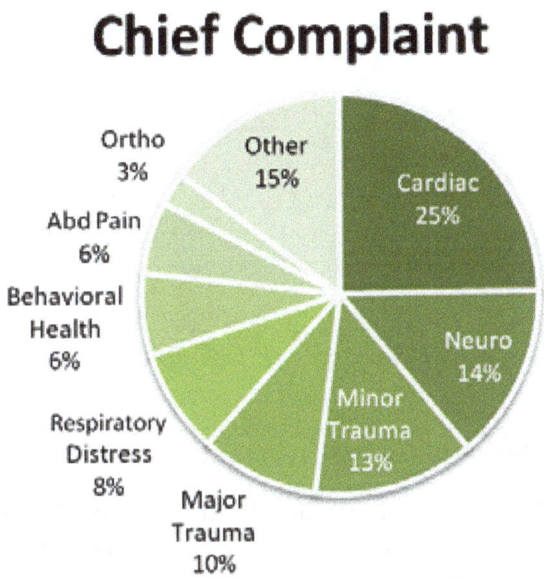


**Figure 7.** illustrates the frequency of problems handled by the eEmergency program

The *e*Emergency program has illustrates the frequency of problems handled by the eEmergency program expanded to include the initiation of several quality improvement programs with major clinical effect on the region. One example includes what is called the "Chest Pain Initiative." Because the *e*ED is often involved in cases before the local provider has arrived, important diagnostic tests and critical therapies can be initiated that in the past may have been delayed. As an example the program has documented improvement in "door to ECG" times. After implementation of *e*ED project, the median time to ECG has improved and now exceeds the Centers for Medicare and Medicaid Services (CMS) standard of ten minutes as shown in Figure 8.

Another component of the illustrates the improvement in median time to ECG for patients with chest pain presenting to emergency departments in the region due to assistance from eEmergency services.Chest Pain Initiative was improvement in aspirin administration. After the *e*ED project was implemented, participating sites were noted to have 100 percent compliance with established guidelines for aspirin administration. Historically, these hospitals reported compliance as low as 67 percent[6]. Other important outcomes impacted included significant decrease in the time to transfer and the increase in use of thrombolytics for care in the appropriately screened and eligible candidates. This number is at 100 percent.

6 Avera Health Quality Department Data (2011).

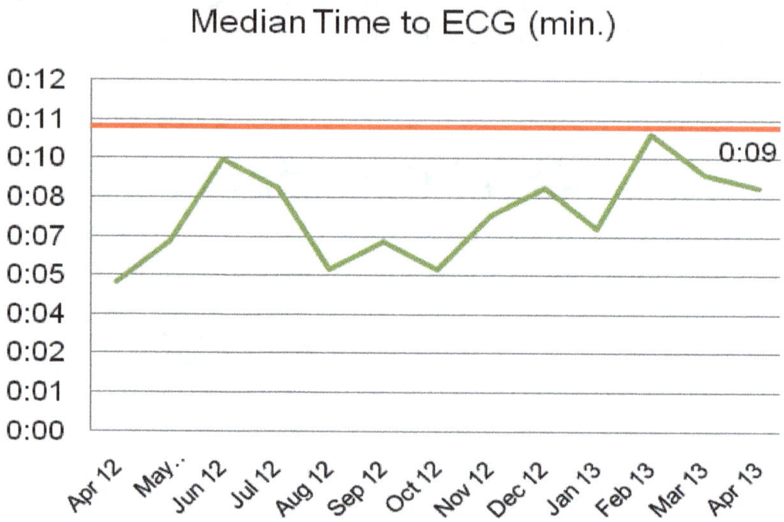


**Figure 8.** illustrates the improvement in median time to ECG for patients with chest pain presenting to emergency departments in the region due to assistance from eEmergency services.

***e*Long Term Care (*e*LTC)** has developed as an outgrowth of *e*ED, and uses telemedicine technologies to improve long term care staff and residents' access to providers and specialty services in a manner that is high quality, convenient, and low cost. The goal of the program is to provide urgent care services to residents of long term care facilities in an effort to prevent emergency department visits and hospital admissions. This program was launched as a pilot project in January 2012 at four sites, and is currently available in six sites. In the first year of pilot, 120 residents were seen by the eLTC provider. Of these, 30 percent (36 encounters) resulted in an avoided a transfer to the emergency department or clinic. As an additional component of the service, specialist care via *e*Consult is available to residents in participating facilities. Grant support to be described below has assisted in innovating in this branch of telemedicine.

***e*Access in Correctional Facilities** has also developed as an outgrowth of *e*ED. In this program, telemedicine technology is used to provide physician-directed urgent care services to inmates, resulting in a reduction of unnecessary and costly transfers. This pilot was launched in May 2012 at four sites. In the first twelve months of service, 372 patients have been served, with thirty-two percent of those encounters resulting in an avoided transfer. The distribution of complaints handled by the virtual physicians was similar to one shown above for the *e*Emergency program as a whole.

### 2.2. Major lessons learned and challenges

Credentialing and licensure for all these telemedicine services requires considerable amount of time and perseverance. Avera *e*CARE™ medical providers are licensed in every state where *e*CARE services are provided. In addition, medical providers must apply for, and be granted, medical privileges in each hospital in which services are provided. Nursing licensure is no less challenging. Several states in which *e*CARE services are provided participate in the Nurse Licensure Compact. In these states, licensure in one participating state covers the nurse when he or she is working in other participating states. South Dakota, Iowa, Nebraska, and North Dakota are all compact members. Separate full, unrestricted nursing licenses are needed in Minnesota, Montana, and Wyoming. Nursing staff is not required to apply for any privileges in any of the hospitals currently served.

Two different processes are used for credentialing and privileging, the traditional process that has been in place for many years, and a newer telemedicine application process. Approximately fifty percent of hospitals receiving *e*CARE services have adopted the telemedicine credentialing/privileging process. The other fifty percent have chosen to continue with the traditional route for a variety of reasons including preference for the existing method and the unsure nature of state and federal survey teams' reception of this new process.

The *e*Pharmacy staff of hospital-trained pharmacists are licensed in each state where *e*Pharmacy services are provided. Licensure is highly regulated by each state's Board of Pharmacy. Most of these states require a separate written exam before granting a license. Credentialing and privileging is not required for pharmacists.

### 2.3. Funding Sources

Avera Health member hospitals and clinics have long been financially supportive of the telemedicine mission. Through the innovative thinking of Avera leaders, telemedicine has been considered a strategic part of Avera's future and has been budgeted for accordingly. In addition to internal financial support, various granting agencies have provided funding for the implementation and growth of many *e*CARE programs. These agencies have ranged from the local, state and federal government, foundations of publicly traded companies, as well as private local and national foundations. Without this generous support, telemedicine expansion on such a broad scale would have been difficult, if not impossible. We will summarize some of *e*CARE's past grant awards and funding opportunities below.

The United States Department of Agriculture (USDA) has funded seven grants exceeding $2.7 million to expand various Avera *e*CARE™ programs. In addition, private foundations focused on rural healthcare have provided financial resources to operationalize some a variety of *e*CARE programs. One particular grant from a private foundation has allowed for greater collaboration between individual Avera *e*CARE™ services. *e*CARE services that were once scattered across a large medical campus are now able to function as a fully integrated virtual hospital, housed in a state-of-the-art building miles from any traditional hospital walls. This new location allows Avera to provide telemedicine based care in a much more cohesive and supportive manner. This new super-hub is called the Avera *e*Helm™. The *e*Helm serves as an incubator for new and innovative telemedicine programs and services by allowing and facilitating dialog and cross-fertilization of existing telemedicine experts.

In 2012, an Avera community hospital was awarded a grant from the Health Resources and Services Administration (HRSA) Office of Rural Health Policy to expand the *e*Long Term Care program to an additional sixteen centers.

### 2.4. Awards

Avera's telemedicine efforts have been recognized by several national health organizations looking to reform and improve health care. In 2009, Avera was awarded the American Telemedicine Association's President's Institutional Award for leadership in telemedicine. Avera has received thirteen "HealthCare's Most Wired" awards from a consortium that includes McKesson, AT&T, and Care Tech Solutions, in cooperation with the College of Healthcare Information Management Executives, the American Hospital Association, and Health and Health Network (H&HN) magazine. Avera also won one of three 2011 & 2012 "Most-Wired Innovator" awards and was recognized for this accomplishment at the 2011 and 2012 American Hospital Leadership Summits. Avera *e*CARE was recognized as a finalist for the Monroe E. Trout Premier Cares award in January, 2012, and was nominated for a Catholic Health Association of the United States award in 2013. *e*CARE has also been recognized internally for its impact on quality of care, and has received three Avera Quality Congress awards; one for *e*Pharmacy, one for *e*Emergency and another for the *e*Emergency Chest Pain Initiative.

## 3. The future –A paradigm shift

The proliferation of different virtual health services in Avera's comprehensive telemedicine program is illustrated in Figure 9. Telemedicine can be used to supplement each phase of the health care continuum. Telemedicine has evolved in the North Central Plains region as a program that supports the entire continuum from primary care, emergency care, critical care, multiple pharmaceutical interventions, and a nascent follow-up program in long term care facilities.

**Figure 10** illustrates the illustrates the complete continuum of telemedicine services which now exist and are co-located in a single hub such as the Avera eHelm which coordinates and enhances patient care "air traffic control" model of telemedicine utilization, where telemedicine providers serve as back up for the other components of the continuum. While this may be the case in some urban settings, rural areas might utilize telemedicine in a formal role in direct patient care, leading a local medical team from a remote location. Remote telemedicine care may actually provide total first line diagnosis and therapies in the near future.

To this end, illustrates the important "air traffic control" or back up capability of telemedicine for each phase in the health care continuum.Avera *e*CARE™ is planning for a major shift in healthcare delivery in the future.

A paradigm shift in health care delivery is being driven by the expansion of telemedicine services. The progression of innovation in telemedicine, especially in remote areas (rural parts of the United States, Third World Countries, Emerging Nations), which cannot develop a full medical infrastructure on their own, will turn to "The Virtual Hospital, The New Doctor's Office, and the New Continuity Service", all expansions of mature telemedicine centers.

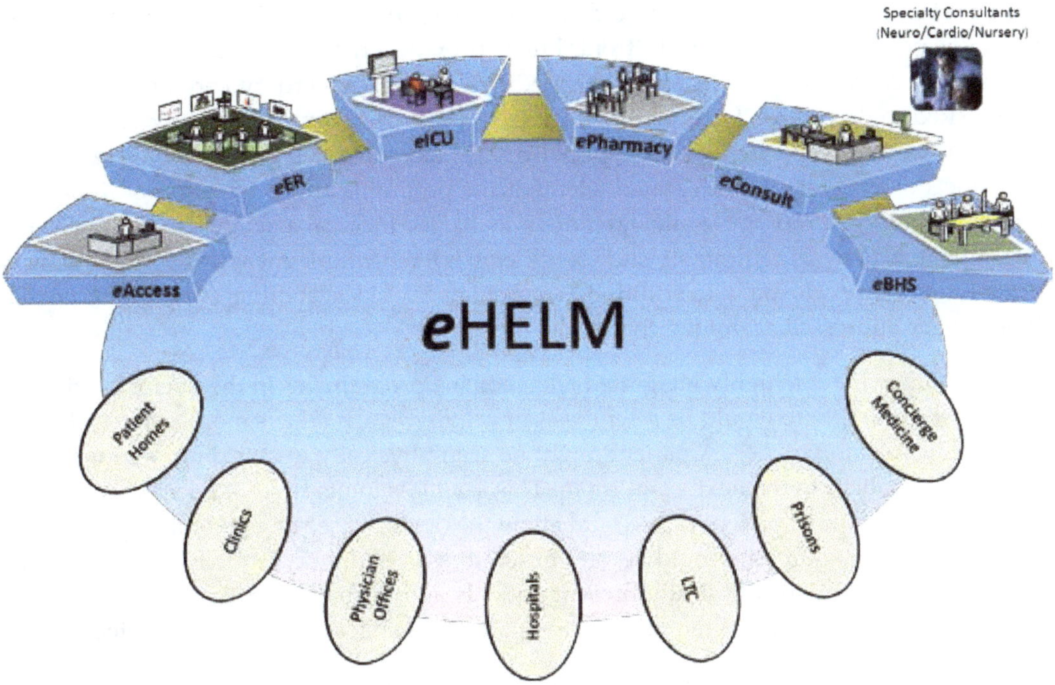


**Figure 9.** illustrates the complete continuum of telemedicine services which now exist and are co-located in a single hub such as the Avera eHelm which coordinates and enhances patient care.

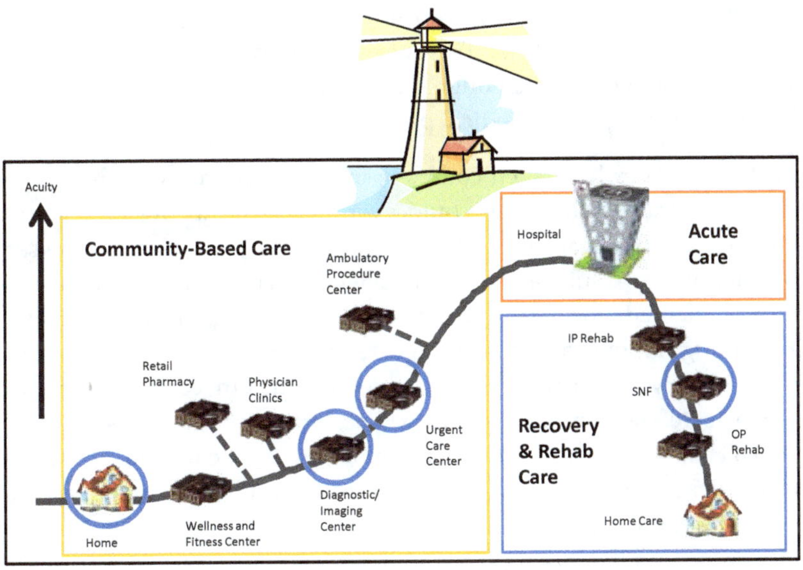


**Figure 10.** illustrates the important "air traffic control" or back up capability of telemedicine for each phase in the health care continuum..

Instead of increased numbers of brick and mortar tertiary centers to which patients travel, now there is the possibility of a virtual electronic hub to provide tertiary hospital services to remote sites as they currently exist. In effect, telemedicine brings the tertiary care hospital to the patient. Reduced costs of transfer of patients, improved patient and family satisfaction, increased access to specialists and especially rare sub-specialist consultation are all the byproducts of a robust and integrated telemedicine program. Implementation of improved wireless (cellular) technology to allow remotely controlled medical machines such as mechanical ventilators, dialysis equipment, and robotic care is likely imminent as an augmentation of such a tertiary care *e*Hospital. In addition, the challenges of local staffing, supply, and power all need to be addressed as unique challenges.

Another trademark of a highly integrated telemedicine program lies in the doctor's office. In a specialist's office there would be a synthesis of activity which allows more active inclusion of telemedicine into practice. A patient might be seen physically in an exam room next to a telemedicine patient in the next exam room. This seamless integration of telemedicine work stations into the flow of patient care would allow the doctor to see any patients regardless of their location. Physician time could be, and in some cases is, divided equally and seamlessly between time spent with physically present patients and virtual patients. In the future, the physician may also be located remotely seeing patients at all locations via telemedicine.

Electronic continuity services could include nontraditional settings such as long term care facilities, correctional facilities, and expanded telemedicine home-based services. In these new and dynamic locations the goal of telemedicine is to continue to monitor compliance with discharge instructions, meticulously supervise proper medication intake at home or in the facility in which the patient resides, and to ensure timely follow up with the primary medical provider and any needed specialists. This system would be designed to prevent errors, relapses, or delays in follow up which might lead to unnecessary emergency visits, hospitalizations, and premature relapses in medical problems.

Finally,**Figure 11** illustrates how such complete telemedicine services may expand beyond health systems and rural neighbors. It could even result in global extension of successful telemedicine systems of medical care. A telemedicine program with multiple services could be located together in a core such as the Avera *e*Helm™. These hubs could just as easily and efficiently provide telemedicine care to the ends of the earth and beyond as they could in the same city or building. Home care, concierge care, doctor's office care, medical home care, urgent care, emergency department care, behavioral health care, general hospital care, specialty hospital care (behavioral health, cardiac, orthopedic), intensive care, long term hospital care (LTHC), and others could be connected to a core like the Avera *e*Helm™ providing telemedicine care and coordination with its multiple primary care and specialty allied health members, nurses, and physicians.

In summary, to illustrates a model of global care coordinated by multiple electronic telemedicine programs coordinated by a core of expert telemedicine caregivers located in a core such as the Avera eHelm™.date more than 153,000 patients have been touched by at least one Avera *e*CARE™ service. More than 165 hospitals and clinics across a 495,000 square mile service use

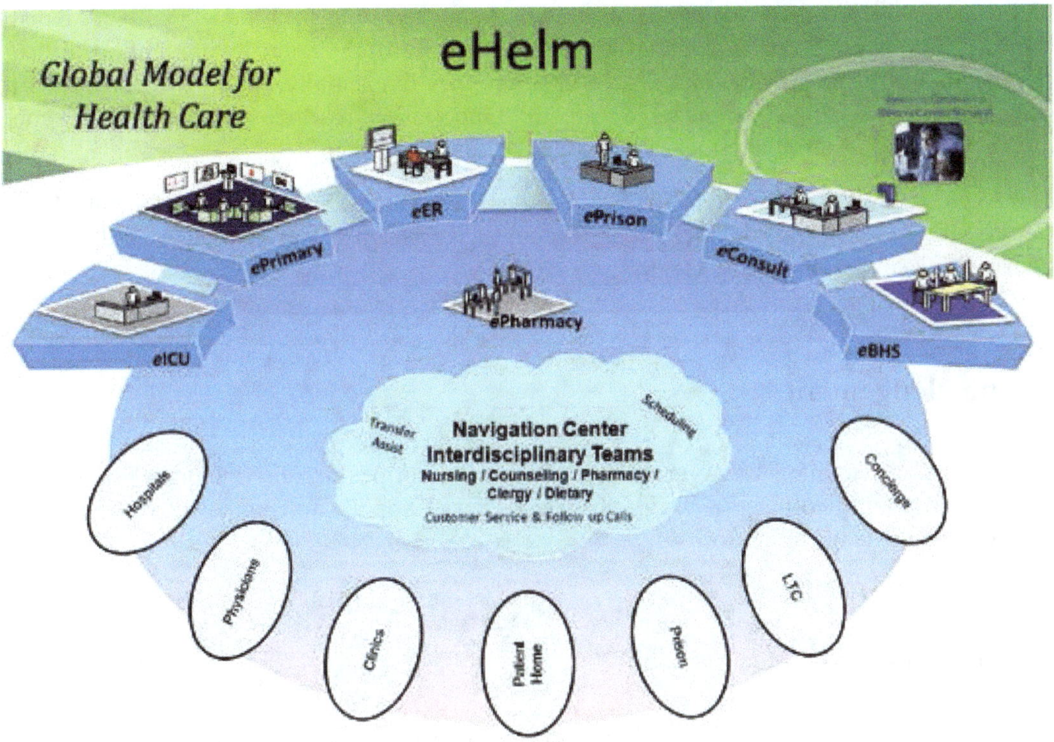


**Figure 11.** illustrates a model of global care coordinated by multiple electronic telemedicine programs coordinated by a core of expert telemedicine caregivers located in a core such as the Avera eHelm™.

at least one Avera *e*CARE™ service. At the present 650 providers are served by Avera eCARE™. The total financial impact has been greater than 55 million dollars.

The future goals of Avera *e*CARE™ includes a plan to create virtual support for hospitals, clinics, long term care facilities and other nontraditional care locations to provide access to care at the same level of quality available in urban settings. In addition, Avera is exploring a robust home monitoring and coaching system of care that enables providers to interact with chronically ill patients in their home environments. These steps will create a virtual support for patient centered medical homes.

In conclusion, the success of these multiple diverse telemedicine programs in the rural region of the North Central United States has been a result of trying to meet the needs for health care in this area. Telemedicine has been well received due to many factors, including the remoteness of many communities, the frequently inclement weather which impairs urgent face-to-face health care, the lack of health care resources in the agricultural economy, and the extremely low number of specialty and subspecialty providers located these states. The success of Avera *e*CARE has not gone unnoticed. Many have asked to learn how to duplicate some or all of Avera models of comprehensive telemedicine.

Today and in the future, Avera will continue to leverage technology to connect with our North Central USA population, to engage the people of this rural region in prevention and in provision of care and services on the go and where they live. Finally, Avera will partner with stakeholders who will join in the advancement of innovation, research and policy for telemedicine practice and reimbursement.

The Avera *e*Care™ Research Group also includes: Jay Weems, Srivedi Gangineni MD, Scott Deppe MD, David Kovaleski, MD, Sarah Kappel CCRN, Tami Schnetter CCRN, Andrea Darr Pharm.D., Deanna Larson RN, David Erickson MD.

## Acknowledgement

The authors wish to thank the Avera *e*Care™ Research Group which also includes: Jay Weems, Srivedi Gangineni, Scott Deppe, David Kovaleski, Sara Kappel, Tami Schnetter, Andrea Darr, Deanna Larson, David Erickson

## Author details

Edward T. Zawada Jr[1,2], Dana Buus[3], Don Kosiak[4], Pat Herr[5] and Michael Heisler[2,6]

1 Avera Health Intensivists/eICU, USA

2 Department of Internal Medicine, University of South Dakota Sanford School of Medicine, South Dakota, USA

3 Avera Health, Sioux Falls, South Dakota, USA

4 Avera Health eServices, Sioux Falls, South Dakota, USA

5 Avera eICU, Avera Health, Sioux Falls, South Dakota, USA

6 Avera eICU, South Dakota, USA

## References

[1] Zawada ET Jr, Kapaska D, Herr P, Heisler M.Avera *e*-CareTM, a Comprehensive Telemedicine Program for the Rural North Central Region of the United States, In "Advances In Telemedicine: Applications In Various Medical Disciplines and Geographical Regions. Georgi Graschew and Theo A. Roelofs, editors. In Tech, Rijeka Croatia, 2001, 255-279.

[2] Zawada ET Jr, Kapaska D, Herr P, Aaronson M, Bennett J, Hurley B, Bishop D, Dagher H, Kovaleski D, Melanson T, Burdge K, Johnson T, Avera *e*ICU® Research Group: Prognostic outcomes after the initiation of an electronic telemedicine intensive care unit (*e*ICU®) in a rural health system. SD Journal of Med 59(9):391-393, (2006).

[3] Zawada Jr ET, Herr P, Larson D, Fromm R, Kapaska D Erickson D: Impact of an ICU telemedicine program on a rural health system. Postgraduate Medicine May (2009). , 121(3), 160-170.

[4] Zawada Jr ET, Gangineni S, Herr P, Heisler M, Deppe S Workload update on the most rural tele-intensivist program. Chest (2012). 142(4):548A.

[5] Lilly, C. M, Fisher, K. A, Ries, M, Pastores, S. M, Vender, J, & Pitts, J. A. Hansen III W: A national ICU telemedicine survey, validation and results. Chest (2012). , 142(1), 40-47.

# 10

# Short Range Technologies for Ambient Assisted Living Systems in Telemedicine: New Healthcare Environments

Silvia de Miguel-Bilbao, Jorge García,
M. Dolores Marcos and Victoria Ramos

## 1. Introduction

The increasing average age of people and the consequent rise of chronic diseases will result in a growth in the need for assistance and healthcare within the coming years. Nevertheless, this is not the only challenge that developed countries face regarding healthcare services. There is an increasing demand for outpatient care accessibility, maintaining and restoring health, as well as maximizing the independence of patients [1], [2].

While the broader field of telemedicine and/or telehealth has been used in various forms for many years, Ambient Assisted Living (AAL) systems in Telemedicine are a relatively recent innovation [3] and an emerging area of interest to service providers and consumers [4]. Smart environment is a rapidly evolving domain focused on providing personal care settings with the primary intent of supporting the patient rather than office visits with health professionals. AAL is used in a wide sense and encompasses the use of audio, video and other telecommunication technologies to evaluate patient status at a distance [5], [6]. Remote healthcare monitoring systems could aid in reducing costs and alleviating the shortage of healthcare personnel [1].

Additionally, the Internet has experienced a large growth over the past three decades, evolving from a network of a few hundred hosts to a platform linking billions of "things" globally [7]. The growth of the Internet shows no signs of slowing down and it has steadily become the cause of a new pervasive paradigm in computing and communications. This new paradigm enhances the traditional Internet into a smart Internet of Things (IoT) created around intelligent interconnections of diverse objects in the physical world. This approach enriches the AAL environment and offers new possibilities for healthcare [2].

Wireless connectivity is a feature of IoT, and is becoming increasingly used in AAL systems with intensive use of Short Range Devices (SRD) such as Radio Frequency Identification (RFID), Ultra Wide Band (UWB), Near Field Communications (NFC), Wireless Local Area Networks (WLAN), Bluetooth, ZigBee, telealarm buttons (social alarms) or domotic devices. These systems involve sensors, computing and communication devices working in increasingly dense electromagnetic environments. One emerging approach to improve the wearability of continuous ambulatory monitoring systems is to improve body-attached sensors with built-in wireless telemetry, thus freeing the user from having to carry a data recorder.

For these telemetry systems, it is likely that a large number of wireless links coexist in the same area sharing the electromagnetic (EM) environment [8]. Electromagnetic Fields (EMF) are present everywhere in our environment and will continue to increase. In this way, our environment will be surrounded by multiple mobile and stationary devices, communicating wirelessly, and working together. The level and frequency pattern of that exposure is continuously changing as technological innovation advances. Exposure to the general public cannot be avoided, since various devices emitting low-level EMF are almost omnipresent in the environment, including wearable devices attached to clothes or directly to the body. Electromagnetic Interference (EMI) can be a serious problem for any electronic device, but working with medical devices can have life-threatening consequences. Practical commercial deployment of these wireless networks requires measurements of the Electromagnetic Compatibility (EMC), as a guarantee of lack of interferences 24 hours a day, seven days a week.

## 2. Antecedents / background

Improvements in medical technology and healthcare have helped people to live longer and with a better quality of life. Nowadays, our societies are facing new challenges in terms of economically and socially supporting their ever more costly welfare systems and increasing elderly population and chronic patients. The future of health care provision will see an exchange from centralized health care services, provided in doctors' offices, clinics, and hospitals, to ubiquitous and pervasive health monitoring in everyday life. The reason for this development is twofold. Firstly, demand for better, more comprehensive and proactive health care and health provision is steadily increasing. Long-term unobtrusive monitoring of biomedical signals to enable early-stage diagnosis of health issues represents a key component in proactive health care. Secondly, there is the requirement to mitigate increasing health care costs caused by the demographic changes of an aging society. By providing health services at a patient's home where the cost is lowest (as opposed to expensive clinical environments), large cost reductions seem to be feasible while at the same time providing a better quality of life [9]. New medical technologies and improvements in health information systems have benefited medical supply ordering and management, patient record administration, medical diagnosis, and the provision of patient services [10].

In recent years we are seeing great advances in all areas of technology from low-power electronics, Short Range Devices and sensor technologies to the development of new and original wired and wireless communication. These advances have already led to the development of new small-sized wireless medical and environmental sensors that are capable of monitoring the human body as well at its environment in a more efficient way. These advances in sensing, communication technologies and in software engineering make it possible to build new solutions for wearable healthcare systems and ubiquitous healthcare smart homes. With these systems, elderly people and those with pre-existing health conditions can remain in their own home, while healthcare providers can remotely monitor and advise them to improve their well being and provide them with quality healthcare.

Over the last few years, the number of short range systems has increased in residential environments. These systems provide a great variety of emerging applications such as tracking and mobile telecare and welfare, with the possibility of the inclusion of many types of conventional alarms (gas, smoke, flood, etc...). Short Range technologies provide direct benefits when applied to a healthcare environment. The main objective of these SRD is to communicate emergency situations due to domestic accidents or health emergencies. These are low-cost information gathering and dissemination devices and facilitate fast-paced interactions among objects themselves (vehicles, cell phones, habitats, habitat occupants), as well as the objects and people in any place and at any time [11]. The special implication of these devices with welfare and safety requirements involves a special interest in its operating conditions as well as in promoting correct habits of usage.

With the rapid advances in increasing computational performance while allowing for ever smaller integration sizes, on-body networks of wirelessly connected computing devices is becoming a reality. The vision of ubiquitous health (U-Health) care is addressed by this Body Area Network (BAN) and Body Sensor Network (BSN) technology [12]. As is shown in Figure 1, a network of interconnected Wireless Sensor Nodes (WSNs) in or around the body monitors a range of biomedical signals to assist in the detection and diagnosis of health - related problems.

In the emergent IoT approach, a wide range of SRD is used. Smart applications and services to cope with many of the challenges individuals and organizations face in their everyday lives, such as environmental and personal health remote monitoring systems. These applications would change the way societies and especially our healthcare system function and thus would have a big impact on many aspects of people's lives in the years to come. IoT is not a mere extension of today's Internet or Internet system. It represents intelligent end-to-end systems that enable smart solutions, and, as such, covers a diverse range of technologies, including sensing, communications, networking, computing, information processing, and intelligent control technologies. Furthermore, technical advances in miniaturization and wireless communications have enabled applications of wireless sensing and biomonitoring, using devices that are now available for general use by healthcare professionals, patients and caregivers [7], [9].

These solutions could significantly reduce the cost of welfare systems while maintaining existing hospitals and dedicated centers for people who cannot benefit from these Information and Communications Technology (ICT) solutions. U-Health Smart Home, a home equipped with ICT to support people directly in their homes, has been identified by governments and

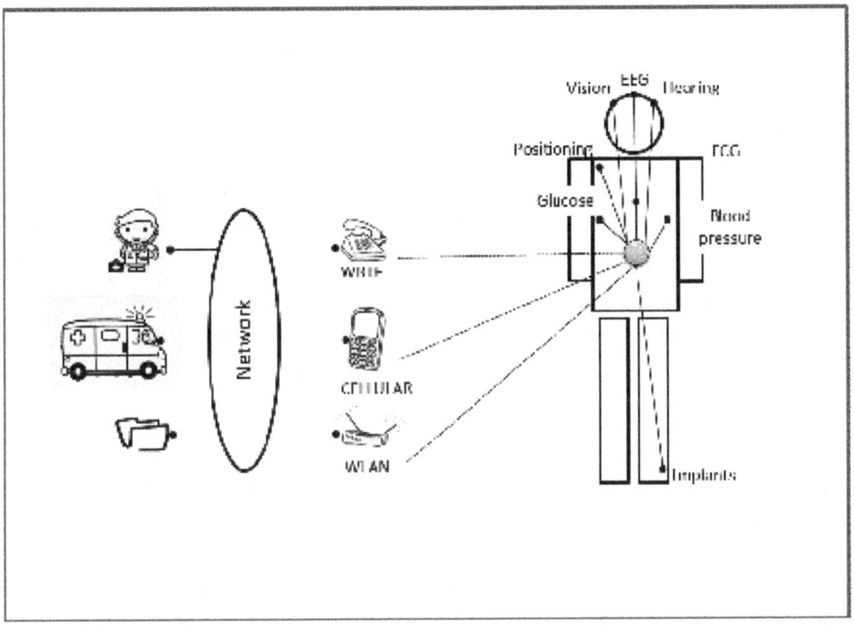


**Figure 1.** Ubiquitous health monitoring: a Body Area Network (BAN), wireless sensor nodes, monitoring biomedical signals and remote health assistance (WRTF: wired telephony service)

medical institutions as an important step toward financial savings, as well as a technologically and socially acceptable solution to maintain the viability of the welfare system. However, there are several obstacles to the acceptance of these solutions, some are technological, and others are more related to human acceptance in terms of comfort and business value.

## 3. Current state of knowledge and main objectives

### a. Research objectives

Given the current pace of implementation, this work reviews the literature regarding the use of SRD in healthcare, both systematically and comprehensively, following an innovation decision framework. We provide a brief introduction on these technological options, the current challenges, and the improvements that occur as a result of the use of this new technology. Then we analyze the specific uses of SRD technology in different areas of healthcare. The potential benefits are evaluated as a driver that will promote its adoption, and possible barriers to their acceptance are identified [13].

In this work the EM conditions have been analyzed and the radiation patterns of several models of social alarm devices have been obtained. Given the increasing use of domiciliary telealarm devices, and the non-existence of previous studies of the working conditions and the emission levels, this paper analyzes two of the aspects that have to be considered to assure a proper, reliable and safe usage of these systems. The first is the compatibility with other communication networks and implanted electric devices. The second is the compliance with exposure levels threshold, to quantify and analyze the risk of exposure caused by the use of these devices.

**b. Current state of knowledge**

For some years now short range technology has been considered a very promising option to cope with healthcare monitoring challenges. Consequently, this work aims to show the new technological advances and which factors might explain the penetration rate in healthcare.

The appearance of smart phones has been the major developmental breakthrough in the field of wireless personal area networks (WPAN). This has conditioned to a large extent the proliferation of devices in AAL systems that use the aforementioned smart Phones as a gateway to the network.

Factors like, accessibility, price, processing and communication capacity, as well as the use of cameras, navigation systems, such as the Global Positioning System (GPS), and accelerometers allow for a great flexibility in the development of further applications. The increasing use of operating systems, such as, Android, iOS, Symbian or Windows Phones that use the Software Development Kit (SDK) allow the development of certain applications to became easier and easier. As a result, networks that are compatible with the smart phones (Bluetooth, Wi-Fi o NFC) are currently the most frequently used by devices that are found within personal area networks in the healthcare environment.

Within the area of AAL three types of wireless networks need to be considered, Wi-Fi networks, domestic networks and networks made up of social alarm devices (SAD). Wi-Fi networks because of their widespread usage, reduced price and operability with other such as PCs, tablets or smart phones are a very attractive proposition for network usage within assisted environments, without forgetting their main advantage, that of internet access. Disadvantages could be the high energy consumption and time required to establish a connection.

With regard to SAD, they are perhaps today the most frequently installed device within elderly households. Within Spain it is estimated that there are currently around 300.000 SAD and that 4% of Europeans of more than 65 years of age, have access to a device of this type [14]. The platforms of SAD are suitable for integration with other devices within the assisted environments. SAD work on a frequency of 869.2-869.25 MHz and operate under the guidelines of the Commission Implementing Decision of 8 December 2011 (2011/829/EU) [15]. Currently, as well as wristband and chain alarms there are devices to detect falls, to monitor lifestyle, to monitor biological parameters, to detect technical alarms (such as smoke alarms, flood alarms or gas emissions), medicine dispensers and many other systems and technical aids.

Within the household wireless systems the Z-Wave technology stands out. In comparison to Wi-Fi, the device runs on batteries and the speed of transmission is lower, from 9.6 Kbps to 40 Kbps. Z- Wave operates in Europe on a wavelength of 868 Mhz.

As is shown in Table 1 with regards to the possible wireless communication options the vast majority use Bluetooth for data communication, differentiating between those that use the conventional form of Bluetooth and those using the newer low consumption version. You can see that there are several devices that are certificated by Continua, which ensure compatibility of data between platforms. Far behind, we can find those that use Wi-Fi as a form of wireless communication and finally you can find some that operate with Zigbee o with ANT.

| Device Type | Model | Connectivity | Image | Autonomy | Memory | URL |
|---|---|---|---|---|---|---|
| Blood glucose | Allmedicus Gluco AGM300 | Bluetooth Health Device Profile (HDP)[1] | 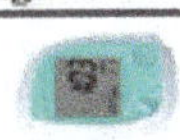 | 2*AAA batteries / 5000 tests | 250 tests | www.allmedicus.com |
| Oxygen Saturation | Nonin 9560 | Bluetooth V2.0 Secure Simple Pairing (SSP), HDP[1] | 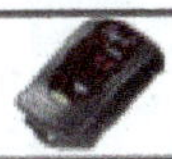 | 2*AAA batteries / 600 spot checks | 9560 tests | www.nonin.com |
| Blood Pressure | iHealth IH-BP7 | Bluetooth V3.0+ Enhanced Data Rate (EDR), Class 2 SPP | 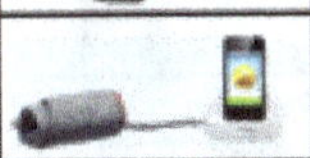 | 1*3.7V battery Li-ion/ 100 measur. per charge | .... | www.ihealth99.com |
| Blood Pressure | A&D UA-767 PBT-C | Bluetooth V2.1, Class 1, HDP[1] | 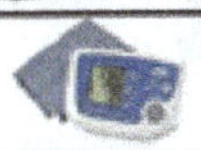 | 4 *AA alkaline batteries. / 300 uses | 40 measur. | www.aandd.jp |
| Blood Pressure | Omron BP792IT | Bluetooth V2.1+ EDR, Class 2, HDP[1] | 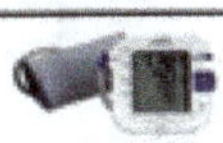 | 4 *AA alkaline batteries. / 300 uses | Up to 84 per user | www.healthcare.omron.co.jp |
| Blood Glucose & Blood Pressure | Fora DUO D40 a/b/g | Bluetooth HDP / GPRS | 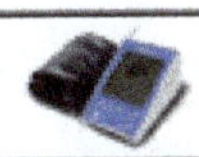 | 4 *AA alkaline batteries, recharg. batt. / | 864 tests | www.foracare.ch |
| Ear Thermometer | Fora IR20b | Bluetooth | 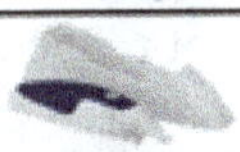 | 2*AAA / 1000 tests | 10 measur. | www.foracare.ch |
| Spirometer | SDI Astra 300 | Bluetooth V2.0 | 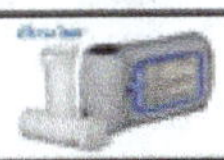 | 2*1,5V alkaline batteries / .... | 1100 tests | www.sdidiagnostics.com |
| Spitopmetry and Oximetry | MIR SpiroBank II | Bluetooth | 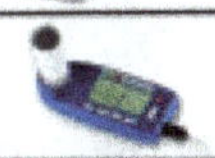 | 4*AAA & CR2032 / 10 years Mem-Batt. | 6000 tests | www.spirometry.com |
| Peak Flow meter | Corscience A M1 +BT | Bluetooth | 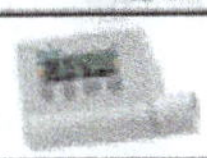 | 3 * AAA /.... | 490 tests (approx) | www.corscience.de |
| Peak flow meter | Vitalgraph Asma-1 BT | Bluetooth | 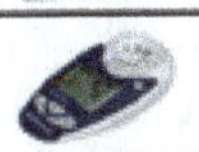 | 2*AAA /.... | 600 tests | www.vitalograph.com |
| ECG 12ch | Corscience BT-12 | Bluetooth SPP Class 2 | 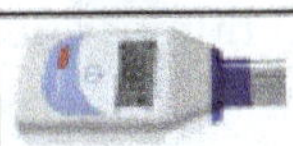 | 2*AA batteries / used constantly: 14 h approx. | .... | www.corscience.de |
| ECG 1ch | Corscience CorBELT | Bluetooth | 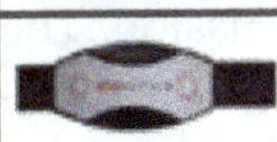 | 2*AA Batteries / used constantly 24 h approx | .... | www.corscience.de |
| ECG 6ch | SECA CT321 | Bluetooth dongle | 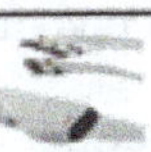 | 2 rechargeable L-Ion batteries / .... | .... | www.seca.com |
| Monitor (17 Health Parameter) | VESAG Health Watch | IEEE 802.15.4 ZigBee | 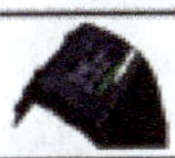 | .... / 60 to 72 hours standby time | .... | www.vesag.com |
| Monitoring device: ECG, Heart Rate ... | Zephyr BioHarness 3 | Bluetooth V2.1 + EDR Class 1 | 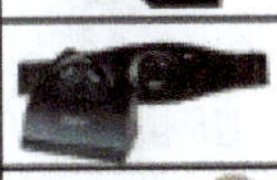 | lithium cell / transmitting 24 h | 500 hours | www.zephyr-technology.com |
| Heart Rate, Respiration Rate. | Isansys LifeTouch HRV011 | ANT Ultra low-power wireless (2.4GHz) | 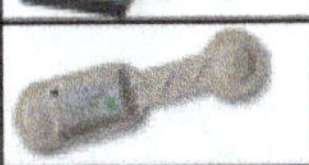 | .... / up to 5 days | .... | www.isansys.com |
| Heart Rate | Polar H7 HR | Bluetooth Smart 4.0 | 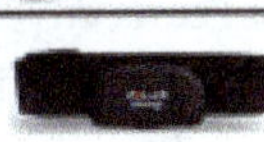 | CR 2025 battery / 200 h | .... | www.polar.fi |

| Device Type | Model | Connectivity | Image | Autonomy | Memory | REF |
|---|---|---|---|---|---|---|
| Pedometer | Omron HJ-721IT | Bluetooth V2.1+ EDR, Class 2, HDP[1] | 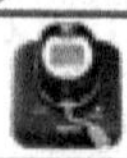 | lithium battery CR2032 / approx. 6 | mem 41 days | www.healthcare.omron.co.jp |
| Weigh Scale and BMI | Omron BF-206BT | Bluetooth V2.1+ EDR, Class 2, HDP[1] | 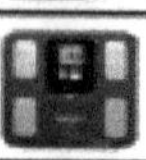 | 4*AA alkaline batteries / .... | approx. six months | www.healthcare.omron.co.jp |
| Weigh Scale and BMI | Fora W310b | Bluetooth | 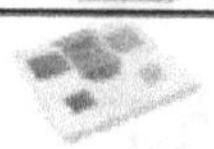 | 4*AAA / .... | 135 measur. | www.foracare.ch |
| Weigh Scale | iHealth Scale | Bluetooth | 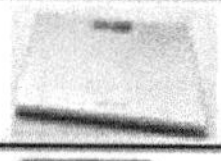 | 4*AAA batteries / .... | 200 measur. | www.ihealth99.com |
| Weigh Scale | Fitbit Aria | Standar 802.11b WI-FI | 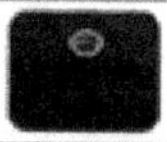 | 4*AA / six months | .... | www.fitbit.com |
| Weigh Scale | A&D UC-321PBT | B/T ver 2.1 Class 1 SSP HDP[1] | 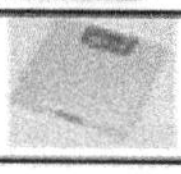 | 4*AA alkaline batteries / 300 measurements | 25 measur. | www.aandd.jp |

**Table 1.** Comparative table of healthcare and wellness devices. [1] Continua Certified.

Regarding the use of Zigbee, and although not reflected in this table, you can find numerous examples of research project initiatives that have developed devices orientated towards healthcare or assisted environments and that use Zigbee as a channel for communications, however, it has to be noted that very few of these initiatives have reached the commercial markets.

In the following paragraphs, we will compare low energy Bluetooth, ANT and Zigbee.

ANT is an initiative that operates on a low power proprietary protocol, works on a 2.4 GHz frequency, and supports the following network topologies: point to point, tree, or mesh network topologies with a range of between 1 and 30 meters, reaching hundreds of meters or kilometers depending on the typology and number of nodes in the network. With regard to the consumption, it is estimated to be in terms of microamperes in latent mode (sleep) and 18 mA in wake mode (wake up) and in transmission. The transmission rates can reach 1 Gbps, but to maintain real lower consumption transmissions, only a few bytes per second are estimated with a possible lifespan of over three years.

Zigbee uses the standard IEEE 802.15.4 on a frequency of 2.4 GHz, as with ANT it can support point to point, tree, or mesh network topologies with a range of between 1 to 100 meters and reach extensive areas using mesh typology. With regard to consumption we are speaking of around 35 mA in transmission and in terms of microamperes when in sleep mode. The rate of transmission can reach 250 Kbps and have a lifespan of up to six months.

Finally, Bluetooth Low Energy (BLE) a feature of Bluetooth 4.0 under the standard IEEE. 802.15.1 within a short range (up to 50 meters) can only support peer to peer and star typology, and as a result can not establish a meshed network, with a data transmission speed that can reach up to 100 Kbps. It is possible to reach low consumption levels of around 25 mA in transmission, and microamperes when in the sleep mode. The lifespan of the battery may be calculated in terms of tens of days.

## 4. Methods

### a. Review of literature

The ratio of penetration of SRD and its real effectiveness in healthcare remain unknown. This work reviews technological advances on SRD, produced from 2001 to 2011, to be applied in healthcare scenarios and mainly in AAL ones.

The research methodology employed for examining the adoption of SRD in healthcare has been divided into four phases: literature collection, categorization of the selected papers, analysis of the publications included in every category and results.

**Search strategy**

Both automatic and manual searches were carried out on professional databases including EMBASE, MEDLINE and PUBMED in order to identify relevant articles published between 2001 and 2011. The keywords used in the searching areas of title, keywords and abstract were a combination of 'short range device (or devices)', 'short range technology (or technologies)', 'radiofrecuency, 'rfid (and synonyms)', 'bluetooth', 'near field communication', 'wlan', 'uwb' and finally 'humans'. The number of papers initially located was 653. After eliminating duplicates and other inaccurate results, 378 were excluded and 275 were finally taken into account. Other systematic reviews carried out by different authors some years or months before were also very useful in identifying and including relevant studies not located by search engines.

Publication types reviewed were: Article, Article in Press, Conference Abstract, Conference Paper, Conference Review, Editorial, Erratum, Letter, Note, Review and Short Survey. Editorials, Letters, and Opinion Papers were excluded as well as those studies which dealt with ethical and legal aspects. No restrictions were imposed on the quality of the study design.

**Data synthesis**

Two authors independently reviewed the selected papers in order to classify them into one of the following categories at least:

- Electromagnetic compatibility
- Electromagnetic health risks
- Electromagnetic effects on the biological tissues
- Monitored environments
- Ambient assisted living
- Technological assessment

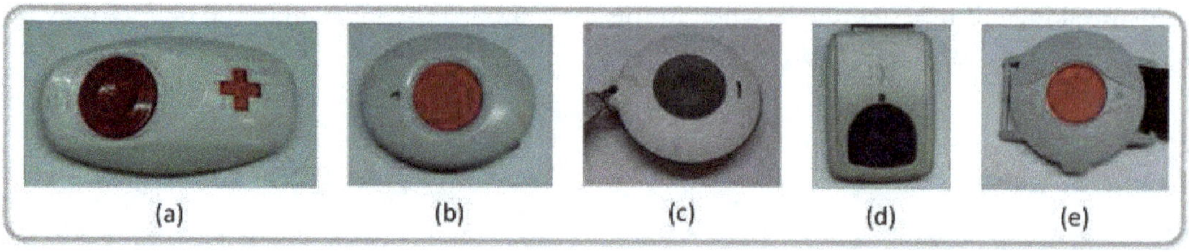

**Figure 2.** Selected models of social alarm devices: (a) AMIE+ Tunstall, (b) Neat Atom, (c) TX4 Bosch, (d) S37 TeleAlarm and (e) System 5000 Smart Call.

A more careful reading of the summaries showed that selected papers not always matched with the focus of this review. The found papers using search engines contained the words we were looking for but they were not always in the proper context. Search engines usually work using orthographical criteria and not semantic ones and this is a great weakness in automated searches.

**b. Measurements: electromagnetic laboratory evaluation**

The systems of social alarm devices consist of two operational units: the buttons that are worn by the users typically hung over the neck or attached at the wrist, and the fixed unit that is connected to the home phone. When the user is in a distress situation, he can push the button, a radio frequency signal will be transmitted to the fixed unit and an emergency phone call will be made to the monitor centre.

The buttons transmit a signal that typically consists of three pulses (depending on the model) at the frequency of 869.21 MHz. These are emissions in domestic settings that can affect the electromagnetic environments and can involve the increase in the exposure to electromagnetic fields of users, patients, medical workers and people in general.

Laboratory measurements have been carried out to characterize and analyse the RF emissions of the more extended social alarm devices. The objectives were to obtain the radiation pattern in order to identify the position when the electric field is at a maximum, and to calculate the power density and the Equivalent Isotropically Radiated Power (EIRP) for each of the tested devices.

The electric field strength and other parameters of the emissions of the device under testing have been measured to examine the compliance with exposure guidelines.

The performed environmental study of the working conditions of the social alarm devices helps to quantify the exposure of assisted people and to analyse the EMC of networks and equipment that operate in the surrounding areas.

For this work five models of social alarm devices were chosen from among the most frequently used in telecare monitoring activities. These devices AMIE+ Tunstall, Neat Atom, TX4 Bosch, S37 TeleAlarm and System 5000 Smart Call, are shown in Figure 2.

The measurements were performed in a semianechoic chamber, shown in Figure 3 and Figure 4. The room has dimensions of 9,76 m x 6,71 m x 6,10 m, the walls are lined with a foam based radiofrequency absorber material (RANTEC Ferrosorb300) specified to have a reflection/absorption coefficient of -18 dB at the frequency of 869.21 MHz.

All of the measurements during this work were made in the far field region with respect to the sources. At 869.21 MHz, the wavelength is about 34 cm, which means the reactive near field extends to around 5.5 cm from the source (based on the usual $\lambda/2\pi$ criterion, where $\lambda$ is the wavelength). The antennas of the social alarm devices are no more than around 5 cm in size, and they are integrated inside the casing device. Hence, the radiating near field extends no further than around 1.5 cm at 869.21 MHz (based on the usual $2D^2/\lambda$ criterion, where D is the maximum source dimension).

The devices tested were mounted on a manual positioning device with an EMCO 1060 motor, allowing the device to be rotated and permitted the measuring antenna to sample the radiation pattern at any angle. All the measurements were performed in vertical and horizontal polarizations; a positioner with an EMCO 1051 motor allows the changes of the position of the measuring antenna that is a VBAA-9144 Schwarzbeck biconical antenna with a frequency range of 80 MHz - 1 GHz. The instruments and devices used to obtain the radiation pattern are shown in Figure 3.

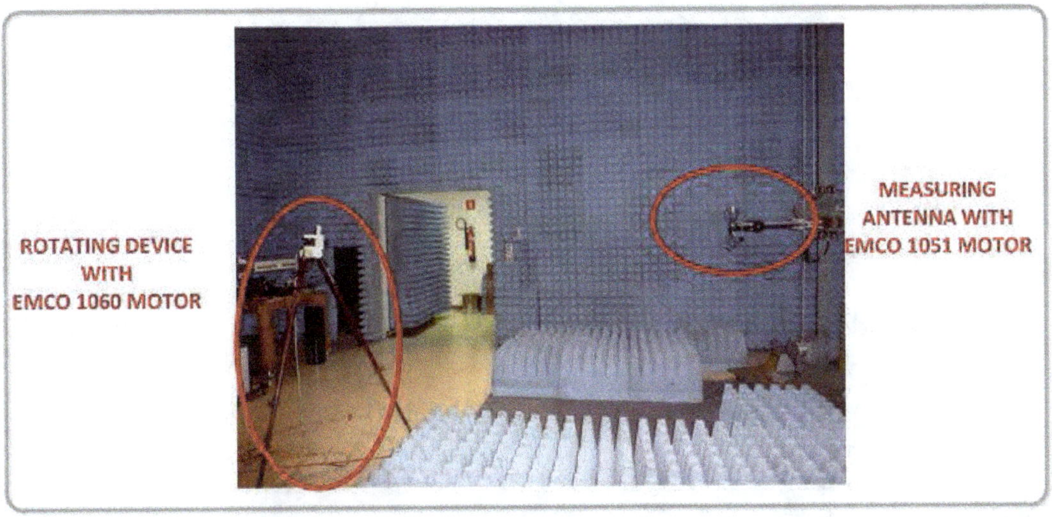


**Figure 3.** Measuring antenna and positioning devices to obtain the radiation pattern inside the anechoic chamber.

The radiation pattern of the models (a) AMIE+ Tunstall, and (b) Neat Atom are shown in Figure 4.

After obtaining the radiation pattern, the position of each tested device at which the electric field strength is maximum was fixed. In that position the electric field strength was measured as a function of distance in horizontal and vertical polarization in the far field region in steps of 10 cm, from 0.2 m to 1.7 m. The positioning device used to determine the distances was a

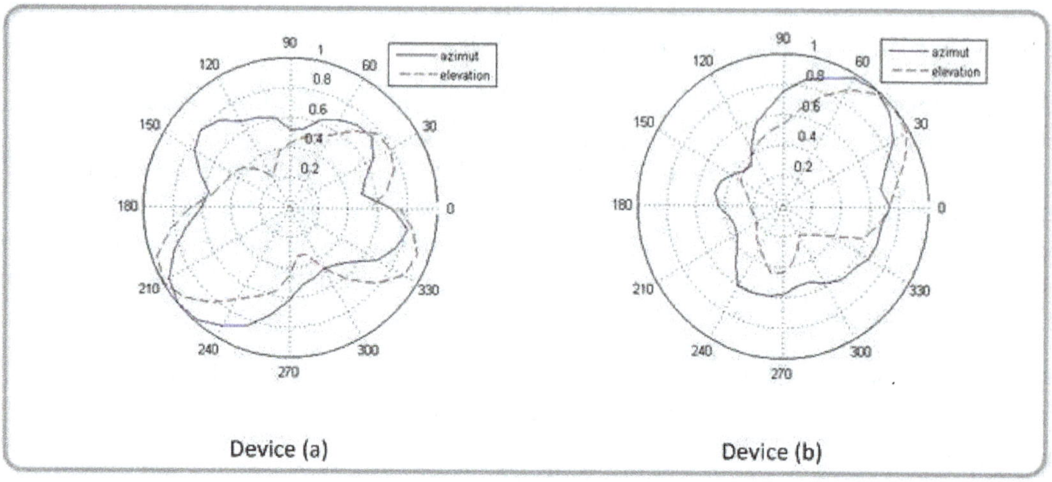


**Figure 4.** Radiation pattern of two models of social alarm devices: (a) AMIE+ Tunstall, and (b) Neat Atom.

FSM 016, with an HD10 controller to move it automatically. This positioning device is shown in Figure 5.

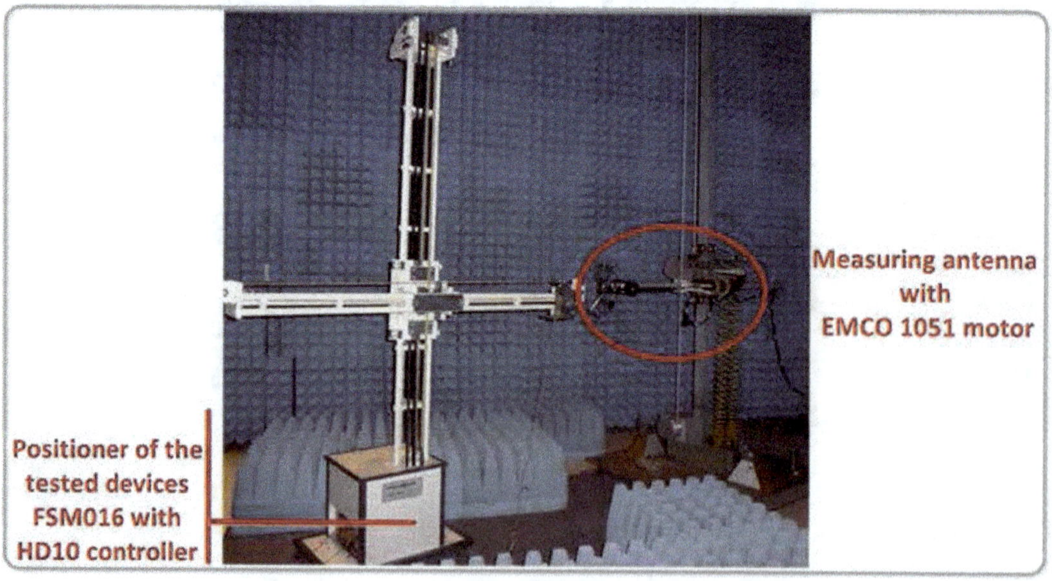


**Figure 5.** Measuring antenna and positioners required for the E-field measurements inside the anechoic chamber.

The measurements were carried out with an EMI Test Receiver ESIB26, Rhode & Schwartz with a frequency range of 20 Hz - 26.5 GHz. The EMI test receiver calculates the electric field strength taking into account the antenna factor and the cable attenuation, according to the following equation [16]:

$$E = V + AF + ATT \tag{1}$$

Where E is the electric field strength (dBuV/m), V is the measured voltage (dBuV), AF is the antenna factor ($dBm^{-1}$), and ATT is the cable attenuation (dB). After obtaining the horizontal and vertical components, the total field strength was calculated. The power density was derived using the following equation:

$$S = EH = \frac{E^2}{377} \tag{2}$$

Where the unit of S is $W/m^2$ and E has now been converted to linear units. The EIRP of each tested device was calculated for comparison with the emission limit of 16.4 mW set by standard regulations [15][17]. EIRP is the power that would have to be emitted if the antenna were isotropic in order to produce a power density equal to that observed in the direction of maximum gain of the actual antenna.

The EIRP is obtained from the power density as follows:

$$EIRP = 4\pi r^2 S_{\max} \tag{3}$$

Where EIRP is in units of W, r is the distance to the antenna in meters, and $S_{max}(r)$ is the maximum power density measured at each distance in $W/m^2$. The EIRP was calculated using the maximum measurement of power density, so the measurements of the electric field strength were realized in the direction of maximum radiation.

**c. Compliance with exposure levels threshold**

This research addresses the characterization of EM environments that are actually present in households, taking into account an analysis of the potential safe usage of domestic telemedicine systems. The data had been analysed with regard to potential risks and operational disturbances in accordance with existing European standards.

The field strength recorded from the tested devices have been compared with the corresponding International Commission on Non-ionizing Radiation Protection (ICNIRP) reference levels values defined for the general public depending on the working frequency [18].

It is also useful to compare the obtained levels with the thresholds for the safety and basic performance of the electromedical equipment. The International Electrotechnical Commission (IEC) Standard IEC 60601-1-2 [19], sets a minimum immunity level of 3 (V/m) for non-life supporting devices.

After calculating the parameters that characterize the emissions of the social alarm devices under testing, the results recorded are compared with the limit values set by the national and international bodies: Commission Implementing Decision of 8 December 2011 amending

Decision 2006/771/EC on harmonisation of the radio spectrum for use by short-range devices (2011/829/EU) [15], and the Spanish National Table of Spectrum Location (ITC/332/2010) [17].

## 5. Results

### a. Review of literature

Although most of the papers collected only partially cover the subject matter, the research performed for this chapter clearly demonstrates the high number of publications related to SRD in healthcare during recent years.

The number of papers seems to have increased significantly since 2001 as Figure 6 shows. The 248 papers finally included in our review were classified into six categories.

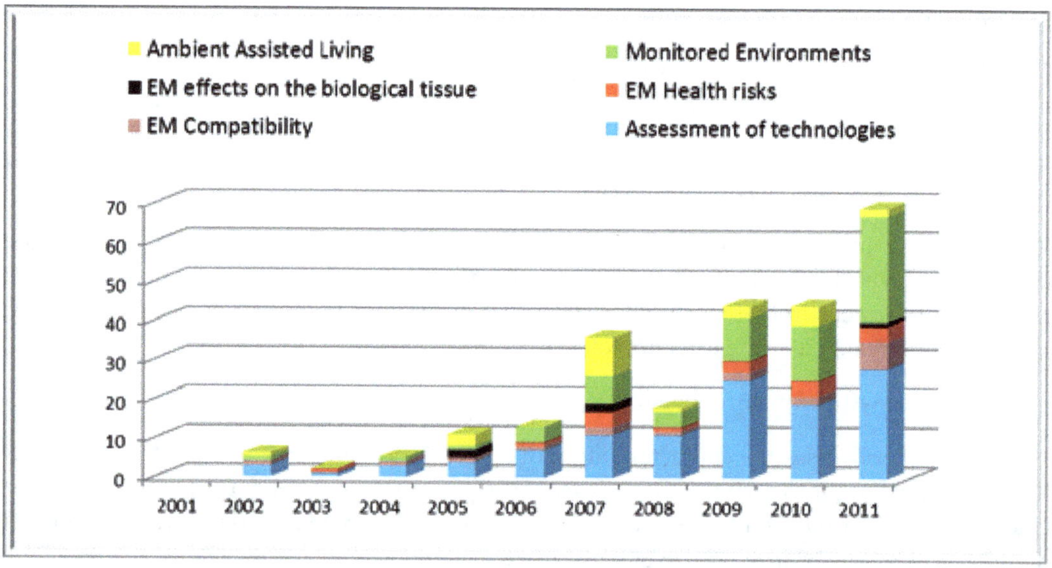


**Figure 6.** Papers which mention SRD technology in healthcare from 2001 to 2011 (Npapers: 248)

However, it is important to note the lack of publications which evaluate the effectiveness of SRD in real healthcare scenarios and most of the studies found only cover technological issues as is shown in Figure 7.

In this work, the two categories which are of most interest to the authors are AAL and monitored environments. Both characterize more complex scenarios, where SRD are combined with sensors to work together in a wireless network, finally connected to remote information repositories of data and software, as presented in Figure 1. Reducing hospital admissions and length of stay are main objectives in order to save economic and human resources, as well as to improve a patient's quality of life. However, most of these outpatients are elderly, or have

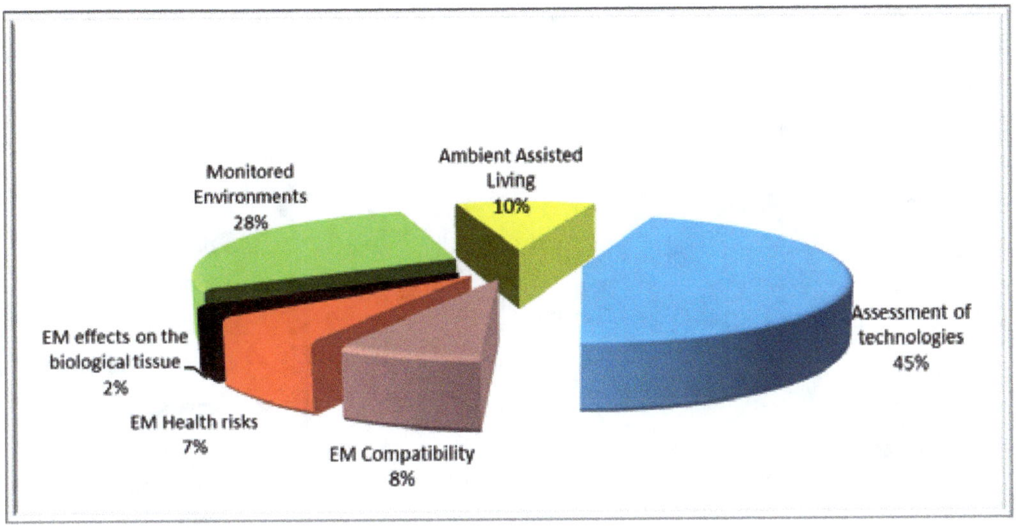


**Figure 7.** Applications Areas in terms of functionality (Npapers: 248)

a temporary or permanent disability, and many have no caregivers to help and technological advances can be very useful to fulfill that goal. From 2007, as shown in Figure 8, the number of papers dedicated to these two categories has been increased.

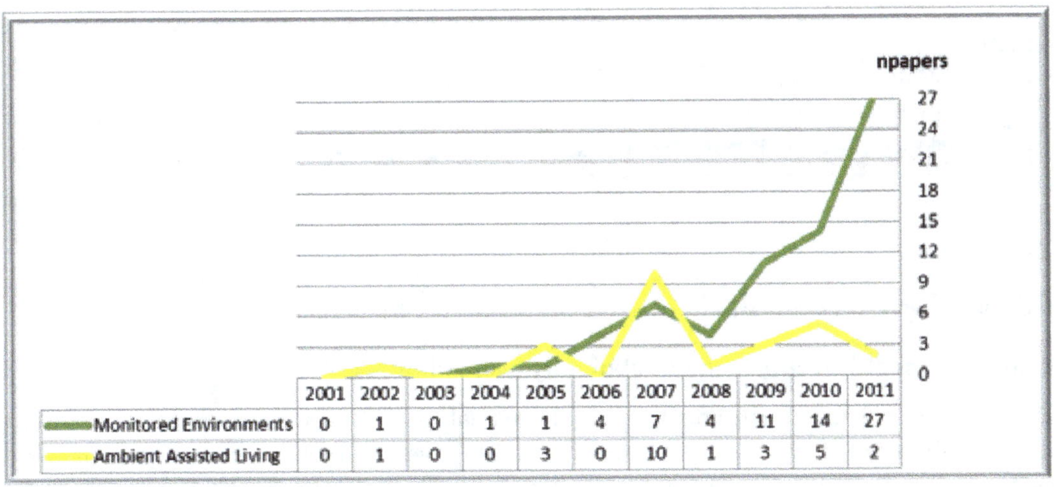


**Figure 8.** Papers dedicated to AAL and monitored environments (Npapers: 95)

Figure 9 shows the different technologies that can provide useful help to patients, healthcare professionals, caregivers and families in emergent healthcare environments. There is a lack of published papers in the years 2001 and 2003.

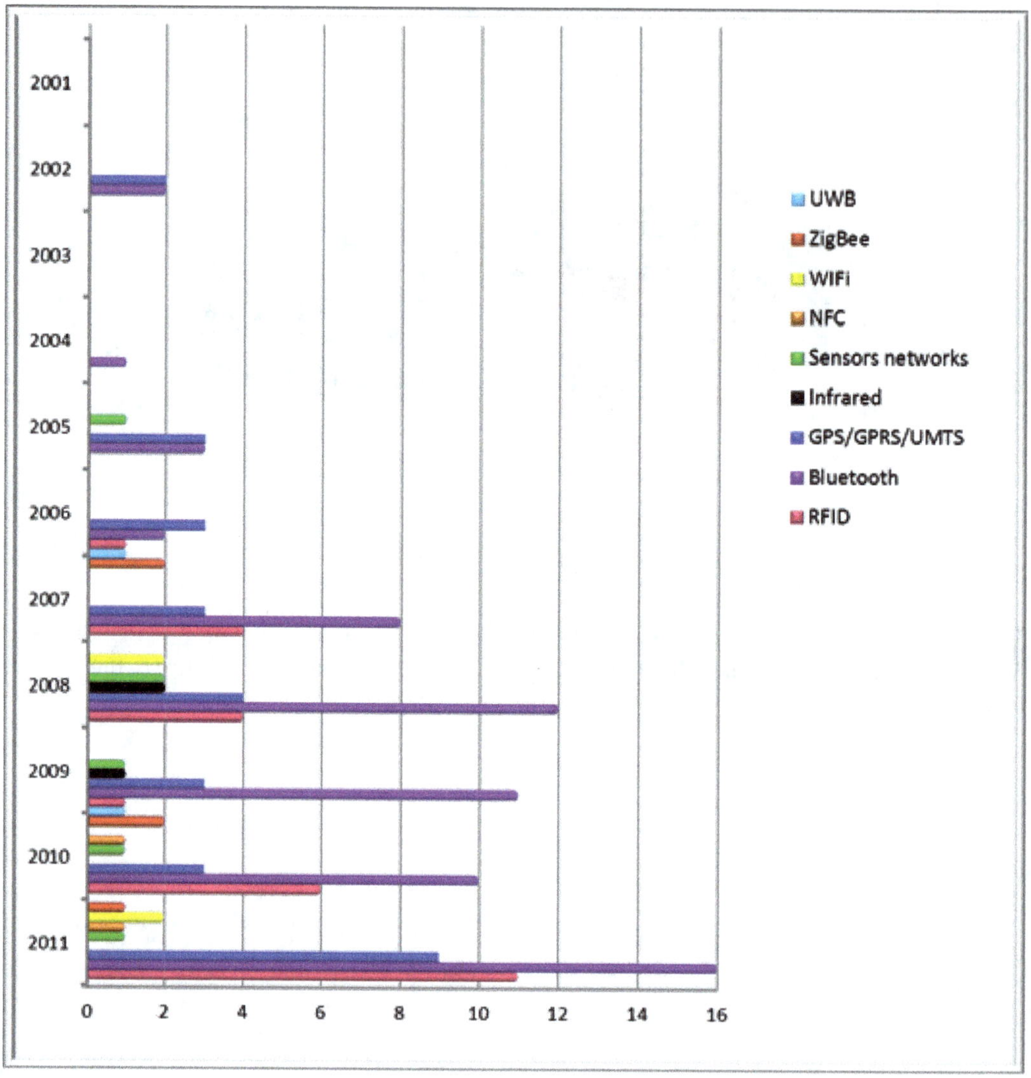


**Figure 9.** Technologies shown in papers for healthcare environments (Npapers: 95)

## b. Measurements: electromagnetic laboratory evaluation

Different types of social alarm devices have been analyzed taking into account their emission features, the type of wireless technology, etc... This work presents a comparison of these systems in terms of their working conditions, and parameters that provide information about the emission levels.

Figure 10 shows the variation of the power density as a function of the distance for the tested devices operating at 869.21 MHz. The power density calculated from an EIRP equal to 16.4 mW limit is shown for comparison. The ordinate axis is represented in logarithmic scale to improve the comparison between the obtained results and the set limit of 16.4 mW. Overall, the power density plots calculated from maximum electric field strength as a function of distance broadly follow the expected inverse-square dependence on the distance.

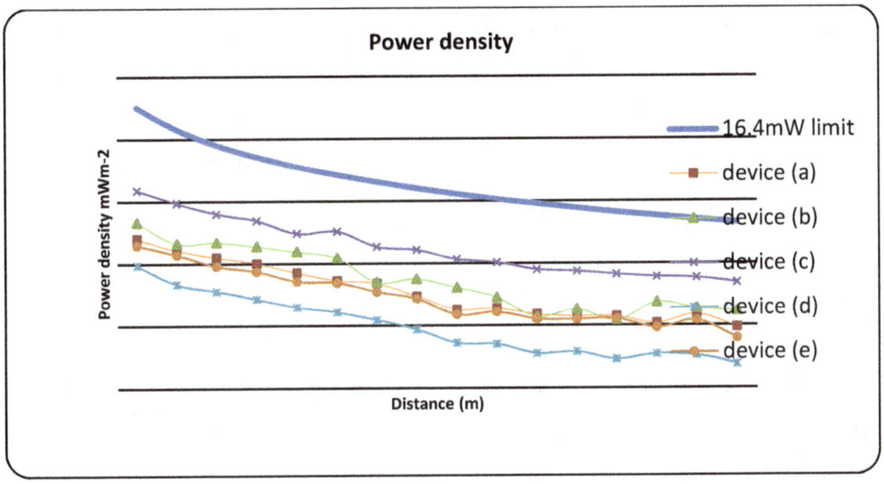


**Figure 10.** Variation of the power limit and the EIRP limit in function of distance for the five tested alarm devices: (a) AMIE+ Tunstall, (b) Neat Atom, (c) TX4 Bosch, (d) S37 TeleAlarm and (e) System 5000 Smart Call.

Table 2 shows the values of the maximum electric field strength (E), power density (S), and EIRP as a function of the distance, for two of the selected models of the social alarms devices, (a) AMIE+ Tunstall, and (b) Neat Atom.

**c. Compliance with exposure levels threshold**

ICNIRP guidelines contain reference levels expressed as values of the electric field strengths and power density that can be compared with measured or calculated values. All the field strengths recorded in this study are well below the corresponding ICNIRP reference level of 40 V/m defined for the general public at the working frequency (869.21 MHz) [18]. It means that electric field strength levels in healthcare home environments are apparently safe according to the health and safety requirements on the exposure of patients, professionals and the general public for protection against possible health effects from nonionizing radiation. The exposure levels thresholds stablished by the ICNIRP are shown in Figure 11.

The reference levels are not intended as limits, but are designed in such a way that complicance with them should ensure compliance with more fundamental basic restrictions.

One prominent concern to take into account is the possible interferences with medical devices. The IEC electromedical devices standard, IEC 60601-1-2 (IEC, 2002), permits radiated-immunity testing of non-life-supporting and life-supporting equipment from 80 MHz to 2,5 GHz, and safety distance limits for patient-coupled devices. This standard sets a minimum immunity level of 3 V/m for non-life supporting devices [19]. Examining the results, the maximum value of the electric field is much lower than the 3 V/m.

| D(m) | E(mV/m) | S(mW/m²) | PIRE(mW) | E(mV/m) | S(mW/m²) | PIRE(mW) |
|---|---|---|---|---|---|---|
| | **Device (a)** | | | **Device (b)** | | |
| 0,2 | 310,662 | 0,256 | 0,129 | 419,038 | 0,466 | 0,234 |
| 0,3 | 249,879 | 0,166 | 0,187 | 283,527 | 0,213 | 0,241 |
| 0,4 | 219,518 | 0,128 | 0,257 | 289,373 | 0,222 | 0,447 |
| 0,5 | 196,383 | 0,102 | 0,321 | 267,815 | 0,190 | 0,598 |
| 0,6 | 164,764 | 0,072 | 0,326 | 243,292 | 0,157 | 0,710 |
| 0,7 | 142,712 | 0,054 | 0,333 | 215,788 | 0,124 | 0,761 |
| 0,8 | 134,910 | 0,048 | 0,388 | 138,447 | 0,051 | 0,409 |
| 0,9 | 105,952 | 0,030 | 0,303 | 146,854 | 0,057 | 0,582 |
| | **Device (a)** | | | **Device (b)** | | |
| **D(m)** | **E(mV/m)** | **S(mW/m²)** | **PIRE(mW)** | **E(mV/m)** | **S(mW/m²)** | **PIRE(mW)** |
| 1 | 83,361 | 0,018 | 0,232 | 125,115 | 0,042 | 0,522 |
| 1,1 | 85,096 | 0,019 | 0,292 | 104,006 | 0,029 | 0,436 |
| 1,2 | 76,252 | 0,015 | 0,279 | 72,701 | 0,014 | 0,254 |
| 1,3 | 73,644 | 0,014 | 0,306 | 83,463 | 0,018 | 0,392 |
| 1,4 | 73,285 | 0,014 | 0,351 | 68,100 | 0,012 | 0,303 |
| 1,5 | 64,293 | 0,011 | 0,310 | 94,780 | 0,024 | 0,674 |
| 1,6 | 75,860 | 0,015 | 0,491 | 84,643 | 0,019 | 0,611 |
| 1,7 | 59,532 | 0,009 | 0,341 | 81,043 | 0,017 | 0,633 |

**Table 2.** Maximum electric field strength, power density, and EIRP for two models of the tested devices: (a) AMIE+ Tunstall, (b) Neat Atom

The recorded values of EIRP are well below the level that would be expected based on 16.4 mW, set by the national and international regulations: Commission Implementing Decision of 8 December 2011 amending Decision 2006/771/EC on harmonisation of the radio spectrum for use by short-range devices (2011/829/EU) [15], and the Spanish National Table of Spectrum Location (ITC/332/2010) [17], so the tested social alarm devices operate in safe conditions under the set limits of EIRP.

## 6. Discussions

This research identifies relevant studies which exemplify the penetration of SRD in new healthcare environments in real work flows. The evaluation of the methodological quality of studies has not been an easy task because of the heterogeneity of the papers included in the

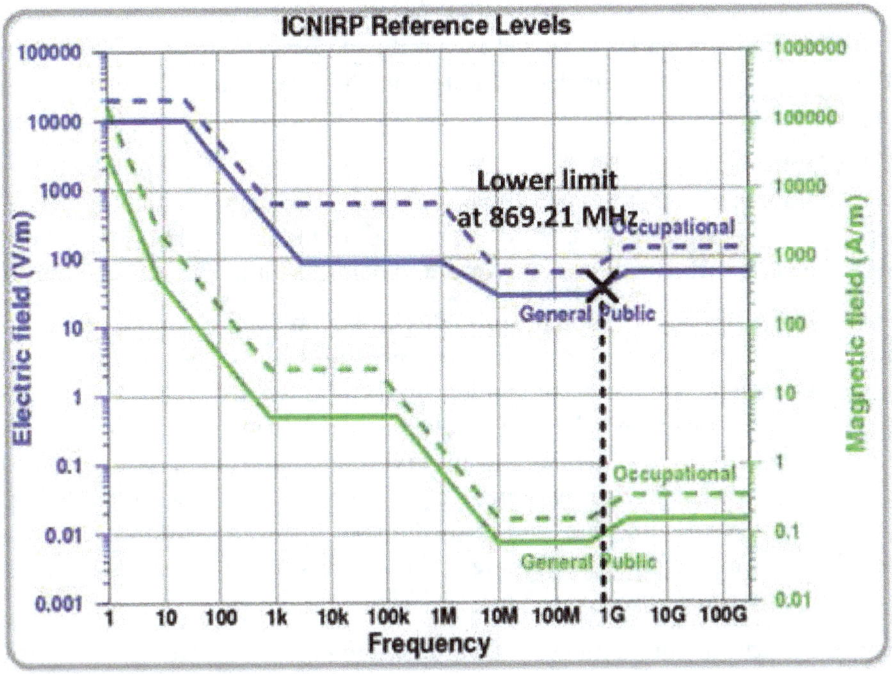


**Figure 11.** ICNIRP reference levels and the lower limit at working frequency of social alarm devices (869.21 MHz)

review. There are a lack of published papers in the years 2001 and 2003, as is shown in Figure 6. Most of the papers included only partially cover the subject matter.

The research performed for this chapter clearly demonstrates the high number of publications on technology assessments. However, despite the large number of studies found, there is a lack of publications evaluating effectiveness of SRD and most of the studies only cover technological assessment issues as can be observed in Figure 7. The absence of homogeneous criteria among authors to choose keywords to describe their papers may have an undesirable consequence: an indeterminate number of papers may have been omitted by search engines.

After reviewing the works it can be stated that wireless sensor nodes will play a key role in enabling the ubiquitous and proactive health monitoring and health care services of the future. To achieve the small form factors required, the reduction of node power consumption eliminates the need for large batteries and increases the energy autonomy of the node, hence reducing the amount of maintenance required. In this work several short range technologies for biomedical monitoring have been described in detail.

Future SRD and wireless sensor network applications in the health care domain are likely to require an even greater amount of data derived from a multitude of different sensors. The algorithms employed within these applications will become computationally more complex, resulting in a higher processing effort. Also, depending on the use of case scenarios, multi-sensory applications put higher demands on radio transmission. At the same time, the new care environments should operate on very small energy budgets, occasioanly using energy provided by harvesting devices alone, rendering power and energy-aware wireless sensor node design even more important. As well as this, the sensors need to be carried conveniently without disturbing the users' normal way of life: small in size, with low power consumption, and using wireless communications.

The fact that in the field of healthcare applications the most studied technology is Bluetooth, as shown in figure 9, and that the percentage of studies dedicated to the assessment of the technology is higher than any other, leads to an important lack of publications on EM risk exposure and EMC between wireless networks and medical equipment.

The use of SRD in assisted environments provides a lot of benefits and an important advance in the monitoring of patients and the elderly, improving the efficiency and the quality. But these successful factors may be accompanied by drawbacks if thresholds of exposure to electromagnetic fields are exceeded and if wireless networks cause degradation in electronic medical devices, which could potentially result in deaths, serious injuries, or administration of inappropriate treatment. The study of these critical successful factors can guide not only in the promotion, but also in the prevention in the use of SRD in healthcare applications. Therefore, the new implemented healthcare solutions must consider issues with respect to EMC and regulatory compliance.

Concretely, the conclusion of the analysis of Figure 7 and Figure 9 is that there are no previous studies about AAL and monitored environments based on social alarms devices operating at 869.21 MHz, and even less about the evaluation of the EMF levels in healthcare environments, despite the fact that these social alarm devices are very widely spread in the monitoring of daily activities of the elderly.

Therefore, one of the main objectives of this study is to quantify the exposure of people, and to analyse the compatibility between equipment and networks in monitored environments by social alarms devices. The electric field strength and the EIRP are well within the guidelines set by the ICNIRP, the IEC, and the thresholds set by standard regulations. It means that electric field strength levels in healthcare home environments are apparently safe according to the operational, health, and safety requirements on the exposure of patients, professionals and the general public for protection against possible health effects from nonionizing radiation.

Although one of the findings of this study is the development of an environmental study of the working conditions of the social alarm devices, it is also important to consider the absorption of radiofrequency energy in the body of a person that wears the device. ICNIRP guidelines are also expressed in terms of specific absorption rate (SAR), measured in W/Kg, in the body tissues. To address this, a parallel study should be carried out to measure the localized SAR arising from social alarm devices in the people that wear them.

## 7. Conclusion

On the whole, this chapter presents an overview of the current literature regarding the ratio of penetration as well as their real effectiveness. It provides physicists, patients and healthcare providers with information about parameters, effectiveness and the safety of SRD related to healthcare applications. The subject's content provides useful data for technology implementers in this growing field of AAL. Pervasive healthcare has been widely approved to be the next generation form of healthcare, in which distributed, patient-centric and self-managed care is emphasized compared to the more traditional hospitalized, staff-centric and professional managed care. The integration of SRD with other pervasive computing technologies such as communications protocols and wireless sensor networks is leading to further innovative applications in the telemedicine area, particularly for ubiquitous persistent monitoring of elderly or disabled people, as well as for patient follow-up during the rehabilitation phase where self-management of medication is prevalent. In recent years, many efforts have been made to develop contactless, portable sensors for continuous vital signs monitoring. But as of now, there are no standards for the system's size, architecture or performance.

Poor compliance for treatment, rehabilitation protocols and medication has become a well-known problem all over the world and causes worsening of disease, death and an increase in healthcare costs. In this context, AAL offers new possibilities to support outpatients in their daily routine to allow an independent and safe lifestyle without caregivers. The objects are capable of identifying, locating, sensing and connecting, and thus can lead to new forms of communication between people and things and things themselves. The development of real smart objects should be the next step, including ingestible or subcutaneous sensor tags.

These functional advantages can be overshadowed if the exposure thresholds are exceeded or if the use of SRD causes malfunction in other medical devices.

Given the increasing use of domiciliary telealarm devices, and the non-existence of previous studies about the working conditions and the emission levels, this paper analyzes two of the aspects that have to be considered to assure a proper, reliable and safe usage of social alarm devices operating at 869.21 MHz. The first is the compatibility with other communication networks and implanted electric devices. The second is the compliance with exposure levels threshold, to quantify and analyze the risk of exposure caused by the use of these devices.

After selecting the most widely used model devices, the emission levels were measured, saved, processed and analyzed to compare them with the existing standards. The obtained results show that electric field strength levels and the EIRP in healthcare home environments are apparently safe in terms of risk of exposure and EM compatibility.

The presented study provides a global, immediate and accurate vision that can help to avoid EM interferences, and monitor the exposure to EM fields of people using and in the proximity of social alarm devices in home environments.

New health solutions based on any kind of Short Range Technology must consider the issues of electromagnetic compatibility and regulatory compliance. Currently, the degree and type of EMF exposure need to be characterized in household settings, in order to ensure that applications operate properly and exposure guidelines are not exceeded.

## Acknowledgements

Financial support of this research was partially provided by the research grant DGPY 1301/08. Authors want to thank the valuable cooperation offered by the General Direction of Telecommunications and Information Technologies, Electromagnetic Compatibility Services, Madrid, and without which, the work carried out in sections 4.b and 5.b would not have been possible in any way.

## Author details

Silvia de Miguel-Bilbao[1], Jorge García[1], M. Dolores Marcos[2] and Victoria Ramos[1]

1 Health Institute Carlos III, Telemedicine and e-Health Research Unit, Spain

2 Agency Laín Entralgo for Education and Health Research, Madrid, Spain

## References

[1] Carranza N, Ramos V, Lizana FG, García J, del Pozo A, Monteagudo JL. A Literature Review of Transmission Effectiveness and Electromagnetic Compatibility in Home Telemedicine Environments to Evaluate Safety and Security. Telemed J e-Health 2010; 16(7): 530-541.

[2] Koch S. Home telehealth - Current state and future trends. Int J Med Inform 2006; 75(8):565-576.

[3] Hebert MA, Korabek B, Scott RE. Moving research into practice: A decision framework for integrating home telehealth into chronic illness care. Int J Med Inform 2006; 75(12):786-794.

[4] Bensink M, Hailey D, Wootton R. A systematic review of successes and failures in home telehealth: preliminary results. Journal of Telemedicine and Telecare 2006; 12(Suppl.3):8-16.

[5] Louis A, Turner T, Gretton M, Baksh A, Cleland J. A systematic review of telemonitoring for the management of heart failure. Eur J Heart Fail 2003; 5:583-590.

[6] Meystre S. The current state of telemonitoring: A comment on the literature. Telemed J E Health 2005; 11:63-69.

[7] Zheng J, Simplot-Ryl D, Bisdikian C, Mouftah H. The Internet of things. IEEE Commun Mag 2011; 49(11):30-31.

[8] Ramos V, Monteagudo JL. Safety and electromagnetic compatibility in wireless telemedicine applications Chapter 3, Book Advances in Telemedicine: technologies, ena-

bling factors and scenarios. ISBN 978- 953-307-159-6 pp 63 – 84. Edtorial InTech. 2011. Access in http://www.intechopen.com/articles/show/title/safety-and-electromagnetic-compatibility-in-wireless-telemedicine-applications

[9] Hanson MA, Powell HC, Barth AT, Ringgenberg K, Calhoun BH, Aylor JH, Lach J. Body area sensors networks: challenges and opportunities. Computer 2009; 42(1): 58-65.

[10] Reiner J, Sullivan M. RFID in healthcare: a panacea for the regulations and issues affecting the industry? Healthcare Purchasing News. 2005.

[11] Budinger TF. Biomonitoring with Wireless Communications. Annu Rev Biomed Eng 2003; 5: 383-412.

[12] Yang GZ. Body sensors networks. Springer 2006. SBN 978-1-84628-484-7.

[13] Alemdar H, Ersoy C. Wireless sensor networks for healthcare: A survey. Comput. Netw. 2010; 54(15):2688–2710.

[14] ICT&Ageing. European Study on Users, Markets and Technologies. Final Report; Empirica, WRC, European Commission; pp. 8-10, pp. 71-72 ; 2010.

[15] 2011/829/EU: Commission Implementing Decision of 8 December 2011 amending Decision 2006/771/EC on harmonisation of the radio spectrum for use by short-range devices.

[16] NPL. A guide to power flux density and field strength measurement. Middlesex London: National Physical laboratory, UK; The Institute of Measurement and Control; 2004

[17] ITC/332/2010 Order of 12 February 2011, which approves the National Table of Spectrum Allocation.

[18] ICNIRP. Guidelines for limiting exposure to time-varying electric, magnetic, and electromagnetic fields (up to 300 GHz). Health Phys 1998, 74:494 –522.

[19] IEC. International Electrothecnical Commission (IEC) Standard IEC 60601-1-2 Electromedical devices. 2002.

# Permissions

All chapters in this book were first published by InTech Open; hereby published with permission under the Creative Commons Attribution License or equivalent. Every chapter published in this book has been scrutinized by our experts. Their significance has been extensively debated. The topics covered herein carry significant findings which will fuel the growth of the discipline. They may even be implemented as practical applications or may be referred to as a beginning point for another development.

The contributors of this book come from diverse backgrounds, making this book a truly international effort. This book will bring forth new frontiers with its revolutionizing research information and detailed analysis of the nascent developments around the world.

We would like to thank all the contributing authors for lending their expertise to make the book truly unique. They have played a crucial role in the development of this book. Without their invaluable contributions this book wouldn't have been possible. They have made vital efforts to compile up to date information on the varied aspects of this subject to make this book a valuable addition to the collection of many professionals and students.

This book was conceptualized with the vision of imparting up-to-date information and advanced data in this field. To ensure the same, a matchless editorial board was set up. Every individual on the board went through rigorous rounds of assessment to prove their worth. After which they invested a large part of their time researching and compiling the most relevant data for our readers.

The editorial board has been involved in producing this book since its inception. They have spent rigorous hours researching and exploring the diverse topics which have resulted in the successful publishing of this book. They have passed on their knowledge of decades through this book. To expedite this challenging task, the publisher supported the team at every step. A small team of assistant editors was also appointed to further simplify the editing procedure and attain best results for the readers.

Apart from the editorial board, the designing team has also invested a significant amount of their time in understanding the subject and creating the most relevant covers. They scrutinized every image to scout for the most suitable representation of the subject and create an appropriate cover for the book.

The publishing team has been an ardent support to the editorial, designing and production team. Their endless efforts to recruit the best for this project, has resulted in the accomplishment of this book. They are a veteran in the field of academics and their pool of knowledge is as vast as their experience in printing. Their expertise and guidance has proved useful at every step. Their uncompromising quality standards have made this book an exceptional effort. Their encouragement from time to time has been an inspiration for everyone.

The publisher and the editorial board hope that this book will prove to be a valuable piece of knowledge for researchers, students, practitioners and scholars across the globe.

# List of Contributors

**Nino Cristiano Chilelli, Maria Grazia Dalfrà and Annunziata Lapolla**
Department of Medicine (DIMED), University of Padova, Italy

**Sunshine Arnold**
Team Coordinator of the Child Protection Team, University of Florida, USA

**Debra Esernio-Jenssen**
Medical Director of the Child Protection Team, Department of Pediatrics, University of Florida, USA

**Donald M. Hilty and Peter M. Yellowlees**
Telepsychiatric Services, University of California Davis, Sacramento, CA, USA

**Nicole Tarui**
UCLA School of Medicine, USA

**Steven R. Viramontes, Margo D. Kerrigan and David L. Sprenger**
Indian Health Service, USA

**Jay Shore**
University of Colorado Denver American Indian and Alaska Native Programs, USA

**Sarah Moran Michael O' Keefe**
Mater Private Hospital, Dublin, Ireland

**Daniel Dragnev, Usman Mahmood and Manoj Kulshrestha**
Hywel Dda Health Board, UK

**Chris Williams**
Betsi Cadwaldr University Health Board, UK

**Pat Herr**
Avera eICU, Avera Health, Sioux Falls, South Dakota, USA

**Michael Heisler**
Department of Internal Medicine, University of South Dakota Sanford School of Medicine, South Dakota, USA
Avera eICU, South Dakota, USA

**Stefania Corti**
Istituto Auxologico Italiano IRCCS, Psychology Reseach Laboratory, Ospedale San Giuseppe, Verbania, Italy
Department of Psychology, University of Bergamo, Italy

**Gian Mauro Manzoni, Giada Pietrabissa and Gianluca Castelnuovo**
Istituto Auxologico Italiano IRCCS, Psychology Reseach Laboratory, Ospedale San Giuseppe, Verbania, Italy
Department of Psychology, Catholic University of Milan, Italy

**Liezl van Dyk and Cornelius S.L. Schutte**
Department of Industrial Engineering, Stellenbosch University, South Africa

**José Luis Monteagudo, Mario Pascual, Adolfo Muñoz, Pilar G. Sagredo, Ricardo Sánchez de Madariaga and Carlos H. Salvador**
Telemedicine and e-Health Research Unit, Instituto de Salud Carlos III, Madrid, Spain

**Edward T. Zawada Jr**
Avera Health Intensivists/eICU, USA
Department of Internal Medicine, University of South Dakota Sanford School of Medicine, South Dakota, USA

**Dana Buus**
Avera Health, Sioux Falls, South Dakota, USA

**Don Kosiak**
Avera Health eServices, Sioux Falls, South Dakota, USA

**Silvia de Miguel-Bilbao, Jorge García and Victoria Ramos**
Health Institute Carlos III, Telemedicine and e-Health Research Unit, Spain

**M. Dolores Marcos**
Agency Laín Entralgo for Education and Health Research, Madrid, Spain

# Index

www.ingramcontent.com/pod-product-compliance
Lightning Source LLC
LaVergne TN
LVHW080623210926
848485LV00003B/204